Klaus-Dieter Budras / Robert E. Habel

BOVINE ANATOMY

BOVINE ANATOMY

SECOND, EXTENDED EDITION

Professor em. Klaus-Dieter Budras

Institute of Veterinary Anatomy
Free University of Berlin

Professor em. Robert E. Habel

College of Veterinary Medicine
Cornell University, Ithaca

Professor Christoph K.W. Mülling

Institute of Veterinary Anatomy
University of Leipzig

Professor em. Paul R. Greenough

Western College of Veterinary Medicine
University of Saskatchewan, Saskatoon

Dr Anita Wünsche, Dr Silke Buda

Institute of Veterinary Anatomy
Free University of Berlin

Contributions to Clinical-Functional Anatomy
**Rolf Berg, Dörte Döpfer, Reinhard Fries, Peter Glatzel,
Kerstin Müller, Christian Stanek**

Scientific Illustrators
Gisela Jahrmärker, Renate Richter, Diemut Starke

schlütersche

COLLABORATION ON THE ATLAS OF BOVINE ANATOMY

Editors:
Prof. em. Dr. Klaus-Dieter Budras
Prof. em. Paul R. Greenough
Prof. em. Robert E. Habel
Prof. Dr. Christoph K.W. Mülling

Contributions:
Prof. Dr. Rolf Berg, Ross University, St. Kitts, West Indies
PD Dr. Hermann Bragulla, Dept. of Biological Science, Louisiana State University
Dr. Silke Buda, Institut für Veterinär-Anatomie, Freie Universität Berlin
Ass. Prof. Dr. Dörte Döpfer, School of Veterinary Medicine, University of Wisconsin, Madison
Prof. Dr. Reinhard Fries, Dr. Tina Eggers, Institut für Fleischhygiene, Freie Universität Berlin
Prof. em. Dr. Peter S. Glatzel, Tierklinik für Fortpflanzung, Freie Universität Berlin
Prof. Dr. Götz Hildebrandt, Katrin Rauscher, Institut für Lebensmittelhygiene, Freie Universität Berlin
Prof. Dr. Dr. h.c. Horst E. König, Institut für Anatomie, Vetmeduni Vienna
Prof. Dr. Dr. h.c. mult. Hans-Georg Liebich, Institut für Tieranatomie, Ludwig-Maximilians-Universität München
Prof. Dr. Kerstin Müller, Klinik für Klauentiere, Freie Universität Berlin
Prof. Dr. Dr. h.c. Paul Simoens, Fakulteit Diergeneeskunde, Universiteit Gent
Prof. em. Dr. Christian Stanek, Vetmeduni Vienna
Dr. Anita Wünsche, Institut für Veterinär-Anatomie, Freie Universität Berlin

Collaborators on the whole project:
Angela Baumeier
Daniela Bedenice
Christina Braun
Anne-Kathrin Frohnes
Constanze Güttinger
Susann Hopf
Claudia Schlüter
Susanne Poersch
Eva Radtke
Monika Sachtleben
Thilo Voges

Acknowledgement of sources of illustrations:
The figures on p. 23 were drawn by Wolfgang Fricke and published by Dr. Anita Wünsche (1965).
The figure on p. 79 (below) was drawn by Wolfgang Fricke and published by Dr. Wolfgang Traeder (1968).
The figure on p. 80 was modified from Traeder (1968).
The figure on the title page was drawn by Diemut Starke.

© 2011, Schlütersche Verlagsgesellschaft mbH & Co. KG,
Hans-Böckler-Allee 7, 30173 Hannover, Germany
E-mail: info@schluetersche.de

ISBN 978-3-89993-052-8 (Print)
ISBN 978-3-8426-8359-4 (PDF)

Bibliographic information published by Die Deutsche Bibliothek
Die Deutsche Bibliothek lists this publication in the Deutsche Nationalbibliografie; detailed bibliographic data are available on the Internet at http://dnb.de.

Typesetting: Die Feder, Konzeption vor dem Druck GmbH, Wetzlar, Germany
Printing: Schleunungdruck GmbH, Marktheidenfeld, Germany
Binding: Hubert & Co. BuchPartner GmbH & Co. KG, Göttingen, Germany
Printed in Germany

TABLE OF CONTENTS

HOW TO USE THIS BOOK

In all three volumes the illustrations were drawn from dissections especially made for that purpose. The boxed information at the top of some text pages is intended to be a dissection guide for students and to give information on the methods used to make the preparations illustrated. Species characteristics of the ox, in contrast to the dog and horse, are printed in italics. Important terms are printed in bold-face type, and when a number is attached to the name, it corresponds to a number in the adjacent illustration. Less important anatomical features are not mentioned in the text, but are listed in the legends of the illustrations. The descriptions are based on normal anatomy. Individual variations are mentioned only when they have clinical importance. The gaps in the numbering of items in the legends of the skeletal system (pp. 3, 15, 31, 33) are caused by omission of features that do not occur in the ox, therefore are not illustrated, but were listed in the German edition for comparison with the dog and horse.

The cranial nerves are indicated by Roman numerals I–XII. Vertebral and spinal nerves are indicated by Arabic numerals.

Abbreviations

The anatomical/medical terms and expressions occurring in the text are explained and interpreted in "Anatomical Terms". Abbreviations of anatomical terms follow the abbreviations as employed in the Nomina Anatomica Veterinaria (2005). Other abbreviations are explained in the appertaining text, and in the titles and legends for the illustrations. A few abbreviations that are not generally employed are listed here:

Spinal Nerves

n — Spinal nerve
nd — Dorsal branch (br.)
ndl — Lateral br. of dorsal br.
ndm — Medial br. of dorsal br.
nv — Ventral br.
nvl — Lateral br. of ventral br.
nvm — Medial br. of ventral br.
cut. br. — Cutaneous br.

Vertebrae and Spinal Nerves

C — Cervical (e.g. C1—first cervical vertebra or nerve)
Cd — Caudal (Coccygeal)
L — Lumbar
S — Sacral
T — Thoracic

Table of Contents

Chapters with a cross-reference to the *Contributions to Clinical-Functional Anatomy* are identified with a green square and a second page number.

Clinical-Functional Anatomy

The numbers within the green square at the beginning of a paragraph refer to the page number of the *Topographic Anatomy*.

MUSCLE / FIG.	ORIGIN	TERMINATION	INNERVATION	FUNCTION	REMARKS
CAUDAL THIGH MUSCLES (p. 16)					
Gluteobiceps (Biceps femoris) (17.7)	Vertebral head: caud. part of *median sacral* crest and last transverse processes; sacrosciatic lig.; and *tuber ischiadicum.* Pelvic head: tuber ischiadicum	Patella; *lat. patellar* lig.; cran. border of tibia (by fascia cruris and fascia lata); common calcanean tendon	Vert. head: caud. gluteal n. Pelvic head: tibial n.	Extensor of hip and stifle; with caud. part, flexor of stifle; abductor of limb; extensor of hock	Not clearly separ... into cran. and ca... parts; almost co... fusion with glu... supf.
Semitendinosus (17.20)	*Tuber ischiadicum*	Cran. border of tibia, *terminal aponeurosis of gracilis*, common calcanean tendon	*Tibial n.*	In supporting limb: extensor of hip, stifle and hock; in swinging limb: flexor of stifle; also adductor and retractor of limb	No vertebral h... transverse inters... between prox. an... middle thirds.
Semimembranosus (17.18)	*Tuber ischiadicum*	Med. condyles of femur and tibia	*Tibial n.*	In supporting limb: extensor of hip and stifle; in swinging limb: retractor, adductor, and pronator of limb	No vertebral head. Belly divides into two branches

Cross-references

The captions of the anatomical figures in the section "Contributions to Clinical-Functional Anatomy" have been deliberately kept to a minimum because the identification of anatomical details with the aid of the figure tables in the front of the book is straightforward. This effectively fulfils the goal of providing an easily memorable exercise for students. The cross-reference numbers refer to both the plate number in the topographical part of the book and the respective structure (Example: Gluteobiceps [17.7] = Plate page 17, No. 7 in the legends).

The same principle is also used in the special anatomy tables.

* *Collegiate Dictionary*, 1993, 10th ed., Merriam-Webster, Springfield, Mass., U.S.A.

PREFACE TO THE FIRST ENGLISH EDITION (ABRIDGED)

This combination of topographic color atlas and concise textbook of *Bovine Anatomy* is the third volume of a series on the anatomy of domestic mammals. The first edition of the *Atlas and Textbook of the Anatomy of the Dog* appeared 20 years ago. It was followed 12 years ago by the second volume, the *Anatomy of the Horse*. In several German and foreign language editions they aroused world-wide interest. Therefore our next project was an *Atlas and Textbook of Bovine Anatomy* following the proven model and thereby closing a previously existing gap: no comparable work on bovine anatomy was available. The special features of the ox are presented to students in a well-grounded survey of topographic anatomy. **Special anatomy** is summarized as brief data in tables of muscles, lymph nodes, and nerves, with references to the corresponding pages in the text. **Comparative anatomy** is addressed through references to the horse and dog. In addition the text-atlas is intended to provide a valuable introduction to the **Anatomy of the Living Animal**. The authors were concerned with the preparation of a clear and graphic reference book of important anatomical facts for veterinarians in practice and research as well as anyone interested in morphology. This book can also serve as a dictionary of English anatomical nomenclature illustrated in color. An appendix on Applied Anatomy, included in the first and second volumes of the series, was omitted from this edition. Because of its extraordinary relevance for the practical instruction of students it will be provided in the next edition.

Our work on the ox has an unexpected urgency for three reasons: 1. Specialized textbooks for each individual species are required for curriculum revision with the trend to premature specialization and the accompanying formation of species-specific clinics. 2. In the present time of economic and social change, new diseases like bovine spongiform encephalopathy (BSE) attain enormous importance through their catastrophic effects. To determine the neuronal pathways of infection, including the autonomic nervous system, and the lymphatic system, and to judge the risk of noxious substances in the nervous system and in many organs of the body cavities, a graphic survey of bovine anatomy is necessary. 3. A licensed veterinarian is legally qualified to serve in a wide variety of positions: in private practice with small mammals, birds, horses, ruminants, and swine; in public health work to prevent transmission of diseases of animals to man; in governmental control of diseases of livestock; and in teaching and research with many species of experimental animals. To maintain public confidence in the profession, students should be required to master the basic as well as clinical sciences for food animals. This places high demands on teachers and students because a very broad and important body of information must be transmitted even though our teaching time has undergone an ill-advised reduction. Nevertheless, we are forced to accept the challenge, even with our compressed text-atlas, to reach the intended goal – to cover a huge amount of subject matter in the short time available.

This English edition is the responsibility of Professor Habel. His translation and scientific engagement in the production of this atlas and the writing and revision of many chapters are his personal service. His collaboration in the community of authors is a great enrichment. [...]

The provisional completion of our common effort offers the originator and editor, after 30 years of persistent work, the opportunity for a brief reflection. The enormous expense for the production of a book, together with the revision and improvement of many new editions, and the necessity of intensive anatomical preparation of subjects for illustration, were at first greatly underestimated. After overcoming many challenges, the dominant emotion is the joy of an unexpected success that came about through fruitful collaboration with the closest coworkers of our Berlin Institute, with the student body, with the readers, and with German and foreign colleagues across national and continental borders. The experience gained thereby is of inestimable value. The editor feels richly rewarded by the achievement of a professional life-work.

Berlin/Ithaca, May, 2003   The authors

PREFACE TO THE SECOND ENGLISH EDITION

The second edition has been substantially expanded by contributions to clinical-functional anatomy which provide valuable information for students as well as veterinarians in practice. These contributions were prepared in close collegial collaboration between preclinical scientists and clinicians.

In consideration of his advanced age Professor Habel who was responsible for the first English edition turned the responsibility for the second English edition over to Professor Mülling and Professor Greenough.

The manner in which anatomy is taught in a veterinary curriculum has changed and continues to change. In newly designed modern as well as in reformed traditional curricula anatomy is taught integrated with other basic sciences, preclinical disciplines and clinical courses. Functional anatomy is presented within the context of practical and clinical application. For students the presentation and integration of anatomical knowledge with clinical procedures and problems provides the context of application that enhances their learning and facilitates understanding and retention of the acquired knowledge of anatomy. The functional and clinical anatomy as presented in this book provide a solid foundation for clinical examination such as transrectal palpation and other diagnostic techniques including modern diagnostic imaging and for surgical techniques.

In this book students as well as veterinarians in practice will find the anatomical essentials for their daily studies and work as well as valuable information for more challenging cases.

The authors hope that this book will foster further integration of anatomy with clinical teaching and learning in a university setting and at the same time support veterinarians in their professional work.

Berlin, Leipzig, Saskatoon, June 2011   K.-D. Budras, C.K.W. Mülling, P.R. Greenough

ACKNOWLEDGEMENTS

Our thanks are due to Prof. Dr. Dr. h.c. Simoens (Ghent) for his contributions of text and illustrations on the eye of the ox, to Prof.Dr. Dr. h.c. König (Vienna) for his article on the mammary glands, and to Prof. Dr. Dr. h.c. mult. Liebich (Munich) for his collaboration on the article, "Female genital organs". Coauthors Dr. Wünsche, Dr. Buda, and PD Dr. Bragulla also had their part in the completion of the book. We had additional professional support from Professors Dr. Berg (St. Kitts West Indies), Dr. Böhme (Berlin) and Dr. Hashimoto (Sapporo). The many suggestions and the completion of many separate tasks on this atlas by the scientific, student, and technical coworkers of our Berlin Institute (see the list of coworkers) were a great help.

Finally, without the prodigious effort of our excellent artists, Renate Richter, Gisela Jahrmärker, and Diemut Starke, the atlas in its present form would be inconceivable. Susanne Poersch deserves thankful recognition for her careful computer composition, and the coworkers Dr. Claudia Schlüter (nee Nöller) and DVM Thilo Voges for the preparation of subjects to be illustrated, together with computer processing, and for making the Index. Our thanks are also due to the publisher, Schlütersche Verlagsgesellschaft in Hannover, and especially to Dr. Oslage for always providing support and understanding cooperation in the development of this book.

For their highly valuable contributions to the clinical-functional anatomy and for being part of the process of completing this work, we thank the following colleagues: Dr. Silke Buda, Prof. Dr. Rolf Berg, Assoc. Prof. Dr. Dörte Döpfer, Prof. Dr. Reinhard Fries, Prof. em. Dr. Peter Glatzel, Prof. Dr. Kerstin Müller, Prof. em. Dr. Christian Stanek.

TOPOGRAPHIC ANATOMY
CHAPTER 1: THORACIC LIMB
1. SKELETON OF THE THORACIC LIMB

The **thoracic and pelvic limb** of the ox, a heavy herbivore, are quite similar in basic structure to those of the horse.

a) On the **SCAPULA** is a large, half-moon-shaped **scapular cartilage (14)**. The **supraspinous fossa (6)** is remarkably narrow. It is cranial to the **scapular spine (5)**. On the distal end of the spine is a prominent sharp-edged **acromion (8)**, as in the dog.

b) On the proximal end of the compact **HUMERUS** the lateral **major tubercle (25)** and the medial **minor tubercle (29)** are divided into cranial and caudal parts, as in the horse. Distal to the cran. part of the major tubercle is the **crest of the major tubercle (26)**, and distal to the caudal part lies the round **surface for the infraspinatus (26')** where the superficial part of the tendon terminates. The **intertubercular groove (28)** *is covered craniolaterally by the major tubercle, so that it is not visible in lateral view. The intermediate tubercle is insignificant, unlike that of the horse.* On the medial surface of the **body of the humerus (31)** is the raised **tuberosity of the teres major (32')**. Laterally the hooked **teres minor tuberosity (27')** and the crest-like **deltoid tuberosity (32)** stand out. On the distal end of the humerus, the articular surface is the **humeral condyle (35)**. The **lateral epicondyle (38)** and the **medial epicondyle (39)** include areas for attachment of the collateral ligg. and caudal projections for the origins of flexor mm. The caudally located **olecranon fossa (40)** and the cranial **radial fossa (41)** are like those of the horse.

c) The two **BONES OF THE FOREARM (ANTEBRACHIUM)** remain complete, and, except for a **proximal (62')** and a **distal (62")** interosseous space, are joined by syndesmosis in youth and by a **synostosis** in later life. The **radius** is flattened and relatively short. The articular circumference of carnivores is reduced to two small caudal **articular facets (44)** in ungulates. The slightly elevated **radial tuberosity (46)** lies farther distally than in the dog and horse. On the distal end the radius bears the **radial trochlea (48)**, with tendon grooves on the cranial surface, and the **medial styloid process (50)** medially. The proximal end of the ulna, the **olecranon tuber (52)**, is a crest with two tubercles, projecting above the radius. The distal end, the pointed **lateral styloid process (61)**, extends distally beyond the radius, with which it is fused, and articulates with the ulnar carpal bone.

d) The proximal row of **CARPAL BONES** consists of the **radial (63), intermediate (63'), ulnar (64)**, and the thick, bulbous **accessory (65), carpal bones**. Of the bones of the distal row, C I is always missing, C II and C III **(66)** are fused, and C IV **(66)** is a relatively larger, separate bone.

e) Of the **METACARPAL BONES**, **Mc I** and **Mc II** are absent, and **Mc V** is a much reduced, rod-like bone articulating with Mc IV. The weight-bearing main metacarpal bones (**Mc III and Mc IV**) are not completely fused, as shown by the **dorsal** and **palmar longitudinal grooves** with the perforating **proximal** and **distal metacarpal canals**, and by the **intercapital notch (69')** between the two separate distal **heads (capita, 69)**. Internally there is an incomplete bony septum between the marrow cavities. On the proximal **base (67)** the flat articular surface is partially divided by a palmar notch into a larger medial part and a smaller lateral part.

f) The **PHALANGES** form two main **digits (III and IV)** and two **dewclaws (paradigiti II and V)**. The sides of the digits are designated axial and abaxial with reference to the long axis of the limb, and the joints are called, for the sake of brevity, the **fetlock, pastern,** and **coffin joints**, as in the horse. Only on digits III and IV are three phalanges present: the **proximal (70)**, **middle (71)**, and **distal (76) phalanges**. They are somewhat prismatic, being flattened on the interdigital surface. The prominent **abaxial palmar eminence** (see text figure) of the prox. phalanx is a landmark for the fetlock joint. *The dorsal border of the distal phalanx extends from the* **extensor proc. (78)** *to the apex.* The dewclaws, which do not reach the ground, except on soft footing, lack the proximal phalanx, and sometimes also the middle phalanx, and are attached to the main digits by fascial ligaments only.

In small ruminants, the dewclaws often lack phalanges; they are then purely cutaneous structures.

Superficial details of the phalanges of the main digits are similar to those of the horse.

g) The **SESAMOID BONES**. The four **proximal sesamoid bones (83)** are in the palmar part of the fetlock joints, and the **distal sesamoid (navicular) bone (84)** is in the palmar part of each coffin joint. They are not present in the dewclaws.

Digital Bones of the Manus

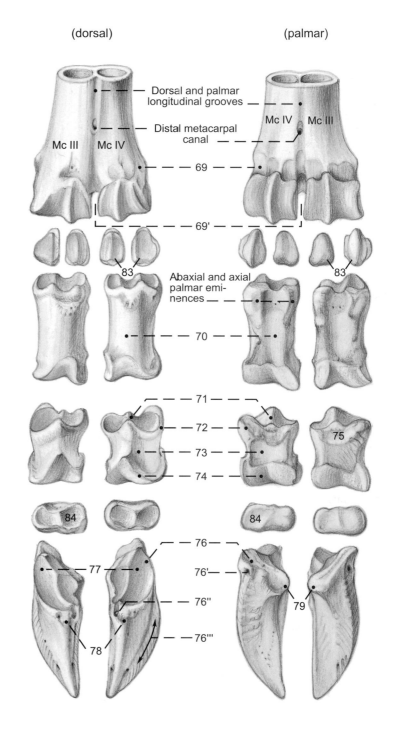

(dorsal)   (palmar)

Dorsal and palmar longitudinal grooves
Mc IV   Mc III
Distal metacarpal canal
Mc III   Mc IV
69
69'
83   83
Abaxial and axial palmar eminences
70
71
72
73   75
74
84   84
76
77   76'
76"
78   79
76'''

Bones of the Thoracic Limb

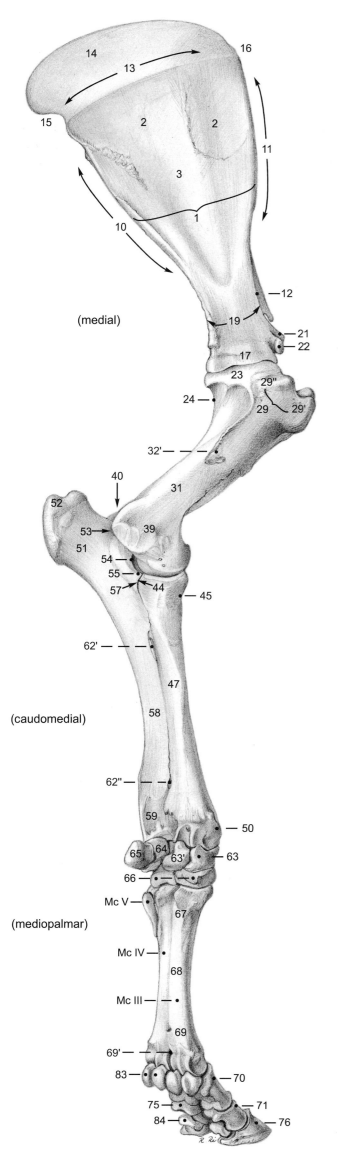

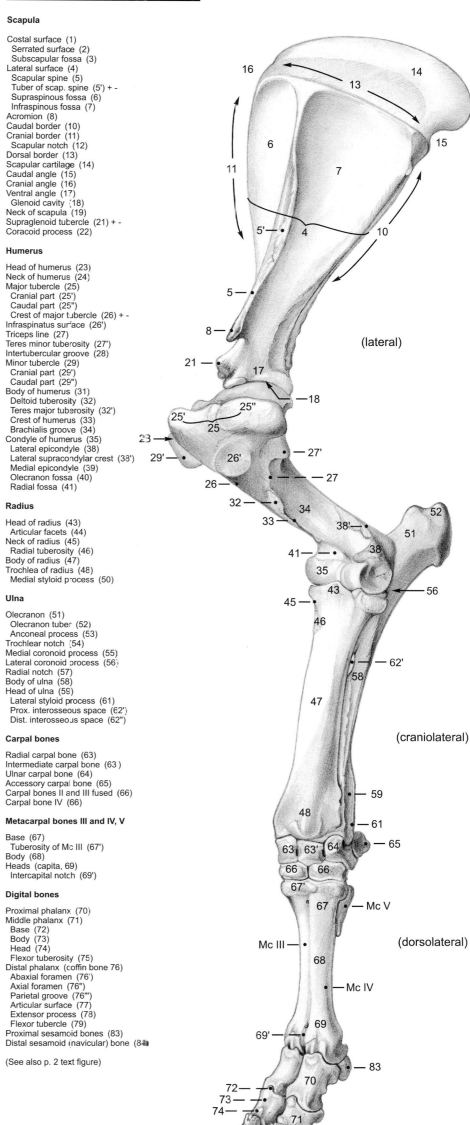

Scapula

Costal surface (1)
  Serrated surface (2)
  Subscapular fossa (3)
Lateral surface (4)
  Scapular spine (5)
  Tuber of scap. spine (5') + -
  Supraspinous fossa (6)
  Infraspinous fossa (7)
Acromion (8)
Caudal border (10)
Cranial border (11)
  Scapular notch (12)
Dorsal border (13)
Scapular cartilage (14)
Caudal angle (15)
Cranial angle (16)
Ventral angle (17)
  Glenoid cavity (18)
Neck of scapula (19)
Supraglenoid tubercle (21) + -
Coracoid process (22)

Humerus

Head of humerus (23)
Neck of humerus (24)
Major tubercle (25)
  Cranial part (25')
  Caudal part (25")
  Crest of major tubercle (26) + -
Infraspinatus surface (26')
Triceps line (27)
Teres minor tuberosity (27')
Intertubercular groove (28)
Minor tubercle (29)
  Cranial part (29')
  Caudal part (29")
Body of humerus (31)
  Deltoid tuberosity (32)
  Teres major tuberosity (32')
  Crest of humerus (33)
  Brachialis groove (34)
Condyle of humerus (35)
  Lateral epicondyle (38)
  Lateral supracondylar crest (38')
  Medial epicondyle (39)
  Olecranon fossa (40)
  Radial fossa (41)

Radius

Head of radius (43)
  Articular facets (44)
Neck of radius (45)
  Radial tuberosity (46)
Body of radius (47)
Trochlea of radius (48)
  Medial styloid process (50)

Ulna

Olecranon (51)
  Olecranon tuber (52)
  Anconeal process (53)
Trochlear notch (54)
Medial coronoid process (55)
Lateral coronoid process (56)
Radial notch (57)
Body of ulna (58)
Head of ulna (59)
  Lateral styloid process (61)
  Prox. interosseous space (62')
  Dist. interosseous space (62")

Carpal bones

Radial carpal bone (63)
Intermediate carpal bone (63')
Ulnar carpal bone (64)
Accessory carpal bone (65)
Carpal bones II and III fused (66)
Carpal bone IV (66)

Metacarpal bones III and IV, V

Base (67)
  Tuberosity of Mc III (67')
Body (68)
Heads (capita, 69)
  Intercapital notch (69')

Digital bones

Proximal phalanx (70)
Middle phalanx (71)
  Base (72)
  Body (73)
  Head (74)
  Flexor tuberosity (75)
Distal phalanx (coffin bone 76)
  Abaxial foramen (76')
  Axial foramen (76")
  Parietal groove (76''')
  Articular surface (77)
  Extensor process (78)
  Flexor tubercle (79)
Proximal sesamoid bones (83)
Distal sesamoid (navicular) bone (84)

(See also p. 2 text figure)

3

2. MUSCLES AND NERVES OF THE SHOULDER, ARM, AND FOREARM

The thoracic limb is skinned down to the hoofs as carefully as possible to preserve the cutaneous nn. and superficial vessels. At the carpus the precarpal subcutaneous bursa should be examined. The skin is carefully cut around the dewclaws to leave them on the limb. In the following nerve and muscle dissection, the pectoral mm. are removed with attention to the cranial and caudal pectoral nn. The blood vessels are spared for their subsequent demonstration. The scapular part of the deltoideus is removed, except for a small stump on the scapula, sparing the cutaneous branch of the axillary n. The tensor fasciae antebrachii is transected at its attachment to the fascia, and the lateral head of the triceps is transected over the superficial branch of the radial n. and reflected distally.

a) The **NERVES AND MUSCLES OF THE SHOULDER AND ARM**. The nerves are supplied by the brachial plexus. The **roots of the plexus (5)** come from the ventral branches of C6–T2. *The number of nerves that arise from the plexus is the same in all species of domestic mammals.*

The **suprascapular n. (8)**, from C6–C7; motor, passes laterally between the cranial border of the subscapularis and the **supraspinatus (1)** and innervates the latter as well as the strongly tendinous **infraspinatus (11)**. The 1–4 **subscapular nn. (4)**, from C7–C8; motor, are the main nerves of the *tripartite* **subscapularis (4)**. Small caudal parts of it are innervated by the **axillary n. (13)**, from C7–C8; mixed. This nerve passes laterally across the cranial border of the tendon of the **teres major (2)**, which it innervates, to the three parts of the deltoideus: **scapular (6)**, **acromial (7)**, and **clavicular (23)** [cleidobrachialis]. The axillary n. also innervates the **teres minor (12)**, emerges through the scapular part of the deltoideus, runs distally on the extensor carpi radialis as the **cranial cutaneous antebrachial n. (30)**, and ends in the proximal half of the forearm. The **thoracodorsal n. (3)**, from C7–C8; motor, ends in the **latissimus dorsi (3)**, the distal stump of which has been retained. The **median n. (14)** C8–T2, forms the axillary loop under the axillary a. with the musculocutaneous n., as in the horse. *The median n. is also bound by connective tissue to the ulnar n. in the upper arm,* and runs at first undivided craniomedially to the level of the elbow joint. The **musculocutaneous n. (9)**, from C6–C8; mixed, gives off the **proximal muscular br.(b)**, which passes between the parts of the **coracobrachialis (16)**, innervating them and the **biceps brachii (26)**. The nerve separates from the median n. in the middle of the arm, and gives off the **distal muscular br. (d)**, which passes deep to the biceps and innervates the **brachialis (21)**. The musculocutaneous n. is continued as the **medial cutaneous antebrachial n. (31)**, which becomes subcutaneous over the lacertus fibrosus (*thin, unlike that of the horse*), and runs distally medial to the cephalic v. The **radial n. (15)**, from C7–T1; mixed, passes laterally between the **medial (19)** and **long (18) heads of the triceps brachii** and gives off branches to them, as well as to the **lateral head (17)**, **tensor fasciae antebrachii (22)**, and **anconeus (25)**. The anconeus is difficult to separate from the lateral head of the triceps, and *an accessory head is incompletely separable from the medial head.* The radial n. follows the spiral course of the brachialis around the humerus from caudal to lateral, and *occasionally it supplies the distal part of the brachialis*, as in the horse. While still under the lateral head of the triceps, the nerve divides into deep (20) and superficial (32) branches.

At the carpal joint the tendon sheaths of the digital extensors, ext. carpi obliquus, and flexor carpi radialis should be examined. The med. and lat. cutaneous antebrachial nerves must be preserved. To demonstrate the nerves and vessels, the pronator teres is transected. The flexor carpi ulnaris and -radialis are transected in the middle of the forearm.

b) **NERVES AND MUSCLES ON THE CRANIOLATERAL SURFACE OF THE FOREARM**. The muscles are innervated by the **deep branch (20)** of the radial n. Its **superficial branch (32)** becomes the occasionally double **lateral cutaneous antebrachial n. (33)**, which runs distally on the extensor carpi radialis, lateral to the cephalic v., with the medial cutaneous antebrachial n. on the medial side of the vein, and gives off several branches to the lateral side of the forearm and carpus. On the metacarpus it divides into dorsal common digital nn. II and III.

The origins of the digital and carpal extensors are predominantly on the lateral epicondyle of the humerus.

The **common digital extensor (40)** has two bellies and two tendons, which cross the carpus in the same synovial sheath. The larger, more cranial one is the **medial digital extensor (proper extensor of digit III)**. Its flat tendon ends mainly on the *extensor process and dorsal surface of the middle phalanx*, but a thin abaxial branch descends vertically to a termination *below the articular margin of the distal phalanx*. At the fetlock joint an axial band of the tendon goes to the proximal end of the *proximal phalanx of the other main digit*. Deep to this band and the tendon, *a fibrous dorsal sesamoid body is embedded in the joint capsule.** Above the pastern joint the tendon is joined by **axial and abaxial (l) extensor branches** of interosseus III. The small caudal belly of the common digital extensor is the **common extensor of digits III and IV**. Its tendon bifurcates above the fetlock joint, and each branch, provided with a synovial sheath, ends on the extensor process of the respective distal phalanx.

The tendon of the **lateral digital extensor (41, proper extensor of digit IV)** receives the extensor branches of interosseus IV (l) and ends in the same way as the medial digital extensor. Each proper extensor has a synovial bursa at the fetlock joint.

The tendon of the large **extensor carpi radialis (35)** is almost surrounded by a synovial bursa on the carpus, and terminates on the tuberosity of Mc III.

The **ulnaris lateralis (38)** [extensor carpi ulnaris] is on the laterocaudal surface of the forearm. It terminates with a *phylogenetically older accessory tendon on the rudimentary Mc V, and with a newer main tendon on the accessory carpal bone, making the muscle a flexor of the carpus.*

The tendon of the **extensor carpi obliquus (39)** [abductor pollicis longus], enclosed in a synovial sheath, runs across the tendon of the extensor carpi radialis and ends on Mc III. *The supinator is absent.*

c) **NERVES AND MUSCLES OF THE CAUDOMEDIAL SURFACE OF THE FOREARM**. The muscles are innervated by the ulnar n. and **median n. (14)** from C8–T2; mixed. The latter courses, accompanied by the brachial a. and v., deep to the **pronator teres (27)** and **flexor carpi radialis (28)**, giving off muscular branches to them and to the **humeral and radial heads** of the **deep digital flexor (34)**. *The pronator quadratus is absent.* The nerve continues in the forearm, accompanied by the median a. and v. It supplies the skin on the medial surface of the carpus and the proximal third of the metacarpus, and, *without division, unlike that of the horse*, passes through the carpal canal on the medial border of the deep tendon of the supf. dig. flexor. In the metacarpus it divides into palmar common digital nn. II and III and the communicating br. to the supf. palmar br. of the ulnar n. Palmar common dig. n. III divides into axial palmar dig. nn. III and IV. The **ulnar n. (10)**, from C8–T2; mixed, while still in the upper arm, gives off the double **caudal cutaneous antebrachial n. (24)** to the caudomedial and caudolateral surfaces of the forearm and carpus. The ulnar n., accompanied by the collateral ulnar a. and v., passes to the caudal surface of the elbow joint. It gives branches to the **flexor carpi ulnaris (29)** and **supf. digital flexor (36, 37)**, as well as to the **ulnar and humeral heads** of the **deep dig. flexor (34)**. Between the flexor carpi ulnaris and ulnaris lateralis it divides into the **dorsal branch (43)**, which in the metacarpus becomes dorsal common dig. n. IV, and the **palmar branch (42)**, which passes through the carpal canal and runs lateral to the tendons of the supf. dig. flexor. It divides into a **deep branch** for the interossei, and a **superficial branch**, which runs distally in the lateral groove between the deep flexor tendon and interosseus IV to form, with the communicating br. of the median n., palmar common digital n. IV.

The supf. dig. flexor is composed of two parts. The tendon of the supf. part passes between the two layers of the **flexor retinaculum (k)**. *The tendon of the deep part passes through the carpal canal with the tendon of the deep flexor. The two tendons of the supf. flexor join in the distal part of the metacarpus.*

4

---
* Habermehl, 1961

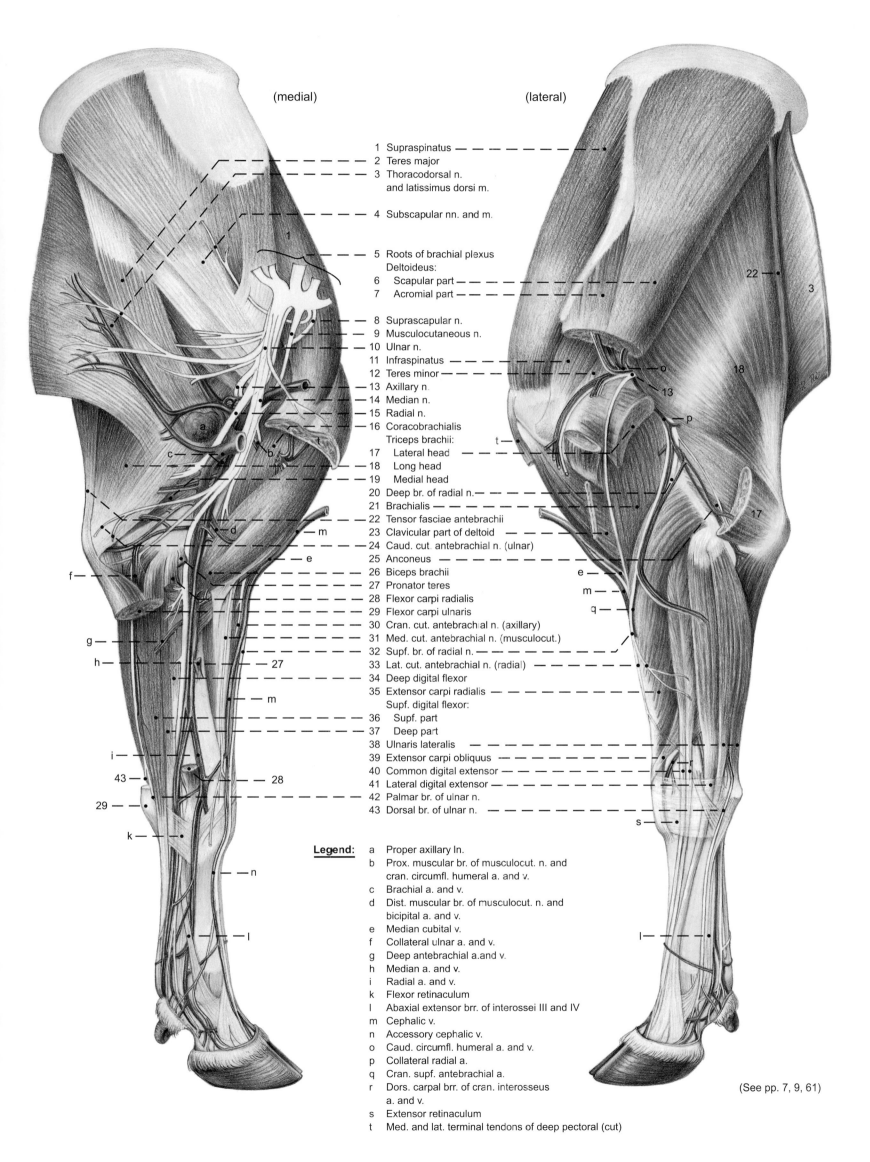

(medial)　　　　　　　　　　　　　　(lateral)

1　Supraspinatus
2　Teres major
3　Thoracodorsal n.
　　and latissimus dorsi m.
4　Subscapular nn. and m.

5　Roots of brachial plexus
　　Deltoideus:
6　　Scapular part
7　　Acromial part

8　Suprascapular n.
9　Musculocutaneous n.
10　Ulnar n.
11　Infraspinatus
12　Teres minor
13　Axillary n.
14　Median n.
15　Radial n.
16　Coracobrachialis
　　Triceps brachii:
17　　Lateral head
18　　Long head
19　　Medial head
20　Deep br. of radial n.
21　Brachialis
22　Tensor fasciae antebrachii
23　Clavicular part of deltoid
24　Caud. cut. antebrachial n. (ulnar)
25　Anconeus
26　Biceps brachii
27　Pronator teres
28　Flexor carpi radialis
29　Flexor carpi ulnaris
30　Cran. cut. antebrachial n. (axillary)
31　Med. cut. antebrachial n. (musculocut.)
32　Supf. br. of radial n.
33　Lat. cut. antebrachial n. (radial)
34　Deep digital flexor
35　Extensor carpi radialis
　　Supf. digital flexor:
36　　Supf. part
37　　Deep part
38　Ulnaris lateralis
39　Extensor carpi obliquus
40　Common digital extensor
41　Lateral digital extensor
42　Palmar br. of ulnar n.
43　Dorsal br. of ulnar n.

Legend:
a　Proper axillary ln.
b　Prox. muscular br. of musculocut. n. and
　　cran. circumfl. humeral a. and v.
c　Brachial a. and v.
d　Dist. muscular br. of musculocut. n. and
　　bicipital a. and v.
e　Median cubital v.
f　Collateral ulnar a. and v.
g　Deep antebrachial a.and v.
h　Median a. and v.
i　Radial a. and v.
k　Flexor retinaculum
l　Abaxial extensor brr. of interossei III and IV
m　Cephalic v.
n　Accessory cephalic v.
o　Caud. circumfl. humeral a. and v.
p　Collateral radial a.
q　Cran. supf. antebrachial a.
r　Dors. carpal brr. of cran. interosseus
　　a. and v.
s　Extensor retinaculum
t　Med. and lat. terminal tendons of deep pectoral (cut)

(See pp. 7, 9, 61)

3. CUTANEOUS NERVES, BLOOD VESSELS, AND LYMPH NODES OF THE THORACIC LIMB

a) The **CUTANEOUS INNERVATION** of the dorsal part of the scapular region is supplied by the dorsal branches of C8 and T1 to T5, which come over the dorsal border of the scapular cartilage. The **supraclavicular nn.** innervate the craniolateral surface of the shoulder and arm, and the **intercostobrachial n.** supplies the caudolateral surface to the level of the olecranon (see text figure).

The small **cranial cut. antebrachial n.** (25, axillary) supplies the arm and extends down to the middle of the forearm. The skin of the forearm is also innervated by the large **lateral cut. antebrachial n.** (27, supf. br. of radial), running on the cranial surface of the extensor carpi radialis lateral to the cephalic v. and accompanied medial to the vein by the **medial cut. antebrachial n.** (30, musculocutaneous). The **caudal cut. antebrachial n.** (7, ulnar) ends at the accessory carpal bone.

The skin of the carpus and metacarpus is innervated on the dorsal surface by the lat. cut. antebrachial n. and its branches: **dorsal common digital nn. II (34) and III (35)**, from the supf. br. of the radial n. The lat. cut. antebrachial n. communicates above the carpus with the medial cut. antebrachial n., which supplies the dorsomedial surface. The dorsolateral surface is innervated by the dorsal br. of the ulnar n. and its continuation, **dorsal common digital n. IV (33)**.

On the palmar surface the skin is innervated by the median n. and its branches, **palmar common digital nn. II (18) and III (17)**, and by the supf. palmar br. of the ulnar n. (p. 9, 8) which receives the **communicating br. (f)** from the median n. and continues as the short **palmar common digital n. IV**.

The digits are supplied by the dorsal and palmar proper digital nn. from the corresponding common digital nn. (See p. 8).

Nerves of the thoracic limb

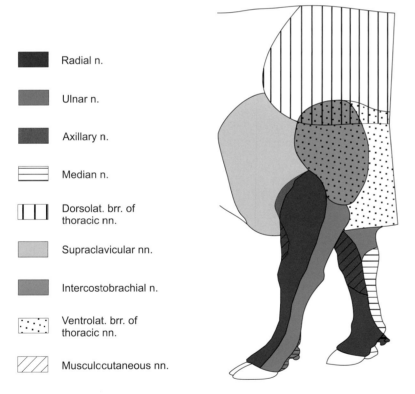

- Radial n.
- Ulnar n.
- Axillary n.
- Median n.
- Dorsolat. brr. of thoracic nn.
- Supraclavicular nn.
- Intercostobrachial n.
- Ventrolat. brr. of thoracic nn.
- Musculocutaneous nn.

b) The **BLOOD VESSELS** of the thoracic limb come from the **subclavian a. and v.** and the external jugular v., from which the **cephalic v. (23)** originates. The latter, as in the horse, but unlike the dog, has no anastomosis with the axillary v. Distal to the cranial border of the first rib, where the subclavian vessels become the **axillary a. and v. (20)**, the latter vessels give off the **external thoracic a. and v. (21)**, as well as the **suprascapular a. and v. (19)** for the lateral muscles of the shoulder and for the shoulder joint, and the large **subscapular a. and v. (1)**, which run along the caudal border of the scapula and supply most of the muscles of the shoulder joint, and the long head of the triceps. One branch of the axillary a. is the **caudal circumflex humeral a. (3)**, which gives off the **collateral radial a. (4)**, from which arises the **cranial supf. antebrachial a. (p. 9, 1)**. This ends in the small **dorsal common digital aa. II and III (p. 9; 9, 12)**. The caudal circumflex humeral v. ends in the region of the

shoulder joint. Distal to the origin of the **cranial circumflex humeral a. (22)** – *the vein comes from the subscapular v.* – the axillary vessels become the **brachial a. and v. (5)**. These first give off the **deep brachial a. and v. (6)** to the caudal muscles of the elbow joint. The next branches are the **collateral ulnar a. and v. (8)**, of which the artery continues indirectly to the *small* **dorsal common digital a. IV**, while the vein ends at the elbow joint, mostly in the caudomedial muscles of the forearm. Distal to the collateral ulnar vessels, the **bicipital a. and v. (24)** arise and supply the biceps. They may originate from the next distal vessels, the **transverse cubital a. and v. (26)**. The last branches of the brachial vessels are the **common interosseus a. and v. (9)**, arising distal to the elbow joint. These divide into the large **cranial interosseus a. and v. (10)** and the *insignificant* **caudal interosseus a. and v. (11)**, *which usually do not reach the carpus.* The cranial interosseous a. and v. pass laterally through the proximal interosseous space and run on the lateral surface of the radius and ulna to the distal interosseous space, *where they are continued by the interosseous brr., passing medially through the space to become the palmar brr. These divide into* **deep and superficial brr. (p. 9. 8)** The ulnar a. and v. are absent, as in the horse. The **cephalic v. (23)**, on the surface of the cleidobrachialis, gives off the **median cubital v. (28)**, a long oblique anastomosis to the brachial v. at its point of transition to the median v. The cephalic v. continues distally on the extensor carpi radialis to the distal third of the forearm, where it gives off the **accessory cephalic v. (32)**. This continues the direction of the cephalic v. to the dorsal surface of the metacarpus and becomes **dorsal common digital v. III (35)**. Inconstant **dorsal common digital vv. II (34)** and IV (33) are given off the main trunk and *end in the distal deep palmar arch*. The cephalic v. turns medially and joins the radial v. above the carpus. The brachial a. and v. are continued medially in the forearm by the **median a. and v. (29)**, which give off in their course several branches: the **deep antebrachial aa. and vv. (12)** to the caudal muscles of the forearm, and the **radial a. and v. (31)** in the middle of the forearm. The sometimes double radial vein receives the cephalic v. proximal to the carpus. At the carpus the radial a. and v. join their respective **dorsal carpal networks**, which also receive the cranial interosseous a. and v. and the dorsal carpal br. of the collateral ulnar a. (without the corresponding v.). **Dorsal metacarpal a. III** comes from the arterial dorsal carpal network. It is accompanied in the dorsal groove of the metacarpal bone by **dorsal metacarpal v. III** from the venous dorsal carpal network. On the palmar surface of the metacarpal bone the radial a. and v. and the deep palmar branches of the cranial interosseus a. and v. form the **deep palmar arches (15)**, which give off the deep **palmar metacarpal aa. and vv. II–IV**. Palmar metacarpal v. II is the direct continuation of the radial v. The continuing median a. and v. pass through the carpal canal on the palmaromedial surface of the deep flexor tendon and the tendon of the deep part of the supf. flexor, to the metacarpus. Here the median a., the supf. palmar br. of the cranial interosseous a., and the supf. palmar br. of the radial a. are connected across the surface of the flexor tendons by the zigzag **superficial palmar arch**, which gives off **palmar common digital aa. II (18)** and IV. **Palmar common digital a. III (17)** is the direct continuation of the median a. distal to the arch, and it is the main blood supply to the large digits. It courses to the interdigital space, crossing the medial branch of the supf. flexor tendon, where the pulse is palpable. It is accompanied by **palmar common digital v. III (17)**. The **interdigital a. and v. (p. 11, 5')** connect the palmar with the dorsal digital vessels. *The palmar common digital veins II and IV originate from the distal deep palmar venous arch.* (See also pp. 8–11.)

c) **LYMPHATIC STRUCTURES.** The large **proper axillary ln. (p. 5, a)** lies caudal to the shoulder joint at the level of the second intercostal space between the thoracic wall and the medial surface of the teres major. Small **axillary lnn. of the first rib** are associated with the axillary vessels on the lateral surface of the rib. *Both groups of lnn. are examined in meat inspection in special cases. In the hanging split carcass the proper axillary node is drawn cranially by the weight of the limb, and may be conveniently found by an incision from the inside of the thoracic wall in the middle of the first intercostal space.* The afferent lymphatics come from the bones, joints, and muscles of the shoulder, and from the arm and forearm. The efferent lymphatics go to the lnn. of the first rib, proper axillary ln., and caudal deep cervical lnn., which are drained on the left side by the thoracic duct and on the right by the right tracheal duct. The lymphatic drainage of the manus goes to the supf. cervical ln.

Arteries, Veins, and Nerves of thoracic limb

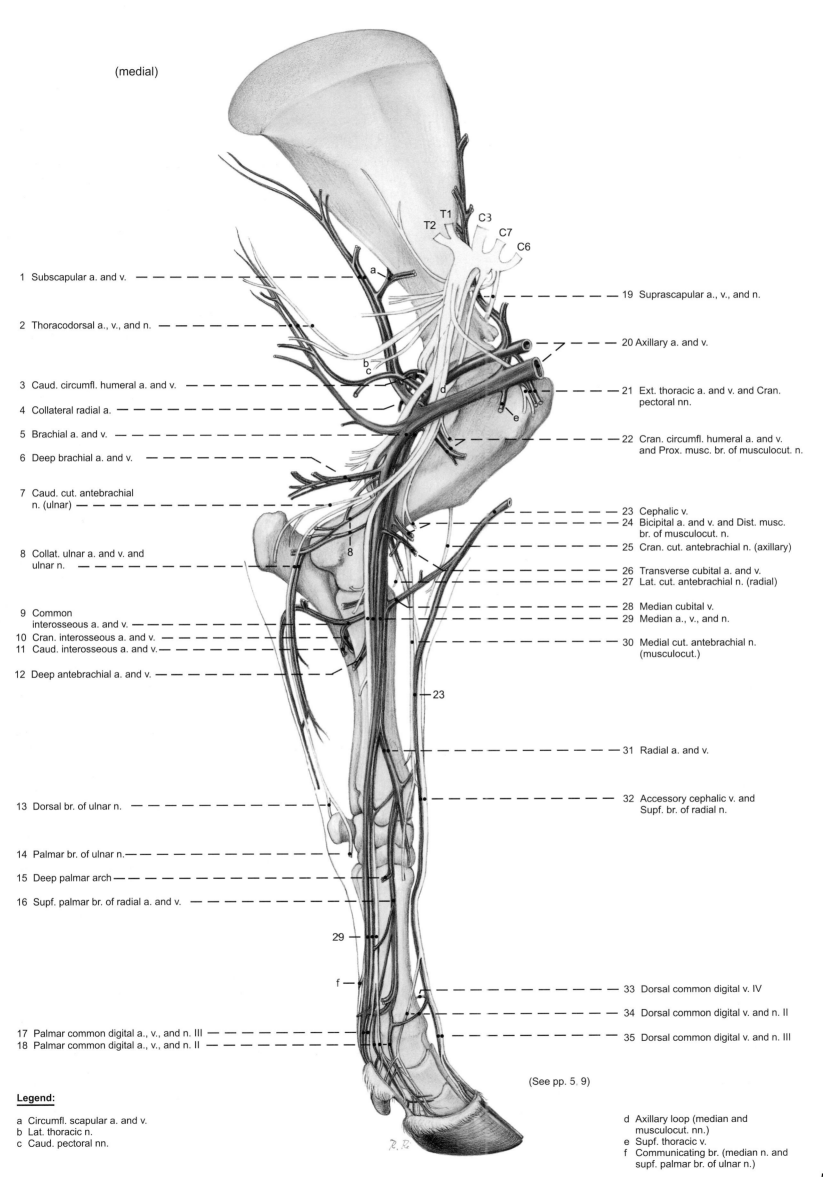

(medial)

T1
T2
C3
C7
C6

1 Subscapular a. and v.

2 Thoracodorsal a., v., and n.

3 Caud. circumfl. humeral a. and v.

4 Collateral radial a.

5 Brachial a. and v.

6 Deep brachial a. and v.

7 Caud. cut. antebrachial n. (ulnar)

8 Collat. ulnar a. and v. and ulnar n.

9 Common interosseous a. and v.

10 Cran. interosseous a. and v.

11 Caud. interosseous a. and v.

12 Deep antebrachial a. and v.

13 Dorsal br. of ulnar n.

14 Palmar br. of ulnar n.

15 Deep palmar arch

16 Supf. palmar br. of radial a. and v.

17 Palmar common digital a., v., and n. III

18 Palmar common digital a., v., and n. II

19 Suprascapular a., v., and n.

20 Axillary a. and v.

21 Ext. thoracic a. and v. and Cran. pectoral nn.

22 Cran. circumfl. humeral a. and v. and Prox. musc. br. of musculocut. n.

23 Cephalic v.

24 Bicipital a. and v. and Dist. musc. br. of musculocut. n.

25 Cran. cut. antebrachial n. (axillary)

26 Transverse cubital a. and v.

27 Lat. cut. antebrachial n. (radial)

28 Median cubital v.

29 Median a., v., and n.

30 Medial cut. antebrachial n. (musculocut.)

31 Radial a. and v.

32 Accessory cephalic v. and Supf. br. of radial n.

33 Dorsal common digital v. IV

34 Dorsal common digital v. and n. II

35 Dorsal common digital v. and n. III

(See pp. 5, 9)

Legend:

a Circumfl. scapular a. and v.
b Lat. thoracic n.
c Caud. pectoral nn.

d Axillary loop (median and musculocut. nn.)
e Supf. thoracic v.
f Communicating br. (median n. and supf. palmar br. of ulnar n.)

7

4. VESSELS AND NERVES OF THE MANUS

> The dissection is done on the embalmed limbs provided and on fresh specimens of the metacarpus and digits. The skin is carefully removed down to the hoofs, preserving the nerves and vessels.

a) The **PALMAR NERVES** come predominantly from the median n., but also from the palmar br. of the ulnar n. (For vessels, see p. 6.)

The **median n. (4)**, accompanied by the **median a. and v.**, passes through the carpal canal, medial to the flexor tendons, to the mediopalmar surface of the metacarpus, where it is covered by deep fascia. (See p. 10.) Here the nerve lies between the *small* **superficial brr. of the radial a. and v. (6)** medially, and the *large* median a. and the *usually double* median v. on the other side. In the middle of the metacarpus the nerve divides under the proximal ligament of the medial dewclaw into palmar common digital nn. II and III. **Palmar common digital n. II (13)** runs in the medial groove between interosseus III and the flexor tendons, accompanied from the distal third of the metacarpus by **palmar common digital a. and v. II (13)**. They divide proximal to the fetlock joint into the **axial palmar a., v., and n. of digit II (18, dewclaw)** and the continuing **abaxial palmar digital a., v., and n. III (19)** for deep digital structures and the dermis of the bulb and wall as far as the apex of the hoof. (Axial and abaxial digital nerves and vessels are understood to be "proper", and this adjective may be omitted.) **Palmar common digital n. III (15)** is usually double. The branches are accompanied on each side by the branches of the also double **palmar common digital v. III**, and between them by **palmar common digital a. III**, proceeding in the direction of the interdigital space (see p. 10).

The **ulnar n.** divides near the middle of the forearm into dorsal and palmar branches. The **palmar br. (p. 7. 14)** crosses deep to the tendon of the flexor carpi ulnaris and runs between the deep part of the superficial digital flexor and the accessory carpal bone. Just distal to the carpus it gives off the **deep br.** to the interossei and continues as the **supf. br. (8)**, which runs in the lateral groove between interosseus IV and the digital flexor tendons, accompanied by the **supf. palmar br. of the cranial interosseous a. (8)**. Distal to the **communicating br. (10)** from the median n., the supf. br. of the palmar br. of the ulnar becomes the short **palmar common digital n. IV**, accompanied by the corresponding a. and v. Proximal to the fetlock joint of the fourth digit they divide into the **axial palmar digital a., v., and n. of digit V (22, dewclaw)** and the **abaxial palmar digital a., v., and n. IV (24)**, with distribution like that of the corresponding structures of digits II and III. *Deep palmar metacarpal nn. like those of the dog and horse do not exist.* Deep **palmar metacarpal aa. and vv. II - IV** from the deep palmar arches run distally on the metacarpal bone and anastomose proximal to the fetlock joint with the supf. palmar vessels (see p. 6).

b) The **DORSAL NERVES** come mainly from the supf. br. of the radial n. (lat. cut. antebrachial n.) and also from the dorsal br. of the ulnar. (Vessels, see p. 6.)

The **dorsal br. of the ulnar n. (5)** emerges between the ulnaris lateralis and the flexor carpi ulnaris, about 2 cm proximal to the accessory carpal bone and runs distally across the bone. It continues on the lateral surface of the carpus to the groove between the metacarpal bone and interosseus IV, where it becomes **dorsal common digital n. IV (7)**. On the dorsolateral surface of the fetlock joint it gives off the small **axial dorsal digital n. V (23)**. (The dewclaws have migrated to the palmar surface from their original lateral and medial positions.) Common digital n. IV is continued by **abaxial dorsal digital n. IV (25)** to the dorsolateral coronary region of the fourth digit.

The **supf. br. of the radial n. (3, lat. cut. antebrachial n.)**, accompanied medially by the **accessory cephalic v. (2)** and the often double **cranial supf. antebrachial a. (1)** passes across the dorsomedial surface of the carpus. Just distal to the middle of the metacarpus the nerve can be palpated on the bone medial to the three digital extensor tendons. Here it divides into **dorsal common digital nn. III (12) and II (9)**. The latter is small. It crosses under **dorsal common digital v. II (11)** if that is present, reaches the medial surface of the fetlock joint with the small **dorsal common digital a. II (9)**, and divides into **axial dorsal digital n. II to the dewclaw (16)**, and **abaxial dorsal digital n. III (17)** to the dorsomedial coronary region of the third digit. *As they cross the fetlock joints the abaxial dorsal and palmar digital nn. course on opposite borders of the abaxial palmar digital v.*

They may be connected by a communicating br. at the level of the proximal phalanx.

The continuing **dorsal common digital a., v., and n. III (12)** cross the tendon of the medial digital extensor (p. 5, 40) and the medial branch of the tendon of the common extensor of digits III and IV (p. 5, 41) to reach the interdigital space where they divide into the **axial dorsal aa., vv., and nn. of digits III and IV**.

There are no deep dorsal metacarpal nn., unlike the system in the metatarsus. Deep dorsal vessels are reduced to the **dorsal metacarpal a. III** and (inconstant) **v. III (p. 11, 4)**, running in the dorsal longitudinal groove of the bone to the interdigital space, where they anastomose with the superficial dorsal common digital vessels.

Arteries and Veins of the Manus (palmar)

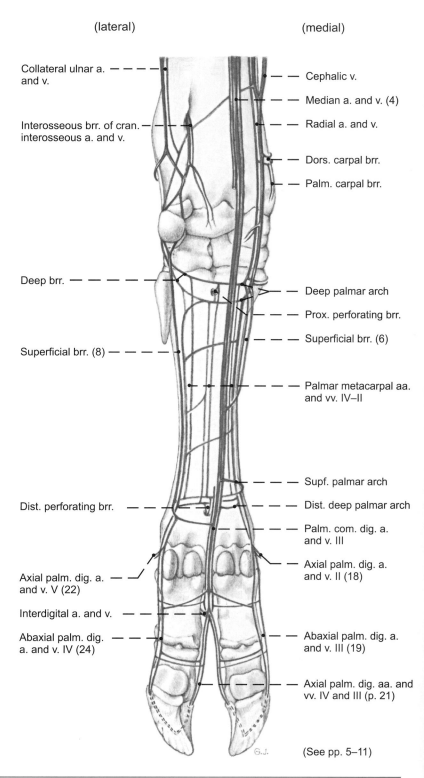

(lateral)   (medial)

Collateral ulnar a. and v.

Cephalic v.

Median a. and v. (4)

Radial a. and v.

Interosseous brr. of cran. interosseous a. and v.

Dors. carpal brr.

Palm. carpal brr.

Deep brr.

Deep palmar arch

Prox. perforating brr.

Superficial brr. (6)

Superficial brr. (8)

Palmar metacarpal aa. and vv. IV–II

Supf. palmar arch

Dist. perforating brr.

Dist. deep palmar arch

Palm. com. dig. a. and v. III

Axial palm. dig. a. and v. V (22)

Axial palm. dig. a. and v. II (18)

Interdigital a. and v.

Abaxial palm. dig. a. and v. IV (24)

Abaxial palm. dig. a. and v. III (19)

Axial palm. dig. aa. and vv. IV and III (p. 21)

(See pp. 5–11)

Arteries, Veins, and Nerves of the Manus

(mediopalmar)   (dorsolateral)

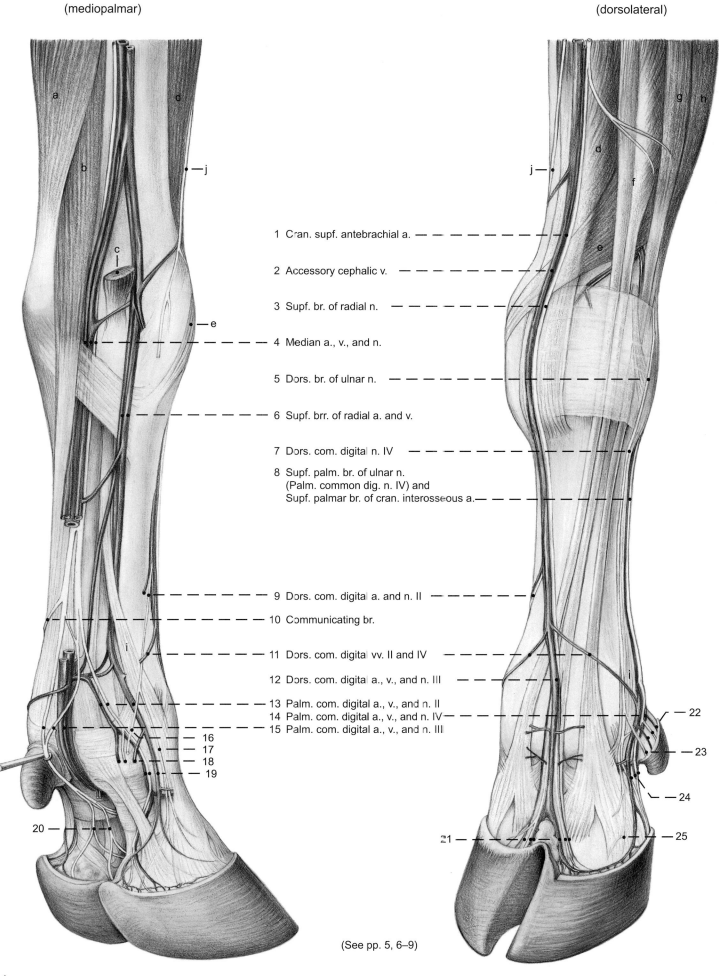

1 Cran. supf. antebrachial a.

2 Accessory cephalic v.

3 Supf. br. of radial n.

4 Median a., v., and n.

5 Dors. br. of ulnar n.

6 Supf. brr. of radial a. and v.

7 Dors. com. digital n. IV

8 Supf. palm. br. of ulnar n.
  (Palm. common dig. n. IV) and
  Supf. palmar br. of cran. interosseous a.

9 Dors. com. digital a. and n. II

10 Communicating br.

11 Dors. com. digital vv. II and IV

12 Dors. com. digital a., v., and n. III

13 Palm. com. digital a., v., and n. II
14 Palm. com. digital a., v., and n. IV
15 Palm. com. digital a., v., and n. III

16
17
18
19

20

21

22

23

24

25

(See pp. 5, 6–9)

5. INTERDIGITAL NERVES AND VESSELS, INTEROSSEI, AND FASCIAE OF THE MANUS

a) The **INTERDIGITAL NERVES AND VESSELS** of the manus come primarily from the **palmar common digital a., v., and n. III** (5), whose branches communicate with the corresponding dorsal nerves and vessels (see p. 8).

On the pes the main blood supply of the digits is the *dorsal metatarsal a. III* (11 and p. 21, 12). This difference is important surgically. The digital vessels and nn. of the pes have the same connections as on the manus. Usually the branches of the double palmar common digital n. III unite for a short distance at the beginning of the interdigital space, and divide again into **axial palmar digital nn. III** (6) **and IV** (7). If there is no common trunk, the branches are continued by the axial palmar digital nn., which give off communicating branches to the **axial dorsal digital nn. III and IV. Palmar common digital a. III** (5) gives off branches to the proximal phalanges. These branches pass between the deep flexor tendon and the bone and anastomose with the abaxial palmar digital aa. A dorsal branch, the **interdigital a.** (5'), anastomoses with the **dorsal metacarpal a. III** (4) and the small **dorsal common digital a. III** (1) and supplies the **axial dorsal digital aa. III** (3) **and IV** (2). Distal to the interdigital a., palmar common digital a. III divides into **axial palmar digital aa. III** (6) **and IV** (7). **Palmar common digital v. III** (5), often double, unites at the middle of the proximal phalanx, where it receives the anastomotic branches of the abaxial palmar digital vv. and gives off the **interdigital v.** (5') and the **axial palmar digital vv** (6, 7). The interdigital v. has connections with dorsal digital vv. corresponding to the arteries. The axial dorsal digital aa., vv., and nn. supply the dorsal coronary and interdigital regions of the third and fourth digits. The axial palmar (plantar) aa., vv., and nn. supply the interdigital deep structures and dermis of the bulb and hoof of the third and fourth digits. (For the supply of the abaxial surface of the digits, see p. 8.) The axial palmar (plantar) a. and v. enter the axial foramen in the distal phalanx and anastomose in the bone with the abaxial palmar a. and v., which enter through the abaxial foramen, to form the terminal arches.

b) The **INTEROSSEI III AND IV** (see p. 18) provide support for the fetlock joints of the ox comparable to that of interosseus III (medius) in the horse. These muscles originate from the proximal end of the metacarpal (metatarsal) bone and the deep palmar (plantar) carpal ligg. In young animals they are relatively fleshy, and in older animals, predominantly tendinous. Interossei III and IV are fused along their axial borders in the metacarpus (metatarsus), but they separate and terminate on the corresponding digits. *In the middle of the metacarpus (metatarsus) the interossei give off the* **accessory lig.**, *which bifurcates and joins the branches of the supf. digital flexor tendon at the level of the fetlock joints in the formation of the* **sleeves** (**manicae flexoriae**) *through which the branches of the deep flexor tendon pass.* Proximal to the fetlock joints each interosseus divides into two tendons (h), each with two **extensor branches** (p. 5, l; p. 9, i). The two tendons are attached to the sesamoid bones (i) of the corresponding digit. A flat **abaxial extensor branch** (g) passes across the surface of the sesamoid bone, to which it is attached, and joins the tendon of the proper digital extensor. The **axial extensor branches** (f) remain fused together until they pass through the intercapital notch in the end of the metacarpal (metatarsal) bone. Then they separate and join the tendons of their respective proper digital extensors. The interosseus, sesamoid bones, and sesamoid ligg. of each digit form a suspensory apparatus which aids the digital flexor tendons in the support of the fetlock joint. In addition, the extensor branches oppose the tension of the deep flexor tendon on the distal phalanx when the weight is on the foot.

c) On the carpus the **FASCIA OF THE MANUS** is thickened dorsally to form the **extensor retinaculum** (p. 5, s) and especially on the palmar surface to form the **flexor retinaculum** (p. 5, k).

On the dorsal surface of the metacarpus (metatarsus) the fascia is thin, but on the palmar surface, in continuation of the flexor retinaculum, it is thick, forming the **proximal ligg. of the dewclaws**. These come from the borders of the metacarpal (metatarsal) bone and have been cut to expose the palmar (plantar) nerves and vessels. At the level of the fetlock joints, the **transverse lig.** connects the dewclaws, and a palpable **distal lig.** runs from each dewclaw to the fascia on the abaxial surface of the coffin joint, resembling in its course the lig. of the ergot in the horse. It also blends with the abaxial end of the distal interdigital lig. (see below). The whole system of ligaments of both dewclaws forms a letter H.

On the fetlock joints the fascia around the digital flexor tendons of each digit is thickened to form the **palmar annular lig.** (12), which joins the **collateral sesamoid ligg.** and the **proximal scutum** – the fibrocartilaginous bearing surface for the flexor tendons, formed on the sesamoid bones and the **palmar (plantar) lig.** between them, and extending proximal to the sesamoid bones.

Distal to the fetlock joint the fascia is reinforced in the **proximal** (13) **and distal** (15) **digital annular ligg.**, attached to the proximal phalanx. The main digits are connected by the proximal and distal interdigital ligg. The **proximal interdigital lig.** (14) is short and thick; it is attached on the axial surfaces of the proximal halves of the proximal phalanges, and is supplemented by the crossed **interdigital phalangosesamoid ligg.** These extend from the sesamoid bones of one digit to the axial tubercle of the proximal phalanx of the other digit. The **distal interdigital lig.** (16) has greater mechanical advantage in resisting the spread of the digits. It consists of superficial and deep parts. The **superficial part** is palpable. Its crossed fibers extend from the abaxial eminence of the flexor tuberosity of the middle phalanx (see p. 3, 71), around the palmar surface of the deep flexor tendon to the navicular bone of the other digit. It serves to hold the deep flexor tendon in place. The crossed fibers of the **deep part** pass from the axial surface of the distal end of the middle phalanx of one digit to the distal phalanx and navicular bone of the other digit. The attachment to the navicular bone is by means of the **distal scutum** – a plate of fibrocartilage that covers the flexor surface of the bone and extends proximal to it. The terminal branches of the deep and supf. flexor tendons have **common digital synovial sheaths**, which begin between the middle and distal thirds of the metacarpus and end just above the coffin joint.

They form **six pouches for each main digit**: two abaxial pouches and one palmar (plantar) pouch proximal to the palmar (plantar) annular lig., two between the two digital annular ligg., and one distal to the superficial part of the distal interdigital lig.

Of the three pouches proximal to the palmar (plantar) annular lig., (I) is between the interossei and the accessory lig.; (II) lies along the accessory lig., partially surrounding the deep flexor tendon; and III is on the palmar (plantar) surface of the supf. flexor tendon. Abaxial (IV) and axial (V) pouches bulge between the two digital annular ligg. The sixth pouch (VI) is distal to the supf. part of the distal digital annular lig. The sheaths of both digits may communicate with each other where they are in contact.

Digital Arteries, Veins, and Nerves

Digit III, left manus, axial surface

Legend:

1 Dors. com. digital a., v., and n. III

2 Axial dors. digital a., v., and n. IV

3 Axial dors. digital a., v., and n. III

4 Dors. metacarpal a. and v. III

5 Palm. (plant.) com. dig. a., v., and n. III

5' Interdigital a. and v.

6 Axial palm. (plant.) digital a., v., and n. III

6' Communicating br. (nerve)

7 Axial palm. (plant.) digital a., v., and n. IV

(axial)

Digit III, right pes, axial surface*

8 Dors. com. digital a., v., and n. III

9 Axial dors. digital a., v., and n. IV

10 Axial dors. digital a., v., and n. III

11 Dors. metatarsal a., v., and n. III

11' Communicating br. (nerve)

Branches to the bulb of the hoof

Branches to the apex of the hoof

(See pp. 5, 7, 9)

(See pp. 17, 21, 23)

Legend:

Tendons:
a Lateral digital extensor
b, c Common digital extensor or Long digital extensor (Med. dig. ext., and common (long) ext. of digits III and IV)

d Supf. digital flexor
e Deep digital flexors Interossei III and IV:
f Axial extensor branches

g Abax. extensor branches
h Tendon to sesamoid bone
i Prox. sesamoid bone of dig. IV
j Dorsal lig.

k Axial common collat. lig.
l Axial collat. ligg.
m Axial palm. (plant.) lig. of pastern joint
n Axial collat. sesamoid lig.

Digital fascia, Fibrous and synovial digital sheaths of manus and pes

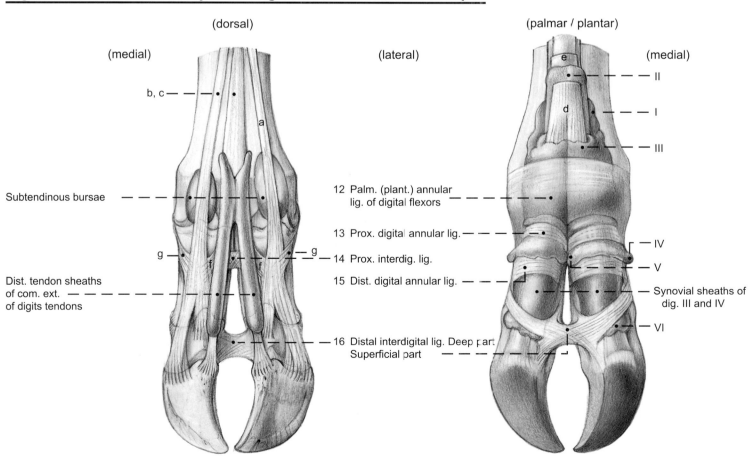

(dorsal)

(medial)

b, c

a

Subtendinous bursae

g — g

Dist. tendon sheaths of com. ext. of digits tendons

(lateral)

12 Palm. (plant.) annular lig. of digital flexors

13 Prox. digital annular lig.

14 Prox. interdig. lig.

15 Dist. digital annular lig.

16 Distal interdigital lig. Deep part
Superficial part

(palmar / plantar)

(medial)

II

I

III

IV

V

Synovial sheaths of dig. III and IV

VI

11

6. SYNOVIAL STRUCTURES OF THE THORACIC LIMB

a) JOINTS OF THE THORACIC LIMB

NAME	BONES involved	TYPE OF JOINT	FUNCTION	REMARKS
I. Shoulder joint	Glenoid cavity of scapula and head of humerus	Simple spheroidal	Restricted to flexion and extension	Infraspinatus and subscapularis act as contractile ligaments
II. Elbow joint		Composite joint		Because the collateral ligg. are attached to the humerus prox. to axis of rotation of the condyle they are stretched in the neutral position of joint and tend to snap it into extension or flexion Pronator teres is feebly muscular.
a) Humeroulnar joint	Humeral condyle and ulna	Simple hinge joint	a–b) Flexion and extension, snap joint	
b) Humeroradial joint	Humeral condyle and head of radius	Simple hinge		
c) Proximal radioulnar joint	Articular circumference of radius and radial notch of ulna	Simple rotating	c) No movement	
III. Distal radioulnar joint:	Absent			Synostosis
JOINTS OF THE MANUS				
IV. Carpal joint		Composite joint		Collateral ligg. have long supf. parts and prox., middle, and distal short deep parts. Med. collat. lig. is stronger. Synovial sac of a) rarely communicates with b); b) and c) always communicate*
a) Antebrachiocarpal joint	Radial trochlea and ulnar styloid process with carpal bones	Composite cochlear	Flexion and extension to 95°	
b) Midcarpal joint	Prox. and dist. rows of carpal bones	Composite condylar	Flexion and extension to 45°	
c) Carpometacarpal joint	Carpal II–IV and metacarpal bones III and IV	Composite plane joint	Little movement	
d) Intercarpal joints	Carpal bones of same row	Composite plane joints	Little movement	
V. Fetlock (metacarpo-phalangeal) joints	Metacarpal III and IV, prox. phalanges, and prox. sesamoid bones	Composite hinge joint	Flexion and extension	The ox has two fetlock joints, whose capsules communicate. In their dorsal walls are fibrocartila-ginous sesamoid bodies.
VI. Pastern (prox. interphalangeal) joints	Prox. and middle phalanges	Simple saddle joint	Flexion, extension, and small lateral and rotational movements	There is no communication between pastern joints. Their dorsal pouches extend to the coffin joint pouches.
VII. Coffin (dist. Interphalangeal) joints	Middle and dist. phalanges and navicular (dist. sesamoid) bones	Composite saddle joint	Flexion, extension, and small lateral and rotational movements	

b) SYNOVIAL BURSAE

The large (up to 8 cm in diameter, Schmidtchen**) **infraspinatus bursa** lies deep to the flat superficial part of the tendon, which terminates on the distinct infraspinatus surface (p. 3, 26') distal to the major tubercle. (The deep part of the tendon ends on the proximal border of the tubercle). The voluminous **intertubercular bursa** on the medial surface of the major tubercle lies deep to the tendon of origin of the biceps and on both sides of it. At the level of the **transverse humeral retinaculum** the bursa surrounds the tendon. As in the horse, the bursa is separate from the joint capsule. The **bursa of the triceps brachii** lies under the terminal tendon on the olecranon tuber. The inconstant **subcutaneous olecranon bursa** lies on the caudal surface of the olecranon in old cattle.

The **subcutaneous precarpal bursa** develops in adults and enlarges with age. It may reach the size of an apple. It extends on the dorsal surface from the midcarpal joint to a point just below the metacarpal tuberosity, covering the termination of the extensor carpi radialis. It usually does not communicate with underlying synovial structures and can be surgically removed when enlarged (hygroma). The **subtendinous bursae of the ext. carpi obliquus, ext. carpi radialis, ulnaris lateralis, and the supf. and deep digital flex-** ors lie under the respective tendons on the medial, dorsal, lateral, and palmar surfaces of the carpal joint.

The **subtendinous bursae of the medial and lateral proper digital extensors** lie dorsally on the fetlock joints. The **navicular bursae** are between the terminal branches of the deep flexor tendon and the navicular bones. Inflammations of the bursae have the same clinical signs as in the horse.

c) TENDON SHEATHS (VAGINAE SYNOVIALES)

On the **dorsal and lateral surfaces of the carpus** the extensor carpi obliquus and the digital extensors have synovial sheaths; the tendons of the ext. carpi radialis and ulnaris lat. do not. On the **medial surface**, only the flexor carpi radialis has a synovial sheath.

On the **dorsal surface of the phalanges** the terminal branches of the tendon of the common extensor of digits III and IV have synovial sheaths. On the **palmar surface** is the **common synovial sheath** of the supf. and deep digital flexor tendons. They are held in position at the fetlock joint and on the proximal phalanx by annular ligg., and in the region of the pastern joint by the supf. part of the distal interdigital lig.

* Desrochers et al., 1997
** Schmidtchen, 1906

Joints, Bursae, and Synovial Sheaths

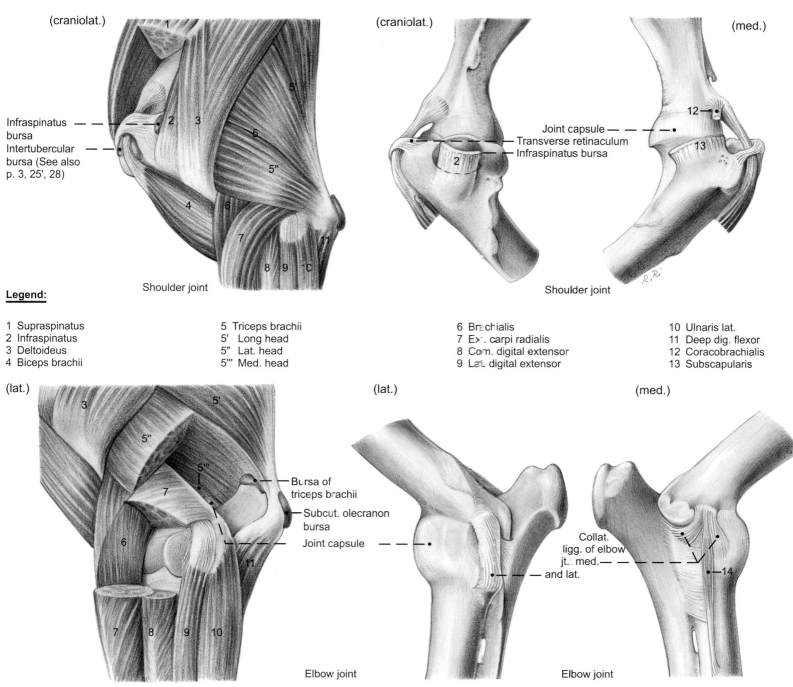

(craniolat.)

Infraspinatus bursa
Intertubercular bursa (See also p. 3, 25', 28)

Shoulder joint

(craniolat.)

Joint capsule
Transverse retinaculum
Infraspinatus bursa

Shoulder joint

(med.)

(lat.)

Bursa of triceps brachii
Subcut. olecranon bursa
Joint capsule

Elbow joint

(lat.)

Collat. ligg. of elbow jt. med. and lat.

Elbow joint

(med.)

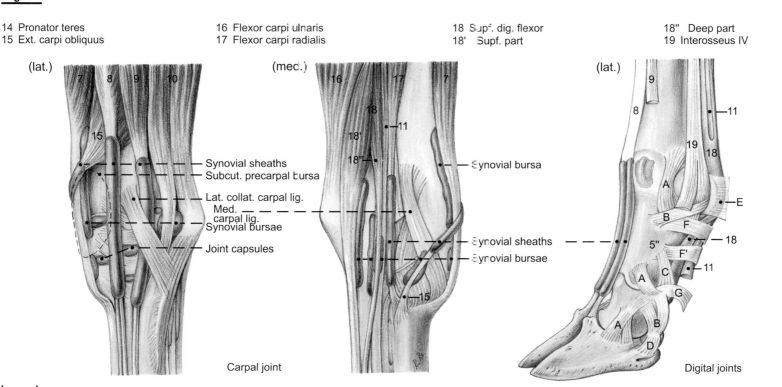

(lat.)

Synovial sheaths
Subcut. precarpal bursa
Lat. collat. carpal lig.
Med. carpal lig.
Synovial bursae
Joint capsules

Carpal joint

(med.)

Synovial bursa
Synovial sheaths
Synovial bursae

(lat.)

Digital joints

13

CHAPTER 2: PELVIC LIMB
1. SKELETON OF THE PELVIC LIMB

The skeleton of the pelvic limb includes the bones of the pelvic girdle, described with the pelvis (pp. 78–79).

a) The **FEMUR** has a proximal **head (1)**, *the articular surface of which presents a condyloid lateral extension on the upper surface of the neck (3)*. The **fovea (2)** is *small and almost centrally located.* The **major trochanter (4)** is, *in contrast to that of the horse, undivided*, and borders a *deep* **trochanteric fossa (5)**. The *rounded caudomedially directed* **minor trochanter (6)** *is connected to the major trochanter by a distinct* **intertrochanteric crest (4')**. The small rounded **tuberosity for the deep gluteal m.** is distal to the major trochanter. *The third trochanter is absent in the ox.* The **body of the femur (8)** is *rounded and relatively slender and straight*, compared to that of the horse. Distolaterally, as in the horse, there is a **supracondylar fossa (13)**, but *it is shallow in the ox*. On the distal end of the femur are the *nearly parallel* **medial (14)** and **lateral (17) condyles**, separated by a deep **intercondylar fossa (20)**. Cranial to the lateral condyle is the extensor fossa. On the cranial surface of the distal end of the femur is the **trochlea (21)**, the medial ridge of which is larger and extends farther proximally, where it is thickened to form a **tubercle (21')**.

The **patella (69)** is a sesamoid bone in the terminal tendon of the quadriceps femoris. The broad proximal **base (69')** has *blunt, rough borders*, and a **cartilaginous process (69''')** for attachment of the **med. parapatellar fibrocartilage (69'''')**, as in the horse. The distal **apex (69'')** is *more acutely pointed than in the horse.*

Left patella

(69''''' Articular surface)

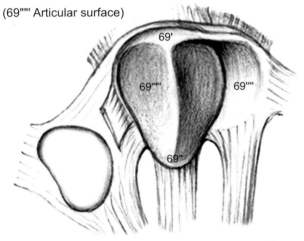

(See p. 29)

b)The **BONES OF THE CRUS (LEG, SHANK)** are the strong tibia and the vestigial fibula, reduced to its proximal and distal extremities.

I. The **tibia** with its **medial condyle (23)** and its laterally extended **lateral condyle (25)** presents *proximal articular surfaces almost on the same level*, between which the **intercondylar eminence (24)** rises. On the **body of the tibia (28)** is the *broad* proximocranial **tibial tuberosity (29)** with the laterally adjacent **extensor groove (27)**. On the distal **tibial cochlea (30)** the articular ridge and grooves are *almost sagittal* like those of the dog, but unlike those of the horse. *The lateral surface of the cochlea has two articular facets for the distal end-piece of the fibula, the lateral malleolus.* The **medial malleolus (31)** has a characteristic distally directed process.

II. *The fibula is more or less reduced, depending on the individual.* The **head of the fibula (32)** *fuses with the lateral condyle of the tibia as a distally directed process*. Rarely is it an isolated bone as in the horse. *A body of the fibula can be present as an exception, but it is usually replaced by a fibrous strand; therefore there is usually no interosseous space in the crus.*

The distal end of the fibula persists as an independent bone, the **lateral malleolus (35)**, *and articulates proximally with the tibia, medially with the talus, and distally with the calcaneus.*

c) The **TARSAL BONES** make up, in proximal, middle, and distal rows, a total of only five bones. The **talus (37)** in the proximal row is *longer and more slender* than in the horse. The ridges of the **proximal trochlea (39)** are sagittal, unlike those of the horse, and articulate with the tibial cochlea medially and with the lateral malleolus. *The proximal trochlea is joined by the roughened* **neck (40)** *to the* **distal trochlea (41')**, *which articulates with the central and fourth tarsal bone. A distal trochlea of the talus is characteristic of the order Artiodactyla, the even-toed ungulates.* The **calcaneus (42)** is *also longer and more slender* than in the horse. Its proximal **tuber**

Left calcaneus

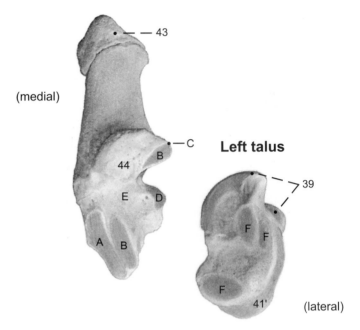

(medial)

Left talus

(lateral)

Legend:

A Artic. surface for T C and T IV
B Artic. surfaces for talus
C Coracoid process
D Artic. surface for malleolus
E Tarsal sinus
F Artic. surfaces for calcaneus

calcanei (43) is *roughened dorsocranially, divided by a transverse crest, and hollowed out in a plantar groove.* The *compact* **sustentaculum tali (44)** is hollowed to form a tendon groove on the plantar surface. *Distally the calcaneus articulates with the central and fourth tarsal bone. The single bone of the middle row, the central tarsal, is fused with the fourth tarsal of the distal row to form one bone*, the **central and fourth tarsal (45')**, *characteristic of Ruminantia. It occupies the full width of the tarsus, and jogs upward proximomedially.* The remaining **tarsal bones** of the distal row occupy the distomedial part of the tarsus. The rounded **T I** is medioplantar. **T II and T III** *are always fused to form one flat bone, also characteristic of Ruminantia.* The **tarsal canal** passes between the two large distal tarsal bones and the mt. bone. It connects with the **proximal mt. canal**, which, unlike the proximal mc. canal, opens on the proximal surface of the base of the mt. bone. The tarsus, metatarsus, and digits are homologous to the human foot (pes) and correspond to the manus of the thoracic limb.

d) The **METATARSAL BONES, PHALANGES, and SESAMOID BONES** of the pes exhibit only minor differences from the bones of the manus. Metatarsal bone III and IV is longer and more slender, and square in cross section; metacarpal bone III and IV is transversely oval. A *small, discoid* **metatarsal sesamoid (70)** *is located proximoplantar to Mt. III in the fused tendons of origin of the interossei.*

Bones of the pelvic limb

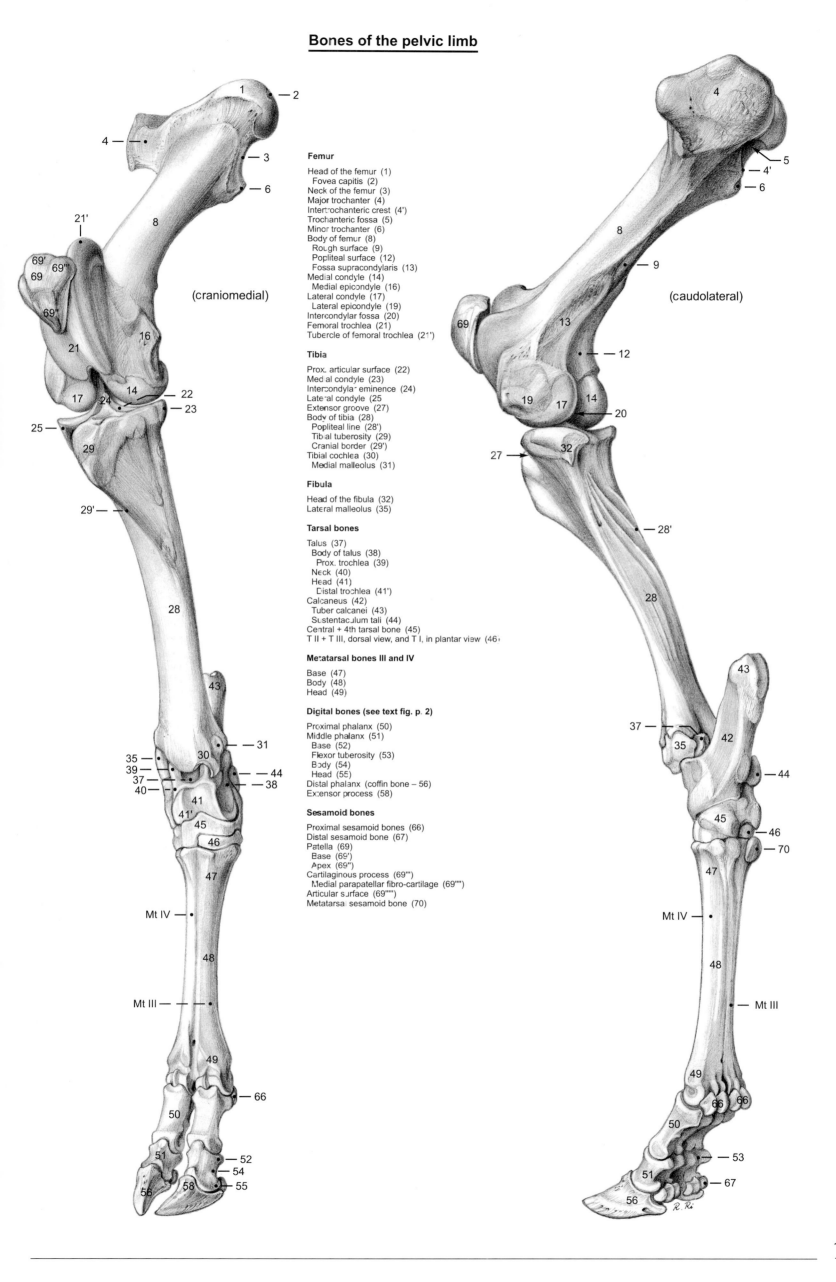

(craniomedial)

(caudolateral)

Femur

Head of the femur (1)
  Fovea capitis (2)
Neck of the femur (3)
Major trochanter (4)
  Intertrochanteric crest (4')
  Trochanteric fossa (5)
Minor trochanter (6)
Body of femur (8)
  Rough surface (9)
  Popliteal surface (12)
  Fossa supracondylaris (13)
Medial condyle (14)
  Medial epicondyle (16)
Lateral condyle (17)
  Lateral epicondyle (19)
Intercondylar fossa (20)
Femoral trochlea (21)
Tubercle of femoral trochlea (21')

Tibia

Prox. articular surface (22)
Medial condyle (23)
Intercondylar eminence (24)
Lateral condyle (25)
Extensor groove (27)
Body of tibia (28)
  Popliteal line (28')
  Tibial tuberosity (29)
  Cranial border (29')
Tibial cochlea (30)
  Medial malleolus (31)

Fibula

Head of the fibula (32)
Lateral malleolus (35)

Tarsal bones

Talus (37)
  Body of talus (38)
    Prox. trochlea (39)
  Neck (40)
  Head (41)
    Distal trochlea (41')
Calcaneus (42)
  Tuber calcanei (43)
  Sustentaculum tali (44)
Central + 4th tarsal bone (45)
T II + T III, dorsal view, and T I, in plantar view (46)

Metatarsal bones III and IV

Base (47)
Body (48)
Head (49)

Digital bones (see text fig. p. 2)

Proximal phalanx (50)
Middle phalanx (51)
  Base (52)
  Flexor tuberosity (53)
  Body (54)
  Head (55)
Distal phalanx (coffin bone – 56)
Extensor process (58)

Sesamoid bones

Proximal sesamoid bones (66)
Distal sesamoid bone (67)
Patella (69)
  Base (69')
  Apex (69")
Cartilaginous process (69"')
  Medial parapatellar fibro-cartilage (69"")
Articular surface (69""')
Metatarsal sesamoid bone (70)

15

2. LATERAL THIGH AND CRANIAL CRURAL MUSCLES WITH THEIR NERVES

The skin of the pelvic limb is removed down to the middle of the metatarsus, with attention to the inconstant subcutaneous calcanean bursa, sparing all of the superficial blood vessels and nerves, and noting the cutaneous nerves. Dorsolaterally on the pelvic limb the muscles of the rump and caudal thigh are demonstrated, and the tensor fasciae latae, gluteus medius, and biceps femoris [gluteobiceps] are severed at their origin and termination and removed. The underlying nerves and vessels, iliacus muscle, the distinct gluteus accessorius with its strong terminal tendon, the gluteus profundus, and the sacrosciatic lig. are preserved.

a) **LATERALLY ON THE THIGH** and on the rump the **cranial gluteal n.** (2) supplies the *especially large and fleshy* **tensor fasciae latae** (5) (which includes the cranial part of the gluteus supf.), *the thin* **gluteus medius** (1), *which causes the characteristic bovine flattening of the rump*, the **gluteus accessorius** (3), (see above, considered a part of the gluteus medius), and the fleshy **gluteus profundus** (4). Each terminal tendon of the deep, middle, and accessory gluteal muscles has a synovial bursa on the major trochanter.

The **caudal gluteal n.** (16) supplies the *vertebral head* of the **biceps femoris [gluteobiceps, 7]**, which includes the caudal part of the gluteus supf. The *ischial head* is innervated by the tibial n. The *vertebral heads of the semitendinosus and semimembranosus, seen in the horse, are absent in the ox.*

The wide **sciatic n.** (17) passes over the gluteus profundus, and, at the hip joint, gives off **muscular brr. to the gemelli and quadratus femoris.** (The internal obturator is absent in the ox.) Here the sciatic n. divides into the common peroneal [fibular] n. cranially and the tibial n. caudally.

The **tibial n.** (19) gives off proximal muscular brr. to the ischial head of the biceps femoris and to the semitendinosus and semimembranosus, which originate from the tuber ischiadicum only, as in the dog.

In the course of the nerve toward the gastrocnemius the **caudal cutaneous sural nerve** (19') is given off in the middle of the thigh and runs with the lateral saphenous v. to the middle of the lateroplantar surface of the metatarsus.

The **biceps femoris [gluteobiceps, 7]** has a large trochanteric bursa on the trochanter major, over which the muscle passes. The bursa is clinically important as a cause of lameness when inflamed. Distal to the trochanter the biceps is divided into two parts as in the dog, but unlike the three parts in the horse. It ends with the fascia cruris on the patella, lateral patellar lig., and the cranial border of the tibia, and has another synovial bursa under its tendon at the level of the femoral condyle (see p. 29). Its tarsal tendon (34) ends on the tuber calcanei.

The **semitendinosus** (20) passes over the medial head of the gastrocnemius and ends, with a synovial bursa, on the cranial border of the tibia and by its tarsal tendon (see p. 19) on the tuber calcanei. *Characteristic of the muscle is a transverse tendinous intersection at the beginning of its middle third.*

The **semimembranosus** (18) is indistinctly divided near the end into a larger part ending on the medial femoral condyle, and a smaller part ending on the medial condyle of the tibia.

b) **ON THE CRUS** the **common peroneal [fibular] n.** (6) sometimes gives off in the middle of the crus a **lateral cutaneous sural n.** (21) toward the hock. The common peroneal n. runs over the lateral head of the gastrocnemius, passes under the peroneus [fibularis] longus, and runs between the latter and the lateral digital extensor to divide in the middle of the tibia into **superficial** (14) and **deep** (9) **peroneal [fibular] nn.** They innervate the flexors of the tarsus and extensors of the digits.

The *fleshy* **peroneus [fibularis] tertius** (10), absent in the dog and entirely tendinous in the horse, originates in the extensor fossa of the femur with the long digital extensor, which it largely covers proximomedially. Its terminal tendon is perforated by that of the cranial tibial and ends on Mt III and Mt IV and under the medial collateral lig. on T II and T III.

The **cranial tibial muscle** (8) *is smaller than in the horse* and is covered by the peroneus tertius and long digital extensor. *It is fused with the vestigial long extensor of digit I.* It is sometimes possible to separate the two tendons, which end on T I and medially on Mt III and Mt IV.

The **peroneus [fibularis] longus** (11), which also occurs in the dog, but not in the horse, is narrow, forms its tendon in the middle of the crus, crosses the tendon of the lateral extensor, passes under the lateral collateral lig., runs across the plantar surface of the tarsus and *ends on T I.*

The **long digital extensor** (13) (See also the cranial tibial m.) *has a superficial lateral belly* (**extensor of digits III and IV**) *and a deep medial belly* (**medial digital extensor, extensor of digit III**).

Both tendons pass under the crural retinaculum with the tendons of the cranial tibial and peroneus tertius; whereas only the long digital extensor tendons pass under the metatarsal retinaculum. They are arranged in the pes like the corresponding tendons of the common digital extensor in the manus. *The tarsal extensor retinaculum of the horse is absent in the ox.*

The **lateral digital extensor** (extensor of digit IV, 12) originates from the lateral collateral lig. of the stifle and the lateral condyle of the tibia. It is a *relatively large muscle* that passes under the tendon of the peroneus longus and laterally over the tarsus to digit IV. Its tendon is arranged here like that of the muscle of the same name in the manus. The **extensor digitalis brevis** (15) *is small*; a peroneus brevis is absent as in the horse.

Pelvic Limb

(lateral)

1 Gluteus medius

2 Cran. gluteal n.

3 Gluteus accessorius

4 Gluteus profundus

5 Tensor fasciae latae

6 Common peroneal n.

7 Biceps femoris

8 Cranial tibial m.

9 Deep peroneal n.

10 Peroneus tertius

11 Peroneus longus

12 Lat. digital extensor

13 Long digital extensor

14 Supf. peroneal n.

15 Extensor digitalis brevis

16 Caudal gluteal n.

17 Sciatic n.

18 Semimembranosus

19 Tibial n.

19' Caud. cut. sural n.

20 Semitendinosus

21 Lat. cut. sural n.

Legend:

22 Iliacus
23 Sacrosciatic lig.
24 Coccygeus
25 Gemelli
26 Quadratus femoris
27 Adductor magnus
   Quadriceps femoris:
28   Rectus femoris
29   Vastus lateralis
30 Gastrocnemius
31 Soleus
   Deep digital flexors:
32   Lat. digital flexor
33   Caudal tibial m.
34 Tarsal tendon of biceps

A Gluteal ln
B Sciatic ln.
C Deep popliteal lnn.

(Nerves and vessels, see p. 21)

(See pp. 19, 21, 23, 29, 67)

17

3. MEDIAL THIGH AND CAUDAL CRURAL MUSCLES WITH THEIR NERVES

> Medially on the thigh the gracilis is detached from the symphyseal tendon and removed, except for a short distal stump. At the tarsus the two retinacula, the tendon sheaths, and the bursae are examined. After demonstration of the tarsal tendons of the biceps and semitendinosus, the medial head of the gastrocnemius is severed near its origin to expose the superficial digital flexor.

a) **MEDIALLY ON THE THIGH** the muscles are innervated by the obturator n. only, or by the femoral and saphenous nn., or by the saphenous and obturator nn.

The **obturator n.** (6) *runs with the obturator v.* medially on the body of the ilium, passes through the obturator foramen, and innervates the following muscles:

The **external obturator** *in the ox has an additional* **intrapelvic part** (7) *that originates inside around the obturator foramen, but is not homologous to the internal obturator of other domestic animals.*

The **adductor magnus (et brevis, 9)** originates from the ventral surface of the pelvis and from the symphyseal tendon as in the horse, *but is more closely bound to the semimembranosus by connective tissue.* It terminates on the caudal surface of the femur, *but does not extend to the epicondyle.*

The **pectineus (et adductor longus, 8)** is more robust than in the horse. Its adductor part is innervated by the obturator n.; its pectineus part by the saphenous n. The tendons of origin come from the iliopubic eminence and pecten pubis, cross the median plane, and form with the tendons of the contralateral pectineus, the bulk of the prepubic tendon. Each pectineus terminates on the caudomedial surface of the body of the opposite femur. The **gracilis** (10) is innervated by the obturator n. supplemented by the saphenous n. It takes origin from the pelvic symphysis and the prepubic tendon. Its tendon forms, with that of the other side, the distinctive symphyseal tendon, which is *bean-shaped in the cow and equilaterally triangular in the bull,* indicating the sex of a split carcass.

At the level of the pecten pubis the **femoral n.** gives off the **saphenous n.** (4) (skin innervation, see p. 20), which not only supplies the last two muscles, but also is the sole innervation of the **sartorius** (3). *This muscle originates by two heads: the cranial one from the tendon of the psoas minor and the iliac fascia, and the caudal one from the body of the ilium dorsocaudal to the tubercle for the psoas minor. The cran. head of the sartorius, the iliopsoas, and the femoral n. pass through the muscular lacuna. The caud. head passes through the vascular lacuna (p. 78).** The femoral n. enters the **quadriceps femoris,** whose *four clearly separate* heads it innervates. The **rectus femoris** (1) and the **vastus lateralis,—medialis** (2), and **—intermedius** conform in origin and termination to the relationships in the horse. (See p. 17.) *The femoral a. and v. and saphenous n. pass between the two origins of the sartorius on their way to the* **femoral triangle.** *The sartorius forms the medial wall of the triangle,* the proximal border of which is formed by the pelvic tendon of the external oblique, the caudal border by the gracilis and pectineus, and the cranial border by the rectus femoris.

b) **ON THE CRUS** the **tibial nerve** (12) gives off its distal muscular brr. to the extensors of the tarsus and flexors of the digits, passes between the heads of the gastrocnemius, and reaches the medial side of the crus, at the distal end of which it divides into the **lateral** (13) and **medial** (14) **plantar nn.**

The **popliteus** (special flexor of the stifle) lies caudal to the stifle joint (see p. 29.4). The **gastrocnemius** (11) originates by two heads from the sides of the supracondylar fossa of the femur and terminates on the calcanean tuber. *It is very tendinous, and an intermediate fleshy tract connects the origin of the lateral head to the terminal tendon of the medial head, which is therefore bipartite. The tendon of the lateral head takes a deeper course and passes through a sheath formed by the tarsal tendons of the biceps and semitendinosus.*** The gastrocnemius tendons (24) *are separate until shortly before their attachment to the tuber calcanei.* The **robust soleus** (see p. 17) *fuses with the lateral head of the gastrocnemius and forms with the two heads the triceps surae.* The **superficial digital flexor** lies between the heads of the gastrocnemius and *is fused with the lateral head* at its origin from the supracondylar fossa. Its thick terminal tendon (22) passes from the deep surface of the gastrocnemius tendon around the medial side to expand superficially over the tuber calcanei, to which it is attached. The spiral groove between the tendons is palpable in the live animal. The tendons of the gastrocnemius and supf. flexor, and tarsal tendons of the biceps and semitendinosus make up

the **common calcanean tendon**—the hamstring of quadrupeds. On the pes the superficial flexor tendon is arranged as in the thoracic limb. The **deep digital flexors** include three muscles as in the horse: the **caudal tibial** (see p. 17) is the smallest; its belly is short and flat and its long narrow tendon lies on the caudal surface of the largest muscle—the **lateral digital flexor** (see p. 17). The tendons of these two muscles pass together over the sustentaculum tali; whereas the tendon of the **medial digital flexor,** as in the horse, passes over the medial surface of the tarsus (p. 29) and joins the other two in the proximal metatarsus to form the common deep flexor tendon, which is arranged as in the thoracic limb.

c) The **INTEROSSEI III AND IV** (see text figure) have the same supportive function for the main digits of the ox as the interosseus medius (III) in the horse. When the weight is on the foot and the fetlock joints are overextended, the interossei, through the sesamoid bones and distal sesamoid ligaments, aid the digital flexor tendons in support of the fetlock joints. Through their **extensor branches** attached to the med. and lat. (proper) digital extensor tendons they oppose the action of the deep flexor tendons on the coffin joints and guarantee that the hoofs are planted on the solar surface. They have the same structure as on the thoracic limb (see p. 10, b). These muscles originate from the long plantar tarsal ligament and the proximal part of the metatarsal bone. In young animals they are relatively fleshy and in older animals predominantly tendinous. Interossei III and IV are fused along their axial borders in the metatarsus, but they separate and terminate on the corresponding digits. *In the middle of the metatarsus the interossei give off the accessory lig., which bifurcates and joins the branches of the supf. digital flexor tendon at the level of the fetlock joints in the formation of the* **sleeves (manicae flexoriae)** *through which the branches of the deep flexor tendon pass.*

Proximal to the fetlock joints each interosseus divides into two tendons, each with two **extensor branches.** The two tendons are attached to the sesamoid bones. A flat **abaxial extensor branch** passes across the surface of the sesamoid bone, to which it is attached, and joins the tendon of the proper digital extensor. The **axial extensor branches** remain fused together until they pass through the intercapital notch in the metatarsal bone. Then they separate and join the tendons *of their respective proper digital extensors.*

(Dorsal aspect)

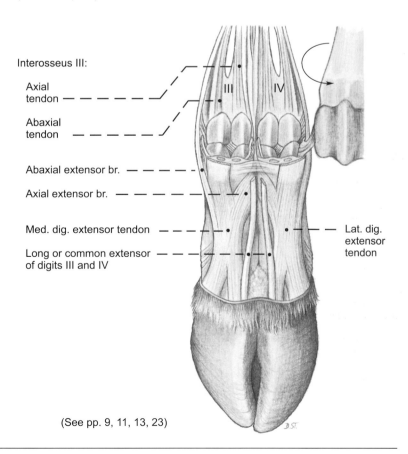

Interosseus III:

Axial tendon

Abaxial tendon

Abaxial extensor br.

Axial extensor br.

Med. dig. extensor tendon

Lat. dig. extensor tendon

Long or common extensor of digits III and IV

(See pp. 9, 11, 13, 23)

* Traeder, 1968
** Pavaux, Lignereux, and Sautet, 1983

Pelvic Limb

(medial)

Quadriceps femoris:

1 Rectus femoris

2 Vastus medialis

3 Sartorius

4 Saphenous n.

5 Deep digital flexor tendons

6 Obturator n. and v.

7 External obturator
(Intrapelvic part)

8 Pectineus
(et adductor longus)

9 Adductor magnus
(et brevis)

10 Gracilis

11 Gastrocnemius

12 Tibial n.

22
23
24

13 Lateral plantar n.

14 Medial plantar n.

Legend:

15 Internal abdominal oblique
16 External abdominal oblique
17 Sacrocaudalis [-coccygeus] ventralis medialis
18 Coccygeus
19 Levator ani
20 Semimembranosus
21 Semitendinosus
22 Superficial flexor tendon
23 Tarsal tendon of semitendinosus
24 Gastrocnemius tendon
25 Peroneus [fibularis] tertius
26 Cranial tibial m.

A Iliofemoral lymph node
B Tuberal lymph node

(Aa. vv. and nn., see p. 21)

(See pp. 17, 21, 23, 29)

4. CUTANEOUS NERVES, BLOOD VESSELS AND LYMPH NODES OF THE PELVIC LIMB

a) The **CUTANEOUS INNERVATION** of the lateral rump and thigh regions is supplied, in craniocaudal order, by the cranial clunial nn. (dorsolat. cut. brr. of L4 to L6), middle clunial nn. (dorsolat. cut. brr. of S1 to S3), and in the region of the tuber ischiadicum and major trochanter by caudal clunial nn. (cut. brr. of the pudendal n., k) and the caudal cutaneous femoral n. (i), *the cutaneous br. of which may be absent*. In addition, the region of the biceps groove is supplied by cutaneous brr. of the tibial n. (p) and the common peroneal [fibular] n. (o). A large area of skin in the craniolateral thigh region is supplied by the **lateral cutaneous femoral n. (3)**. On the medial surface of the thigh the nerves are the **iliohypogastric (1)**, **ilioinguinal (2)**, and **genitofemoral (4)** (see also p. 91).

The innervation of the crus down to the hock is provided mainly medially, but also craniolaterally, by the **saphenous n. (11)**; mainly caudolaterally by the **caudal cutaneous sural n. (24)** from the tibial n., and laterally also by the **lateral cutaneous sural n. (25)** from the common peroneal [fibular] n. The pes (see p. 23) is innervated dorsally by dorsal common digital nn. II–IV from the **superficial peroneal (o")**, and in the interdigital region by dorsal metatarsal n. III (from the **deep peroneal (o')**, see p.11) and plantar common digital n. III (see p. 11). Plantar common digital nn. II–IV are branches of the **medial (29)** and **lateral (28) plantar nn.**

Nerves of the pelvic limb

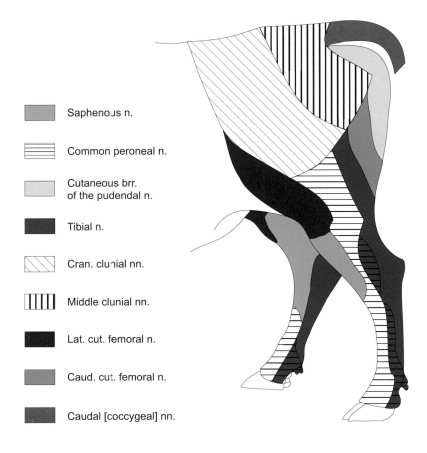

Saphenous n.

Common peroneal n.

Cutaneous brr. of the pudendal n.

Tibial n.

Cran. clunial nn.

Middle clunial nn.

Lat. cut. femoral n.

Caud. cut. femoral n.

Caudal [coccygeal] nn.

b) The **BLOOD VESSELS** of the pelvic limb come primarily from the external iliac a. and v., and to a lesser extent from the **internal iliac a. and v. (14)**. The latter give off, caudodorsal to the body of the ilium, the **cranial gluteal a. and v. (15)** for the gluteal muscles and the *gluteobiceps*. The internal iliac a. and v. terminate in the region of the lesser sciatic foramen by dividing into the **caudal gluteal a. and v. (16)** and the internal pudendal a. and v. The **obturator v. (17)** *originates from the internal iliac immediately after the cranial gluteal v*. An obturator a. is absent as in the dog. The **external iliac a. and v. (13)** leave the abdominal cavity through the vascular lacuna and become the femoral a. and v. While still in the abdomen they give off the **deep femoral a. and v. (18)** with the origin of the arterial **pudendoepigastric trunk (19)**, whereas the **pudendoepigastric v. (19)** may come directly from the ext. iliac v. as in the dog. Distal to the hip joint the deep femoral a. and v. give off

the **medial circumflex femoral a. and v. (20)** to the adductors and caudal thigh muscles. They also give off obturator branches that ascend through the obturator foramen. The medial circumflex femoral v. supplies the **lateral saphenous v. (21)**, which, without an accompanying artery, emerges in the popliteal region between the gluteobiceps and semitendinosus. It runs with the caud. cut. sural n. along the lateral surface of the common calcanean tendon and divides in the distal third of the crus (unlike that of the horse) into a cranial branch and a **caudal branch (27)**. The caudal branch, before it reaches the tarsus, sends an anastomotic br. to the medial saphenous v. Distal to the tarsal joint, the caudal branch is connected with the small lateral plantar v. to form the proximal deep plantar arch. The **cranial branch (26)** runs with the supf. peroneal n. along the dorsolateral surface of the tarsus and, in the distal half of the metatarsus, becomes the dorsal common digital v. III. The insignificant dorsal common digital v. II and the large dorsal common digital v. IV, branch off and terminate in the venous distal deep plantar arch (see p. 23).

The **femoral a. and v. (6)** pass between the two origins of the sartorius into the femoral triangle and give off cranially, between the vastus medialis and rectus femoris, the **lateral circumflex femoral a. and v. (5)** for the quadriceps femoris; then they cross the femur medially toward the popliteal region and give rise to the **saphenous a. (11)** and the **medial saphenous v. (11)**, which emerge around the caudal border of the sartorius and run distally on the gracilis. The artery and vein continue imperceptibly into their respective caudal branches *without giving off cranial branches in the ox*, unlike the dog and horse. The caudal branches descend on the craniomedial surface of the common calcanean tendon, accompanied by the tibial n., to the sustentaculum tali. En route, the venous br. receives the anastomosis from the caud. br. of the lat. saphenous v., and at the level of the tarsal joint the arterial and venous branches divide into the **medial (29)** and **lateral (28) plantar aa. and vv.**

Distal to the femoral triangle the femoral a. and v. give off the **descending genicular a. and v. (7)** to the stifle, and caudally the origins of the **caudal femoral a. and v. (22)** mark the transition between the femoral vessels and the **popliteal a. and v. (23)**. The latter vessels pass between the heads of the gastrocnemius and give off the small **caudal tibial a. and v. (8)** cranial to the popliteus. Distal to that muscle they are continued as the large **cranial tibial a. and v. (10)**. Before these pass distal to the tibiofibular synostosis to the craniolateral surface of the tibia, *they give off the* **crural interosseus a. and v. (9)** *to the deep digital flexors*. These vessels are absent in the dog and horse. On the dorsolateral surface of the tarsal joint the cranial tibial a. and v. become the large **dorsal pedal a.** and the small **dorsal pedal v. (12)**, which, together with the deep peroneal [fibular] n., pass deep to the extensor retinaculum to the metatarsus (see p. 23).

c) The **LYMPH NODES** of the rump and pelvic limb belong to various lymphocenters.

The **deep popliteal ln.**, 3–4 cm long (see p. 17) in the popliteal space between the gluteobiceps and the semitendinosus collects the lymph from the pes and a large part of the crus. The supf. popliteal ln. is absent.

The **sciatic ln.**, 2–3 cm in diameter (see p. 17) lies on the lateral surface of the sacrosciatic ligament at the lesser sciatic foramen and receives lymph from the caudal femoral muscles.

The conspicuous **iliofemoral (deep inguinal) ln.** (see p. 19) drains the pelvis, thigh, crus, and the associated bones and joints. The **subiliac ln.** (p. 67, 5) may reach a length of 10 cm. It drains the skin of the rump, thigh, stifle, and crus. *In meat inspection all of these lymph nodes are examined in retained carcasses*. In addition, the **coxal ln.** (not shown) lies medial to the tensor fasciae latae, and the following lnn. are *present in the ox*, but not in the dog and horse: **gluteal ln.** (see p. 17) *at the greater sciatic notch*, and the **tuberal ln.** (see p. 19) *on the medial surface of the tuber ischiadicum*. The lymph is drained through the sacral, sciatic, iliofemoral, medial and lateral iliac, lnn. and through the lumbar trunks to the cisterna chyli.

Arteries, Veins, and Nerves of the pelvic limb

(medial)

13 External iliac a. and v.

14 Internal iliac a. and v.

15 Cranial gluteal a. and v.

16 Caudal gluteal a. and v.

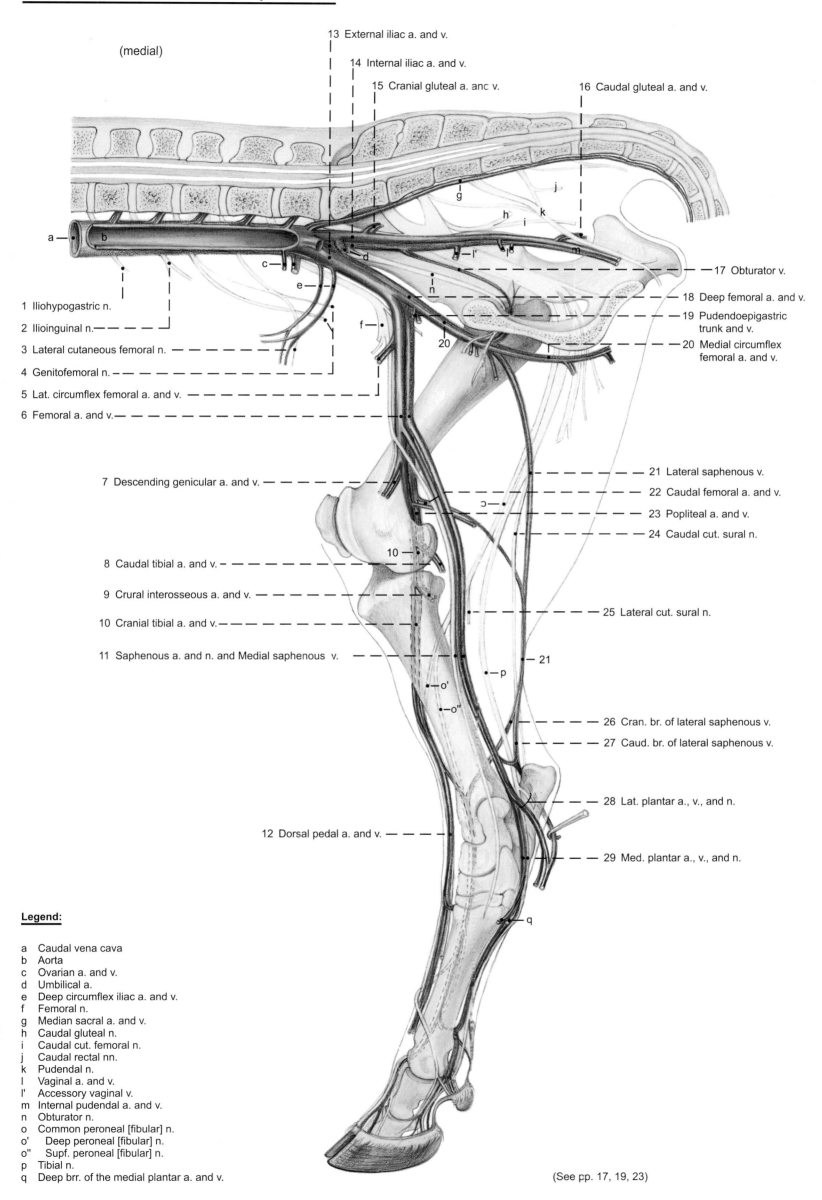

1 Iliohypogastric n.
2 Ilioinguinal n.
3 Lateral cutaneous femoral n.
4 Genitofemoral n.
5 Lat. circumflex femoral a. and v.
6 Femoral a. and v.

7 Descending genicular a. and v.

8 Caudal tibial a. and v.
9 Crural interosseous a. and v.
10 Cranial tibial a. and v.
11 Saphenous a. and n. and Medial saphenous v.

12 Dorsal pedal a. and v.

17 Obturator v.
18 Deep femoral a. and v.
19 Pudendoepigastric trunk and v.
20 Medial circumflex femoral a. and v.

21 Lateral saphenous v.
22 Caudal femoral a. and v.
23 Popliteal a. and v.
24 Caudal cut. sural n.

25 Lateral cut. sural n.

26 Cran. br. of lateral saphenous v.
27 Caud. br. of lateral saphenous v.

28 Lat. plantar a., v., and n.

29 Med. plantar a., v., and n.

Legend:

a Caudal vena cava
b Aorta
c Ovarian a. and v.
d Umbilical a.
e Deep circumflex iliac a. and v.
f Femoral n.
g Median sacral a. and v.
h Caudal gluteal n.
i Caudal cut. femoral n.
j Caudal rectal nn.
k Pudendal n.
l Vaginal a. and v.
l' Accessory vaginal v.
m Internal pudendal a. and v.
n Obturator n.
o Common peroneal [fibular] n.
o' Deep peroneal [fibular] n.
o" Supf. peroneal [fibular] n.
p Tibial n.
q Deep brr. of the medial plantar a. and v.

(See pp. 17, 19, 23)

5. ARTERIES, VEINS, AND NERVES OF THE PES

> The dissection is done as on the thoracic limb (see p. 8).

a) The **PLANTAR NERVES** of the tarsus and metatarsus come from the tibial nerve alone. (See the palmar nerves, p. 8. For blood vessels, see p. 20.)

The **tibial n.** divides into the medial and lateral plantar nn. at the distal end of the crus, as in the dog and horse. The **medial plantar n. (3)** passes over the medial side of the tarsus to the metatarsus, covered by fascia and accompanied by the **medial plantar a. and v.** In the metatarsus it runs in the palpable medial groove between the interosseus and the deep flexor tendon, accompanied by the **superficial branches of the medial plantar a. and v.**, to the distal third of the metatarsus, where it divides with the vessels into **plantar common digital aa., vv., and nn. II (9) and III (8)**.

Plantar common digital n. II (9) and the vessels of the same name give off proximal to the fetlock joint the small **axial plantar digital a., v., and n. II (11)** to the medial dewclaw, and the continuing **abaxial plantar digital a., v., and n. III (17)**. This nerve and the artery on its plantar side cross deep to the distal ligament of the dewclaw, while the more dorsal vein crosses it superficially, to the abaxial bulb and hoof regions of the third digit to the apex.

The large **plantar common digital n. III (8)** turns across the plantar surface of the medial branch of the supf. dig. flexor tendon, crosses the artery of the same name, and runs between this and the medially located vein to the interdigital space. The nerve may occasionally be double, or it may divide over a short distance and reunite. At the middle of the proximal phalanx, it and the accompanying vessels divide into the **axial plantar digital aa., vv., and nn. III (20) and IV (19)**. These supply the axial bulb and hoof regions of the third and fourth digits, as the corresponding abaxial structures do (see also p. 11, upper right fig.).

Before their distribution *the nerves each receive a communicating branch from the junction of the superficial and deep dorsal nn.*, and the **plantar common digital a. and v. III (8)** anastomose at their bifurcation with dorsal mt. a. and v. III via the **interdigital a. and v.** (Compare the corresponding vessels of the manus, p. 10.)

The **lateral plantar n.** accompanied by the **lateral plantar a. and v.**, if present, cross distolaterally deep to the long plantar tarsal lig. and reach the metatarsus (see p. 21). The nerve, after reaching the lat. border of the deep flexor tendon just distal to the tarsus, gives off its **deep branch** to the interossei III and IV and becomes **plantar common digital n. IV (5)**. The latter, accompanied by **plantar common dig. a. IV (5)**, takes a course like that of plantar common dig. n. II, and divides with the vessels into **axial plantar digital a., v., and n. V (10)** and **abaxial plantar digital a., v., and n. IV (18)**, which are distributed as the corresponding structures of digits II and III are. **Plantar common digital v. IV** comes from the **distal deep plantar arch**, and is very short.

A communicating branch betweeen the lateral and medial plantar nn., present in the horse, is absent in the ox. Deep plantar mt. nn., present in the dog and horse, are absent in the ox, as are corresponding nn. in the thoracic limb. The deep plantar vessels, **plantar mt. aa. and vv. II–IV**, vary in size. They are similar to the deep palmar vessels on the manus.

b) The **DORSAL NERVES** of the pes come from the **superficial and deep peroneal [fibular] nn.** (For blood vessels see p. 20.)

The **superficial peroneal n. (2)** is distributed as in the dog, but unlike that of the horse, it supplies superficial digital nn. In the crus it gives off **dorsal common digital n. IV (6)**. This crosses distolaterally, deep to the large **cranial br. of the lat. saphenous v. (2)** and the insignificant supf. br. of the dorsal pedal a., runs lateral to the tendon of the lat. dig. extensor in the proximal half of the metatarsus, and in the distal half crosses deep to the large **dorsal common dig. v. IV (6)**. The nerve then runs on the dorsal side of plantar common dig. v. IV to the level of the fetlock joint, where it divides into the small **axial dorsal dig. n. V (14)** to the lateral dewclaw, and the continuing **abaxial dorsal dig. n. IV (15)** to the dorsolateral coronary and bulbar regions of the fourth digit.

The remaining trunk of the supf. peroneal n. courses medial to the cranial br. of the lat. saphenous v. to the dorsal surface of the metatarsus. Separated by the vein from the parallel dorsal common

dig. n. IV, it divides at the end of the proximal third of the mt. into the large dorsal common dig. n. III and the small **dorsal common dig. n. II (4)**. This crosses obliquely mediodistally over mt. III, without accompanying vessels, to the dorsomedial side of the fetlock joint and divides into **axial dorsal dig. n. II (12)** and **abaxial dorsal dig. n. III (13)**. These nerves are distributed like the corresponding nerves of the fifth and fourth digits. The continuing **dorsal common dig. n. III (7)**, accompanied laterally by **dorsal common dig. v. III (7)**, runs on the tendon of the lateral belly (common extensor of digits III and IV, see p. 16) of the long digital extensor to the interdigital space. Distal to the fetlock joint it divides into **axial dorsal dig. nn. III (21) and IV (22)**. Just before the division it sends a **communicating br.** to the (deep) dorsal mt. n. III (to be described).

The **deep peroneal n.**, accompanied by the *large* **dorsal pedal a.** and the *small* **dorsal pedal v.**, runs on the flexion surface of the tarsus deep to the long and lat. dig. ext. tendons and the **crural and metatarsal extensor retinacula** to the metatarsus. Here the nerve and vessels become **dorsal mt. a., v., and n. III (1)**. They run along the dorsal longitudinal groove on the metatarsal bone to the interdigital space.

Dorsal mt. n. III receives the communicating br. from the dorsal common dig. n. III, and the resulting short common trunk divides into **communicating brr.** to the axial plantar dig. nn.

The dorsal vessels are distributed like the corresponding vessels of the manus. (See p. 11, upper right fig.)

The dorsal and plantar abaxial dig. nn. may be connected by a communicating br. as in the thoracic limb.

Arteries and Veins of the Pes (plantar)

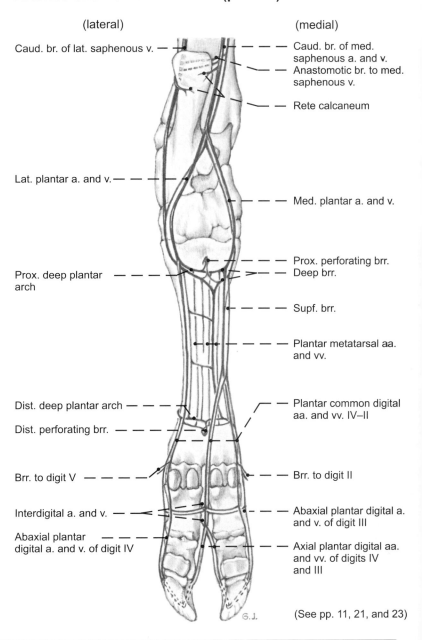

(lateral)   (medial)

- Caud. br. of lat. saphenous v.
- Caud. br. of med. saphenous a. and v.
- Anastomotic br. to med. saphenous v.
- Rete calcaneum
- Lat. plantar a. and v.
- Med. plantar a. and v.
- Prox. perforating brr.
- Deep brr.
- Prox. deep plantar arch
- Supf. brr.
- Plantar metatarsal aa. and vv.
- Dist. deep plantar arch
- Plantar common digital aa. and vv. IV–II
- Dist. perforating brr.
- Brr. to digit V
- Brr. to digit II
- Interdigital a. and v.
- Abaxial plantar digital a. and v. of digit III
- Abaxial plantar digital a. and v. of digit IV
- Axial plantar digital aa. and vv. of digits IV and III

G. J.

(See pp. 11, 21, and 23)

Arteries, Veins, and Nerves of the Pes

(medioplantar)

(dorsolateral)

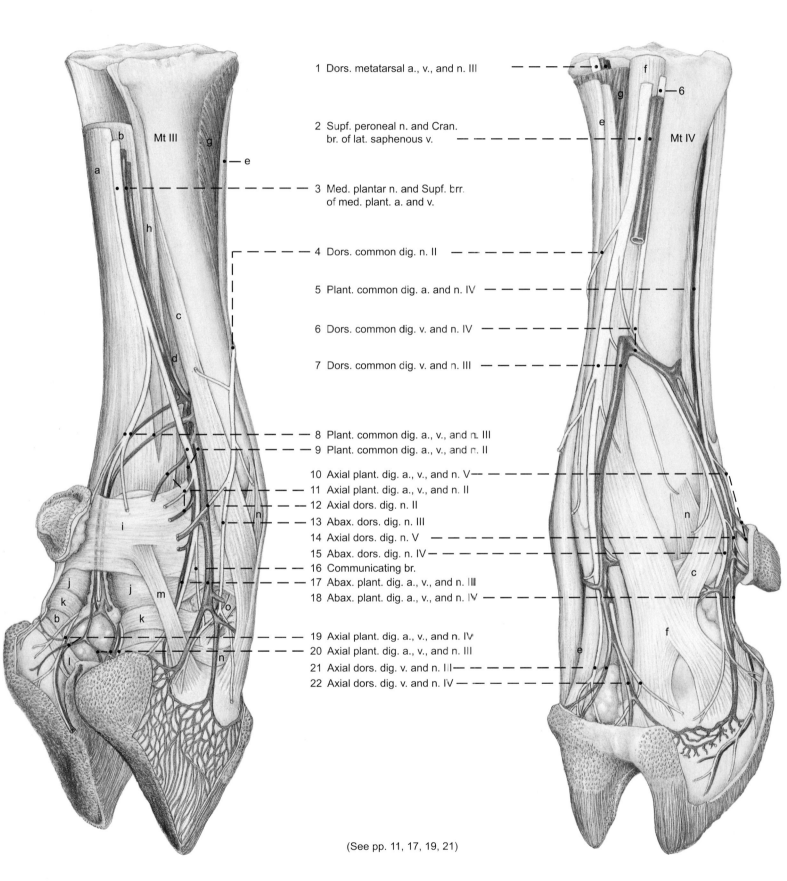

1 Dors. metatarsal a., v., and n. III

2 Supf. peroneal n. and Cran. br. of lat. saphenous v.

3 Med. plantar n. and Supf. brr. of med. plant. a. and v.

4 Dors. common dig. n. II

5 Plant. common dig. a. and n. IV

6 Dors. common dig. v. and n. IV

7 Dors. common dig. v. and n. III

8 Plant. common dig. a., v., and n. III
9 Plant. common dig. a., v., and n. II
10 Axial plant. dig. a., v., and n. V
11 Axial plant. dig. a., v., and n. II
12 Axial dors. dig. n. II
13 Abax. dors. dig. n. III
14 Axial dors. dig. n. V
15 Abax. dors. dig. n. IV
16 Communicating br.
17 Abax. plant. dig. a., v., and n. III
18 Abax. plant. dig. a., v., and n. IV
19 Axial plant. dig. a., v., and n. IV
20 Axial plant. dig. a., v., and n. III
21 Axial dors. dig. v. and n. III
22 Axial dors. dig. v. and n. IV

(See pp. 11, 17, 19, 21)

Legend:

Tendons:
a Supf. dig. flexor
b Deep dig. flexors and
   Interossei III and IV:
c Abax. extensor brr.
d Tendon of interosseus III

Tendons:
e Long dig. extensor
   Com. ext. of digits III and IV
   Medial extensor of dig. III
f Lateral dig. extensor
g Extensor digitalis brevis

h Accessory lig. of interossei
i Plantar annular lig.
j Prox. dig. annular lig.
k Dist. dig. annular lig.

l Supf. part of dist. interdig. lig.
m Dist. lig. of dewclaw
n Collateral lig.
o Abax. plant. lig. of pastern joint

23

6. DERMIS OF THE HOOF

a) **THE HOOFS** are fully developed on both main digits (3 and 4). They are composed of modified skin with a thick, strongly cornified epidermis. The hoof surrounds the skeletal and soft structures of the distal part of the digit. The main hoofs have an elongated half-round form, and together they serve the same function as the equine hoof, giving rise to the false concept of the "cloven hoof."

The terms of direction used on the equine hoof—dorsal and palmar or plantar, as well as proximal and distal—apply to the bovine hoof, but medial and lateral are replaced by axial and abaxial with reference to the long axis of the limb, which passes between the main digits.

The Dewclaws are reduced digits II and V that are attached, without synovial joints, by fascial ligaments at the level of the fetlock joint (see p. 10). They do not reach the ground, except in soft footing. The short conical dewclaws are, in principle, composed of the same modified skin layers as the main hoofs. They usually have only two phalanges, sometimes only the distal one.

The hairless skin covering the end of the digit is distinctly modified in its three layers—subcutis, dermis, and epidermis—compared to the haired skin (common integument). These three layers are modified in different parts of the hoof to form five segments: periople, corona, wall, sole, and bulb (see also p. 27).

The **Subcutis** is absent in two segments (wall and sole), but in the other segments forms relatively firm immovable cushions that consist of a three-dimensional network of transverse, longitudinal, and oblique robust connective tissue fibers with enclosed fat lobules. In the bulb there is an especially thick cushion that absorbs the shock when the foot is planted.

The **Dermis** consists of a deep reticular layer and a more superficial papillary layer. The papillary layer, with the exception of the wall segment, bears dermal papillae. These papillae arise either from a smooth surface or from parallel dermal ridges. The wall segment presents parallel dermal lamellae directed from proximal to distal. In some places (proximally and distally) the lamellae bear a row of cap papillae on their free edge.

The deep layers of the **Epidermis** conform to the dermal papillae and lamellae, producing tubular horn in all segments except the wall, and lamellar horn in the wall segment. (See p. 25, middle and lower figures.)

b) **THE SEGMENTS OF THE HOOF** can be clearly distinguished on the dermal surface when the horn capsule is removed after maceration in warm water. The perioplic segment is next to the haired skin. The coronary and wall segments follow distally. The horn formed in these segments moves from proximal to distal and makes up the **horny wall (paries corneus)**. *This turns from the abaxial surface to the axial surface at the **dorsal border (Margo dorsalis)** of the hoof.* The horn formed in the sole and bulbar segments makes up the ground surface of the hoof. *In clinical practice the entire ground surface is often called the sole.*

I.   The **perioplic segment (Limbus, 1)** is about 1 cm wide. Dorsally and abaxially the subcutis forms a slightly convex **perioplic cushion**, absent on the axial surface. On the palmar/plantar surface it expands and is continuous with the digital cushion in the bulb. The **perioplic dermis (6)** covers the subcutis and bears fine distally directed **perioplic papillae** about 2 mm long and relatively sparse. *Abaxially it is separated by a shallow groove from the dermis of the haired skin.* The **periople (Epidermis limbi, 1)** covers the dermis

and forms **horn tubules (12)** on the dermal papillae. The soft perioplic horn grows distally as the external layer of the wall. It usually does not reach the distal border because it flakes off easily. When moist it is markedly swollen.

II. **Coronary segment (Corona):** The coronary segment is distal to the perioplic segment and *extends to a level about halfway down the hoof,* unlike that of the horse. The subcutis forms the **coronary cushion**, which is wide and only slightly convex. Its width and thickness decrease on both sides of the hoof in the palmar/plantar direction. The **coronary dermis (7)** bears fine conical **coronary papillae**, rounded off at the ends. *At their base they are thicker and project horizontally, whereas the apical portion is inclined distally in the direction of growth. The inflection of the coronary segment that forms part of the bar in the horse is slightly indicated at the abaxial end of the lamellar dermis.* The **coronary epidermis (2)** forms **horn tubules (13)** which correspond to the dermal papillae and make up the middle layer of the wall. *The thickest, mostly unpigmented, tubules are in the middle layer of the coronary horn, whereas thinner tubules in the outer layer and indistinct or distally absent tubules in the inner layer are typical.*

III. The **Wall segment (Paries)** is distal to the coronary segment *and of about equal width. The inflection of the wall that forms part of the bar in the horse is only slightly indicated.* The subcutis is absent from the wall segment. The **lamellar (parietal) dermis (8)** bears proximodistally oriented **dermal lamellae**. *These are smooth; unlike those of the horse, no secondary lamellae are present.* The **wall epidermis (11)** bears **epidermal lamellae (14)** between the dermal lamellae. The epidermal lamellae are cornified in their middle layers to form the horny lamellae. Unfortunately two different meanings of the word wall complicate the description of the hoof. The horny wall (lamina, hoof plate, Paries corneus) is the more common, broader concept. Homologous to the human fingernail, it is the part of the hoof capsule that includes three layers formed by the perioplic, coronary, and wall segments. The wall *segment* might better be called the lamellar segment, keeping in mind the distinction between the lamina and its lamellae.

IV. **Sole segment (Solea):** *In artiodactyls this is a narrow crescent* inside the **white zone (5)**. It is divided into a dorsal **body** and **axial** and **abaxial crura** (see text fig. p. 26). The **subcutis** is absent. The **solear dermis (9)** bears low transverse ridges topped by **dermal papillae**, with the result that the papillae are arranged in rows. The **solear epidermis (3)** contains **horn tubules (15)**.

V.   **Bulbar segment (Torus ungulae):** The bulbar segment lies palmar/plantar to the sole and between its crura. It extends back to the haired skin. The subcutis forms the **digital cushion**, which distinguishes the bulb from the sole. In the apical part of the bulb the cushion is 5 mm thick; in the basal part it is up to 20 mm thick. *These two parts maybe demarcated by an imaginary line connecting the ends of the white zone (see text fig., p. 26).* The digital cushion is covered by the **bulbar dermis (10)**, which bears **dermal papillae**. These arise in part from discontinuous low, wavelike ridges. Upon the dermis lies the **bulbar epidermis (4)**, containing **horn tubules (16)**. The harder bulbar horn between the crura of the sole presents a flat ground surface. This apical portion is more prominent and more obviously part of the bulb in the sheep, goat, and pig. The horn in the base of the bulb is, depending on the state of hoof care, more or less markedly split into scale-like layers of soft-elastic rubbery consistency. (For segments of the hoof, see also p. 27.)

24

Hoof and Dewclaw

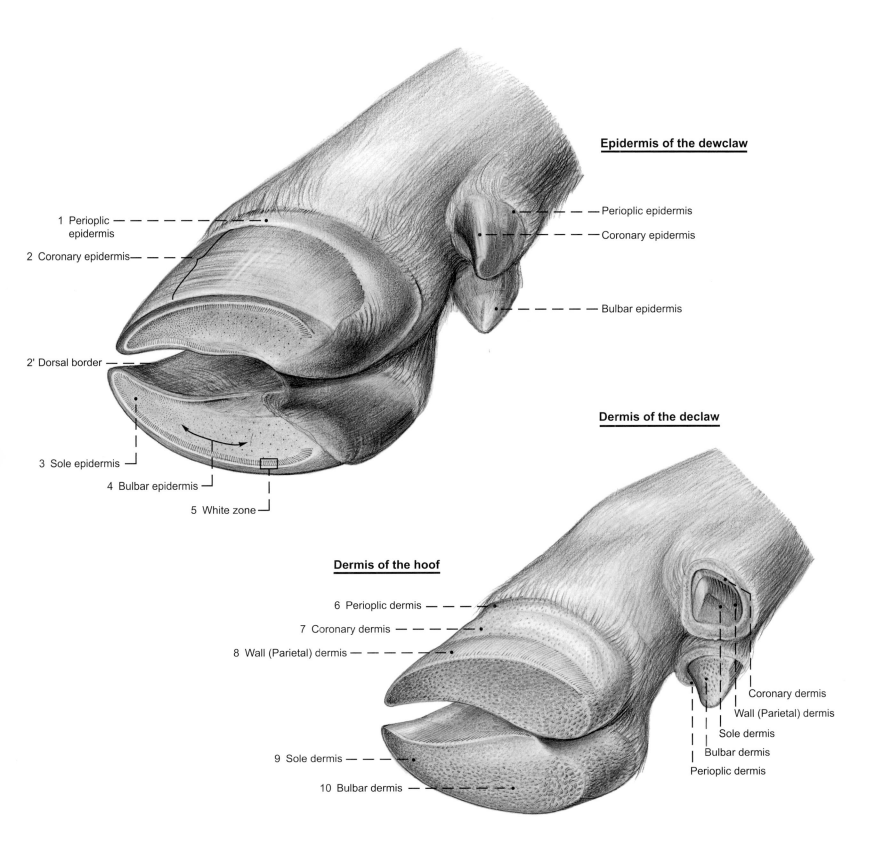

Epidermis of the dewclaw

— Perioplic epidermis
— Coronary epidermis

— Bulbar epidermis

1 Perioplic epidermis
2 Coronary epidermis
2' Dorsal border
3 Sole epidermis
4 Bulbar epidermis
5 White zone

Dermis of the declaw

Dermis of the hoof

6 Perioplic dermis
7 Coronary dermis
8 Wall (Parietal) dermis

Coronary dermis
Wall (Parietal) dermis
Sole dermis
Bulbar dermis
Perioplic dermis

9 Sole dermis
10 Bulbar dermis

Epidermis (Capsule) of the hoof

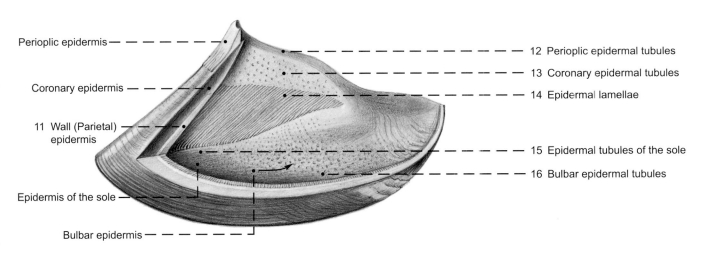

Perioplic epidermis

Coronary epidermis

11 Wall (Parietal) epidermis

Epidermis of the sole

Bulbar epidermis

12 Perioplic epidermal tubules
13 Coronary epidermal tubules
14 Epidermal lamellae

15 Epidermal tubules of the sole
16 Bulbar epidermal tubules

7. THE HOOF (UNGULA)

a) The **HOOF CAPSULE** surrounds: the distal end of the **middle phalanx (C)**, the **distal interphalangeal joint (L)**, and the **distal phalanx (coffin bone, D)** with the **terminations** of the **common dig. extensor tendon (H)** on the extensor process and the **deep dig. flexor tendon (K)** on the flexor tubercle. Also enclosed is the **distal sesamoid (navicular) bone (E)**, which serves as a trochlea for the deep dig. flexor tendon. The **navicular bursa (M)** reduces friction between them.

The **cornified hoof capsule** consists of the lamina (horny wall) with an abaxial part, a dorsal border, and an axial part facing the interdigital space, as well as the horny sole and horny bulb. The capsule has a thickness of about 10 mm in the dorsal part and about 5 mm in the axial part. The growth of the epidermis pushes the cornified masses distally at a rate of about 5 mm per month. After an exungulation the renewal of the entire hoof capsule would require up to 20 months. Horn formation is more intensive in calves than in adults and more active on the pelvic than on the thoracic limb. In the last third of pregnancy and in very high milk production, horn formation is reduced. That is shown on the superficial surface of the hoof by the formation of semicircular grooves.

When cattle are kept on soft footing with little or no possibility of exercise the horn grows faster than it is worn off and therefore the hoofs must be trimmed regularly.

I. The **lamina (Paries corneus)** consists of external, middle, and internal layers, which are bonded together and formed by the perioplic, coronary, and wall segments respectively. The external layer is very thin; the middle layer constitutes the bulk of the lamina; and the internal layer bears the horny lamellae that make up the junctional horn.

II. The junctional horn is part of the **suspensory apparatus of the coffin bone**. This term includes all of the tissues that attach the coffin bone (distal phalanx) to the inside of the lamina. The suspensory apparatus of the coffin bone consists of a connective tissue (dermal) part and an epidermal part. Collagenous fiber bundles anchored in the outer zone of the coffin bone run obliquely proximodorsally in the reticular layer and then in the lamellae of the dermis. The collagen fibers are attached to the basement membrane. The tension is then transmitted through the living epidermal cell layers by desmosomes and bundles of keratin filaments to the junctional (lamellar) horn, which is attached to the lamina. The pressure exerted on the coffin bone by the body weight is transformed by the shock absorbing suspensory apparatus of the coffin bone into tension; the tension is transformed in the lamina to pressure; this pressure weighs upon the ground at the solear border of the lamina. One part of the body weight is not transformed, but falls directly on a support of solear and apical bulbar horn. In the basal bulbar segment the elastic horn and the thick subcutaneous cushion act as a shock absorbing mechanism of the hoof. The chambered cushions work in a manner comparable to the gel cushion system of modern running shoes. With the exception of a nonweightbearing concavity at the axial end of the white zone, the sole and bulb horn form a flat ground surface.

The suspensory apparatus of the coffin bone actuates the **hoof mechanism** by traction on the internal surface of the lamina and by pressure on the sole and bulb. This can be measured with strain gauges. It concerns the elastic changes in form of the hoof capsule that occur during loading and unloading. In weight bearing, the space inside the lamina is reduced, while the palmar/plantar part of the capsule expands and the interdigital space is widened. During unloading, the horny parts return to their initial form and position.

III. The **rate of horn formation** differs greatly among the individual hoof segments. In the coronary segment horn formation is very intensive. In the proximal half of the wall segment the rate of horn formation is low. In the distal half, on the other hand, horn is formed in measurable amounts and at an increasing rate toward the apex of the hoof. (The term sterile bed, used in older textbooks for the wall segment is therefore incorrect.) Proximally in the wall segment the beginnings of the dermal lamellae bear **proximal cap papillae**. From the epidermis on these papillae, nontubular **proximal cap horn** is produced. This is applied to the sides of the proximal parts of the horny lamellae. Distal to the cap horn, as far as the middle of the wall, not much lamellar horn is added. In the distal half of the wall segment the horny lamellae become markedly higher, up to 5 mm, and, beginning with their middle portion, become flanked by amorphous **distal cap horn** that is applied cap-like over the edges of the dermal lamellae. It is formed on the **distal cap papillae** by the living epidermis there (see p. 27, right figure).

Distally on the wall-sole border the almost vertically directed dermal lamellae bend into horizontally directed dermal ridges of the sole segment. At the bend the lamellae are split into **terminal dermal papillae** which have a remarkable diameter of 0.2–0.5 mm. They are covered by living epidermis from which **terminal tubular horn** is formed. As a part of the white zone the terminal horn fills the spaces between the horny lamellae (see p. 27, right figure).

IV. The **white zone** (white line) consists only of horn produced by the wall segment, and presents external, middle, and internal parts. The **external part (a)** appears to the naked eye as a shining white millimeter-wide stripe. It consists of the basal sections of the horny lamellae and the flanking proximal cap horn, and borders the mostly nonpigmented inner coronary horn, which does not belong to the zona alba. The **middle part (b)** of the white zone is formed by the intermediate sections of the horny lamellae with the distal cap horn that lies between them. The **internal part (c)** of the white zone consists of the crests of the horny lamellae and, between them, the terminal tubular horn. They cornify in the distal half of the wall or at the wall-sole border.

The white zone has abaxial and axial crura (b", b'), which lie between the mostly unpigmented coronary horn and the sole horn. The axial crus ends halfway between the apex of the hoof and the palmar/plantar surface of the bulb. The abaxial crus extends farther, to the basal part of the bulb, where the end of the white zone becomes distinctly wider and turns inward. (See p. 25 above and text illustration.) The whole white zone and especially the wider abaxial end are predisposed to "white line disease," which by ascending infection can lead to "purulent hollow wall." The way for ascending microorganisms is opened by crumbling cap and terminal tubular horn, which technical material testing proves to be masses of soft horn.

V. **Horn quality** is the sum of the characteristics of the biomaterial horn, including hardness or elasticity, resistance to breakage, water absorption, and resistance to chemical and microbial influences. Horn quality is adapted to the biomechanical requirements of the different parts of the hoof. Accordingly, hard horn is found in the lamina; soft elastic horn in the proximal part of the bulb. Horn quality can be determined by morphological criteria in combination with data from physicotechnical material testing.

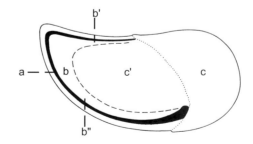

a White zone
Sole:
b Body of the sole
b' Axial crus
b" Abaxial crus
Bulb of hoof:
c Basal part
c' Apical part

Hoof

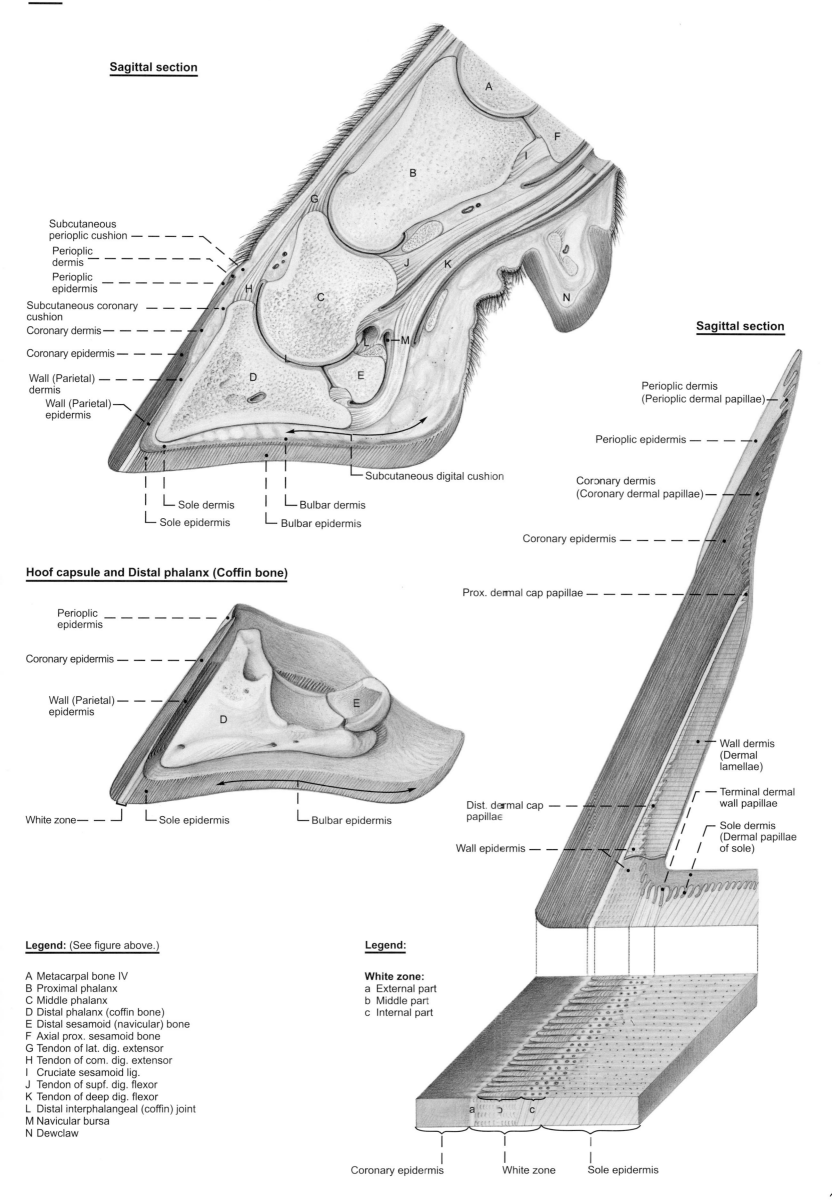

Sagittal section

Subcutaneous perioplic cushion
Perioplic dermis
Perioplic epidermis
Subcutaneous coronary cushion
Coronary dermis
Coronary epidermis
Wall (Parietal) dermis
Wall (Parietal) epidermis

A

B

G

F

I

H

C

J

K

L

M

N

D

E

Sole dermis
Sole epidermis
Bulbar dermis
Bulbar epidermis
Subcutaneous digital cushion

Sagittal section

Perioplic dermis (Perioplic dermal papillae)
Perioplic epidermis
Coronary dermis (Coronary dermal papillae)
Coronary epidermis
Prox. dermal cap papillae
Dist. dermal cap papillae
Wall epidermis
Wall dermis (Dermal lamellae)
Terminal dermal wall papillae
Sole dermis (Dermal papillae of sole)

Hoof capsule and Distal phalanx (Coffin bone)

Perioplic epidermis
Coronary epidermis
Wall (Parietal) epidermis
White zone
Sole epidermis
Bulbar epidermis

D

E

Coronary epidermis
White zone
Sole epidermis

a
b
c

Legend: (See figure above.)

A Metacarpal bone IV
B Proximal phalanx
C Middle phalanx
D Distal phalanx (coffin bone)
E Distal sesamoid (navicular) bone
F Axial prox. sesamoid bone
G Tendon of lat. dig. extensor
H Tendon of com. dig. extensor
I Cruciate sesamoid lig.
J Tendon of supf. dig. flexor
K Tendon of deep dig. flexor
L Distal interphalangeal (coffin) joint
M Navicular bursa
N Dewclaw

Legend:

White zone:
a External part
b Middle part
c Internal part

27

8. SYNOVIAL STRUCTURES OF THE PELVIC LIMB

a) JOINTS OF THE PELVIC LIMB

NAME	BONES involved	TYPE OF JOINT	FUNCTION	REMARKS
I. **Hip joint** (Art. coxae)	Ilium, ischium, pubis in acetabulum, and head of femur	Composite spheroidal	Restricted to flexion and extension	Ligaments: transverse acetabular, labrum acetabulare, lig. of head of femur. Accessory lig. absent.
II. **Stifle** (Art. genus)		Composite joint		
a) Femorotibial joint	Tibial condyles and femoral condyles	Simple condylar	Mainly flexion and extension restricted by ligaments	Ligg.: collateral, cruciate, transverse, meniscotibial, meniscofemoral. Injection: Med. sac, same as II b. Lat. sac in extensor groove of tibia on border of tendon of peroneus tertius; does not communicate with any other sac.*
b) Femoropatellar joint	Femoral trochlea and patella	Simple sesamoid	Tendon guide	Ligg.: med., middle, and lat. patellar, and med. and lat. fem.-patel. Injection: 4 cm. prox. to tibial tuberosity, between med. and middle patellar ligg. Communicates with med. fem.-tibial sac.

III. Prox. tibiofibular joint. Present in exceptional cases only. Usually the rudimentary fibula is fused with the lateral tibial condyle.

IV. Distal tibiofibular joint is a tight joint. Its cavity communicates with the tarsocrural joint.

NAME	BONES involved	TYPE OF JOINT	FUNCTION	REMARKS
V. **Tarsal joint** (hock)		Composite joint		
a) Tarsocrural joint	Tibial cochlea, prox. trochlea of talus, calcaneus, and lat. malleolus	Composite cochlear joint	Flexion and extension, snap joint	The collateral ligg. each have long and short parts. Long plantar lig. is divided into medial and lat. branches. Many other ligg. are blended with the fibrous joint capsule.
b) Prox. intertarsal joint	Distal trochlea of talus, calcaneus, and T IV + T C.	Composite trochlear joint	Flexion and extension	Injection: Into dorsomed. pouch between med. collat. lig. and med. branch of tendon of cran. tibial muscle
c) Dist. intertarsal joint	T C and T I–T III	Composite plane joint	Slight movement	
d) Tarsometatarsal joint	T I–T IV and metatarsal III and IV	Composite plane joint	Slight movement	

e) Intertarsal joints. Vertical, slightly moveable joints between tarsal bones in the same row.

VI. Digital joints. See thoracic limb.

b) SYNOVIAL BURSAE

Of the inconstant bursae, the **iliac (coxal) subcutaneous bursa**, unilateral or bilateral over the tuber coxae, and the **ischial subcutaneous bursa** lateral on the tuber ischiadicum, are clinically important. Of the important bursae related to the major trochanter, the inconstant **trochanteric bursa of the gluteus medius** is on the summit and mediodistal surface of the trochanter. The constant **trochanteric bursa of the gluteus accessorius** is on the lateral surface of the femur just distal to the major trochanter. The clinically important, but inconstant **trochanteric bursa of the biceps femoris** is between the vertebral head of the biceps and the terminal part of the gluteus medius on the major trochanter. This bursa may be the cause of a dislocation of the vertebral head of the biceps behind the major trochanter.

The large, up to 10 cm long, constant **distal subtendinous bursa of the biceps femoris** lies between the lat. femoral condyle and the thick terminal tendon of the biceps attached to the patella and the lat. patellar lig. Occasionally it communicates with the lat. femorotibial joint. When inflamed it produces a decubital swelling on the stifle.

The inconstant **subcutaneous bursa of the lat. malleolus**, when inflamed, produces a decubital swelling on the tarsus.

The multilocular **subcutaneous calcanean bursa** on the calcanean expansion of the supf. digital flexor tendon is also inconstant and occurs only in older animals.

The constant, extensive **subtendinous calcanean bursa of the supf. digital flexor** lies between that tendon and the termination of the gastrocnemius on the tuber calcanei. The **navicular (podotrochlear) bursae** (p. 27, M) between the terminal branches of the deep digital flexor tendon and the navicular bones are like those of the thoracic limb.

c) SYNOVIAL SHEATHS

Dorsally on the hock the tendons of the peroneus longus and the digital extensors are surrounded by synovial sheaths. The sheaths of the digital extensors communicate partially with the sheath of the cranial tibial and the sheath-like bursa of the peroneus tertius. On the **plantar aspect of the hock** the lat. digital flexor and the caudal tibial m. have a common sheath, and the med. digital flexor has a separate sheath. The tendon sheaths **in the digits** are like those of the thoracic limb.

* Desrochers et al. 1996

Joints, Bursae, and Synovial Sheaths of the Pelvic Limb

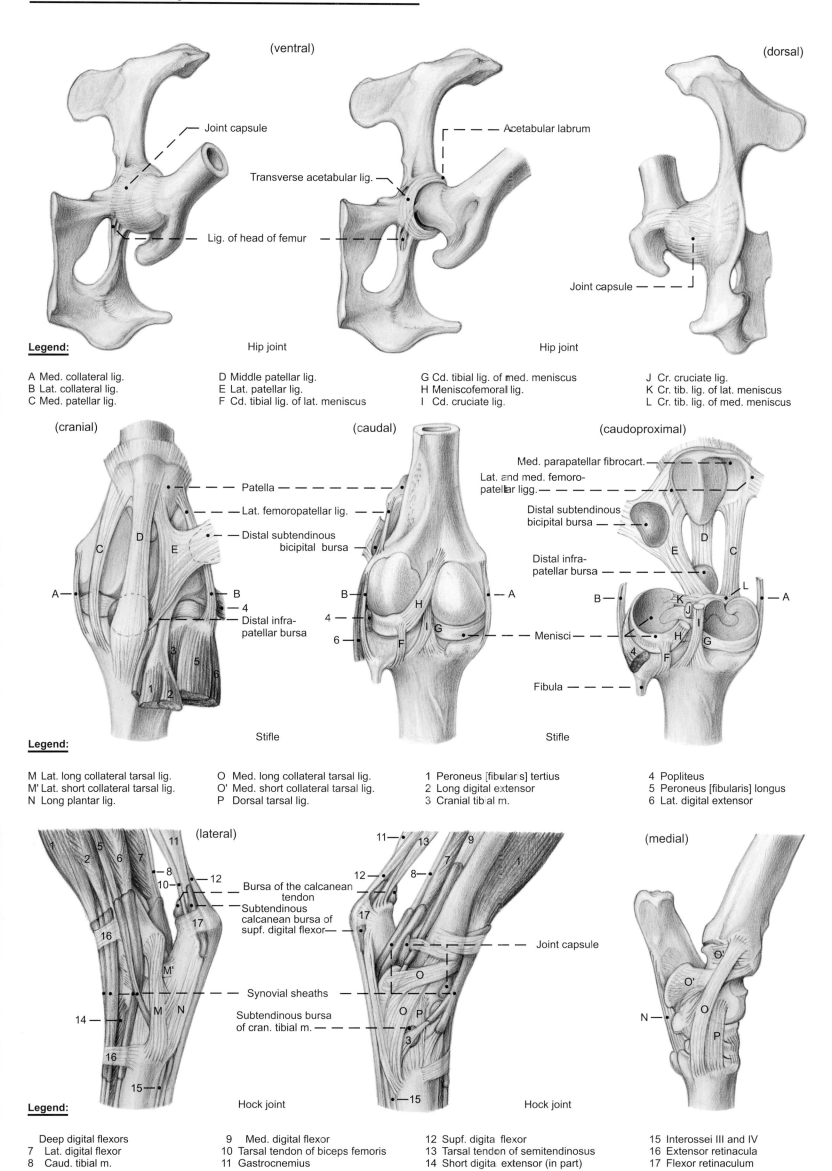

(ventral)

Joint capsule

(dorsal)

Acetabular labrum

Transverse acetabular lig.

Lig. of head of femur

Joint capsule

Hip joint

Hip joint

Legend:

A Med. collateral lig.
B Lat. collateral lig.
C Med. patellar lig.

D Middle patellar lig.
E Lat. patellar lig.
F Cd. tibial lig. of lat. meniscus

G Cd. tibial lig. of med. meniscus
H Meniscofemoral lig.
I Cd. cruciate lig.

J Cr. cruciate lig.
K Cr. tib. lig. of lat. meniscus
L Cr. tib. lig. of med. meniscus

(cranial)

(caudal)

(caudoproximal)

Patella

Lat. femoropatellar lig.

Distal subtendinous bicipital bursa

Distal infra-patellar bursa

Med. parapatellar fibrocart.
Lat. and med. femoro-patellar ligg.

Distal subtendinous bicipital bursa

Distal infra-patellar bursa

Menisci

Fibula

Stifle

Stifle

Legend:

M Lat. long collateral tarsal lig.
M' Lat. short collateral tarsal lig.
N Long plantar lig.

O Med. long collateral tarsal lig.
O' Med. short collateral tarsal lig.
P Dorsal tarsal lig.

1 Peroneus [fibularis] tertius
2 Long digital extensor
3 Cranial tibial m.

4 Popliteus
5 Peroneus [fibularis] longus
6 Lat. digital extensor

(lateral)

Bursa of the calcanean tendon
Subtendinous calcanean bursa of supf. digital flexor

Synovial sheaths

Subtendinous bursa of cran. tibial m.

Joint capsule

(medial)

Hock joint

Hock joint

Legend:

Deep digital flexors
7 Lat. digital flexor
8 Caud. tibial m.

9 Med. digital flexor
10 Tarsal tendon of biceps femoris
11 Gastrocnemius

12 Supf. digital flexor
13 Tarsal tendon of semitendinosus
14 Short digital extensor (in part)

15 Interossei III and IV
16 Extensor retinacula
17 Flexor retinaculum

29

CHAPTER 3: HEAD

1. SKULL AND HYOID APPARATUS

The bovine skull undergoes marked changes in shape as it grows from the newborn calf to the adult—changes that are caused in part by the development of the horns. In the process, the roof of the cranium, the occipital surface, and the lateral surfaces alter their relative positions significantly.

a) On the **CRANIUM**, the roof (Calvaria) *is formed by the rectangular* **frontal bones (I)★.** *They extend back to the caudal surface of the* **intercornual protuberance (3)★■** *where they are fused with the* **parietal (II)■** and **interparietal (III)■** bones. These are united with the **occipital (VI)■●** bone, but no sutures are visible here in the adult. The **external occipital protuberance (31)■●,** the point of attachment of the funicular lig. nuchae, *is about 6 cm ventral to the top of the skull.* The **nuchal line (m)■,** arching laterally from the external occipital protuberance, corresponds to the nuchal crest of the horse and dog. *On the caudolateral angle of the frontal bone is the* **cornual process (3')★■** *with its rough body and smoother neck with vascular grooves.*

Projecting from the middle of the lateral border of the frontal bone is the **zygomatic process (1)★■,** which *joins the* **frontal process (56)★■** *of the* **zygomatic bone (IX)★■.** The **temporal line (k)★** is the dorsal boundary of the **temporal fossa (j)★.** It is a sharp, palpable ridge running from the zygomatic process back to the horn and serves as a landmark for cornual nerve block (see pp. 34, 40, and 53).

b) The **FACIAL ASPECT.** The **facial crest (57')★** begins on the zygomatic bone *and curves across the maxilla to the* **facial tuber (57")★■.** *The often double* **infraorbital foramen (59)★** *is dorsal to the first cheek tooth* (p. 2). Caudal to the **nasoincisive notch (X")★** a fissure persists between the dorsal **nasal bone (X)★** and the ventral **incisive (XII), maxillary (XI), lacrimal (VIII),** and **frontal (I)** bones. The nasal bone has two rostral processes (X').

c) The **FORAMINA** of the skull are important for the passage of nerves and vessels, and for nerve block anesthesia. Caudolaterally on the skull between the occipital condyle (33)■ and the jugular process (36)■ is the double **canal for the hypoglossal n. (35)■.** Dorsal to the petrous temporal bone is the internal opening of the **temporal meatus (e)●.** There is a lateral opening (e)★ in the temporal fossa. *The ox does not have a foramen lacerum; it has an* **oval foramen (45)★■●** *for the mandibular n.,* connected by the **petro-occipital fissure (q')●** *with the* **jugular foramen (q),** which conducts cranial nerves IX, X, and XI. *Before the internal carotid a. is occluded at three months of age, it goes through the fissure.* In the caudal part of the orbit are three openings: from dorsal to ventral, the **ethmoid for. (2)★,** the **optic canal (52)★●,** and the **for. orbitorotundum (44")★** *(the combined orbital fissure and round for. of the horse and dog.)* The *pointed projection lat. to these is the* **pterygoid crest (46)★■.** On the dorsal surface the frontal bone is pierced medial to the zygomatic process by the **supraorbital canal (1")★,** often double, which opens in the orbit. *The palpable* **supraorbital groove (1')★** *runs rostrally and caudally from the* canal.

d) The **MANDIBLE (XVII).** See p. 33.

e) The **HYOID APPARATUS** (Text figure). The **body (basihyoid)** gives off a *stubby* median **lingual process.** The **thyrohyoid** fuses later with the body and articulates with the rostral horn of the thyroid cartilage of the larynx. The **ceratohyoid** articulates with the body and with the *rod-shaped* **epihyoid,** which in turn articulates with the long, flattened **stylohyoid.** The last three joints are synovial. The proximal end of the stylohyoid is joined by the fibrocartilaginous **tympanohyoid** to the styloid process. *The* **angle** *of the stylohyoid is drawn out in the form of a hook.*

Hyoid apparatus

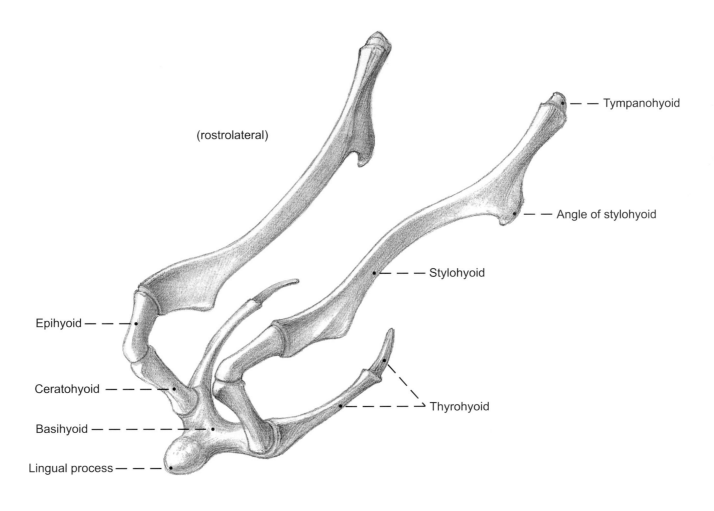

(rostrolateral)

Tympanohyoid

Angle of stylohyoid

Stylohyoid

Epihyoid

Ceratohyoid

Basihyoid

Thyrohyoid

Lingual process

Directions for the use of figures on p. 31: features marked with an asterisk (★)—upper fig.; those marked with a square (■)—lower fig.; those marked with a bullet (●)—p. 33 upper figure; those marked with a rhombus (◆)—p. 33 lower figure.

Cranium

External lamina (a) ●
Diploe (b) ●
Internal lamina (c) ●
Temporal meatus (e) ★ ●
Retroarticular foramen (h) ■
Temporal fossa (j) ★
  Temporal line (k) ★ [External frontal crest]
  Nuchal line (m) ■
  Temporal crest (m') ★ ■
Jugular foramen (q) ●
Petrooccipital fissure (q') ●

Neurocranial bones

I. Frontal bone ★

Zygomatic process (1) ★ ■
Supraorbital groove (1') ★
Supraorbital canal (1") ★
Ethmoid foramen (2) ★
Intercornual protuberance (3) ★ ■
Cornual process (3') ★ ■

II. Parietal bone ■

III. Interparietal bone ■

IV. Temporal bone ★ ■

a. Petrous part (6) ■ ●
Mastoid process (7) ■
Internal acoustic meatus
  Internal acoustic pore (8) ●
Facial canal (9) ●
  Stylomastoid foramen (10) ■
Styloid process (10') ■
  Petrotympanic fissure (12) ■
Cerebellar fossa (13) ●

b. Tympanic part (15) ★
External acoustic meatus
  External acoustic pore (16) ★ ■
Tympanic bulla (17) ■
Muscular process (17") ■

c. Squamous part (18) ★
Zygomatic process (19) ★ ■
Lateral opening of temporal meatus (e) ★
Mandibular fossa (20) ■
  Articular surface (21) ■
  Retroarticular process (22) ■

VI. Occipital bone ■ ●

Squamous part (30) ■
  External occipital protuberance (31) ■ ●
  Internal occipital protuberance (31') ●
Lateral part (32) ■ ●
  Occipital condyle (33) ■ ●
  Condylar canal (34) ■ ●
  Hypoglossal nerve canal (35) ■ ●
  Jugular and paracondylar process (36) ★ ■ ●
Basilar part (37) ■ ●
  Foramen magnum (38) ■ ●
  Muscular tubercle (40) ■ ●

VII. Sphenoid bone ■ ●

Basisphenoid bone
Body (41) ■ ●
  Sella turcica (42) ●
Wing [Ala] (43) ■ ●
  Groove for ophthalmic and maxillary nn. (44') ●
  Foramen orbitorotundum (44") ★
  Oval foramen (45) ★ ■ ●
  Pterygoid crest (46) ★ ■
Presphenoid bone
Body (50) ■ ●
Wing [Ala] (51) ■ ●
  Orbitosphenoid crest (51') ●
  Optic canal (52) ★ ●

Face

Pterygopalatine fossa (A) ■
Major palatine canal
  Caudal palatine foramen (B) ■
  Major palatine foramen (C) ■
Minor palatine canals
  Caudal palatine foramen (B) ■
  Minor palatine foramina (D) ■
  Sphenopalatine foramen (E) ■ ●
Choanae (F) ■
Orbit (G) ★ ■
Palatine fissure (H) ★ ■

Facial bones

VIII. Lacrimal bone ★

Fossa for lacrimal sac (54) ★
Lacrimal bulla (54') ★ ■

IX. Zygomatic bone ★ ■

Temporal process (55) ★ ■
Frontal process (56) ★ ■

X. Nasal bone ★

Rostral process (X.') ★
Nasoincisive notch (X.") ★

XI. Maxilla ★ ■

Body of maxilla (57) ★ ■
  Facial crest (57') ★
    Facial tuber (57") ★ ■
  Infraorbital canal
    Infraorbital foramen (59) ★
  Lacrimal canal (see p. 35 D)
Zygomatic process (63) ★ ■
Palatine process (64) ■
Alveolar process (65) ★ ■

XII. Incisive bone ★ ■ ●

Body of incisive bone (66) ★ ■ ●
Alveolar process (67) ★ ■
Palatine process (68) ★ ■ ●
Nasal process (69) ■ ●

XIII. Palatine bone ■ ●

Perpendicular plate (70) ■ ●
Horizontal plate (71) ■ ●

XIV. Pterygoid bone ■ ●

Hamulus (72) ■ ●

XV. Vomer ●

(rostrodorsal ★)

(caudobasal ■)

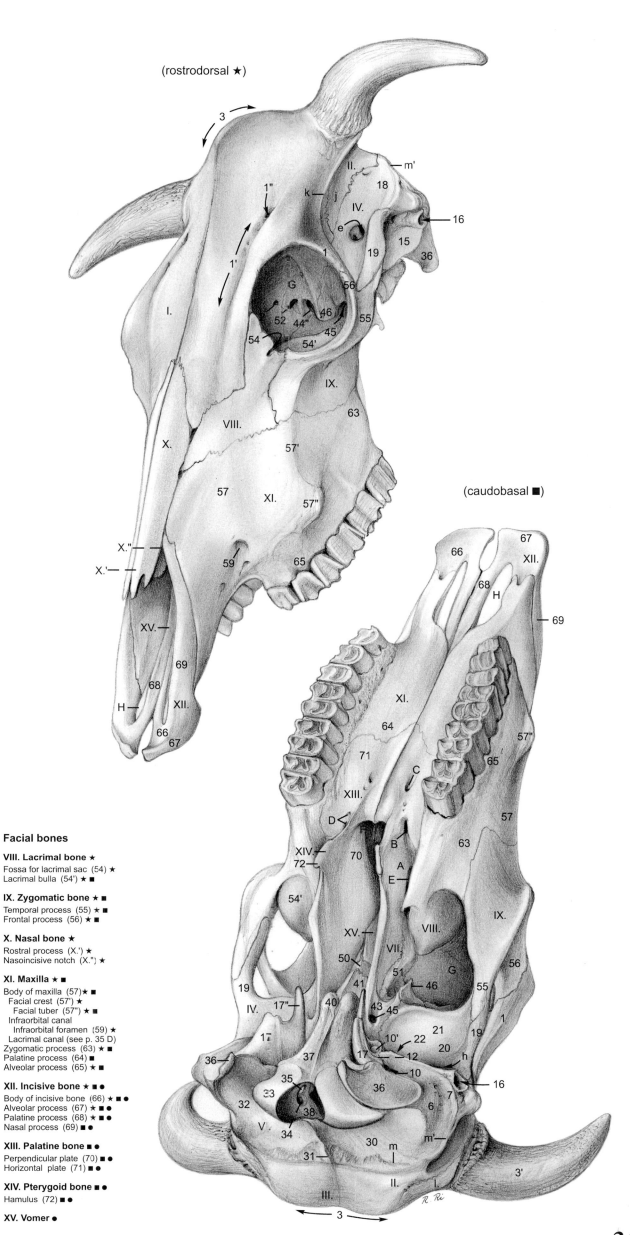

2. SKULL WITH TEETH

DENTITION.

The **formula** for the **permanent teeth** is:

$$2 \left(I\frac{0}{3} C\frac{0}{1} P\frac{3}{3} M\frac{3}{3} \right) = 32$$

where I = incisor, C = canine, P = premolar, and M = molar.

The **formula** for the **deciduous teeth (milk teeth)** is:

$$2 \left(Di\frac{0}{3} Dc\frac{0}{1} Dp\frac{3}{3} \right) = 20$$

where Di = deciduous incisor, Dc = deciduous canine, and Dp = deciduous premolar.

In domestic ruminants the missing upper incisors and canines are replaced by the **dental pad (p. 45, a)** *a plate of connective tissue covered by cornified epithelium.*

The individual **TEETH** have a **crown, neck,** and **root.** They consist of **dentin** (ivory), **enamel,** and **cement.** The five **surfaces** of a tooth are: **lingual, vestibular (labial or buccal), occlusal,** and two **contact surfaces.** The **mesial contact surface** of the incisors is toward the median plane; on all other teeth it is directed toward the incisors. The opposite contact surface is **distal.** *Although the upper incisors and canines are absent after birth, the primordia are present in the embryo.*

The **canine teeth (C)** *have the shape of* **incisors (I1, 2, 3)** *with a definite* **neck** *and a shovel-shaped* **crown;** *therefore they are commonly counted as the fourth incisors.* When these teeth erupt, the crown is covered briefly by a thin pink layer of gingival mucosa, and neighboring teeth overlap, but by the end of the first month they have rotated so that they stand side by side. The permanent incisors erupt at about the following ages: I1, 1½–2 yrs.; I2, 2–2½ yrs.; I3, 3 yrs.; C, 3½–4 yrs. At first the crown is completely covered by enamel; lingual and labial surfaces meet in a sharp edge. The lingual surface is marked by **enamel ridges** extending from the occlusal border about two thirds of the way to the neck. As the tooth wears, the thin lingual enamel is abraded faster than the thick labial plate, keeping the tooth beveled to a sharp edge (see text fig.). The darker, yellowish **dentin** is exposed and forms most of the occlusal surface. The dental star appears, filled with secondary dentin. The lingual border of the occlusal surface is notched between the ridges on the lingual surface. When the tooth wears down to the point where the ridges disappear, the lingual border of

that the first cheek tooth is P2. Between the canines and the premolars in the lower jaw there is a space, the **diastema (J),** with no teeth. The size of the cheek teeth increases greatly from rostral to caudal. The incisors and canines are brachydont teeth; they do not grow longer after they are fully erupted, and they do not have infundibula. The cheek teeth are hypsodont; they continue to grow in length after eruption, but to a lesser extent than in the horse.

The **infundibula** of the cheek teeth develop by infolding of the enamel organ. (See text fig.) When tooth erupts the central enamel of each infundibulum is continuous with the external enamel in a crest. As the crest wears off the infundibulum is separated from the external enamel and the **dentin** is exposed between them. *In ruminants the sections of the infundibula visible on the occlusal surface are crescentic.* The infundibula are partially filled by **cement** and blackened feed residue. The outside of the newly erupted tooth is also coated with cement.

The **upper premolars** have one infundibulum and three roots. The **upper molars** have two infundibula and three roots. The horns of the crescents of all the infundibula of the upper cheek teeth point toward the buccal surface. The **lower premolars (P2, 3, 4)** are irregular in form. P2 is small and has a simple crown, usually without enamel folds. P3 and P4 have two vertical enamel folds on the lin-

(Upper teeth, lingual surface)

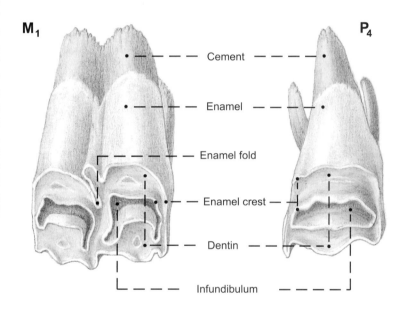

M₁   P₄

- Cement
- Enamel
- Enamel fold
- Enamel crest
- Dentin
- Infundibulum

gual surface. On P4 the caudal one may be closed to form an infundibulum. The lower premolars have two roots. The **lower molars (M1, 2, 3)** have two infundibula and two roots. The horns of the infundibula point toward the lingual surface.

The lower jaw is narrower than the upper jaw, and the occlusal surface of the upper cheek teeth slopes downward and outward to overlap the buccal edge of the lower teeth, but the lateral motion of the mandible in chewing, first on one side and then on the other, wears the occlusal surfaces almost equally.

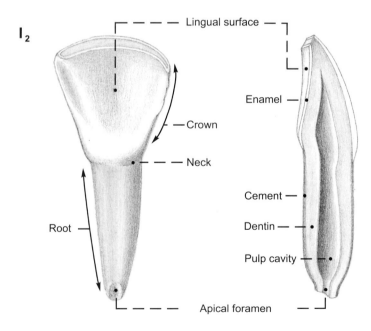

I₂

- Lingual surface
- Enamel
- Crown
- Neck
- Cement
- Dentin
- Pulp cavity
- Root
- Apical foramen

the occlusal surface is a smooth curve and the tooth is said to be level. This usually occurs in sequence from I1 to C at 6, 7, 8, and 9 years. Deciduous incisors and canines are smaller than permanent teeth and have narrower necks. The first premolar is missing, so

Directions for the use of figures on p. 31: features marked with an asterisk (★)—upper fig.; those marked with a square (■)—lower fig.; those marked with a bullet (●)—p. 33 upper figure; those marked with a rhombus (◆)—p. 33 lower figure.

Cranium

External lamina (a) ●
Diploë (b) ●
Internal lamina (c) ●
Temporal meatus (e) ★ ●
Retroarticular foramen (h) ■
Temporal fossa (j) ★
  Temporal line (k) ★ [External frontal crest]
  Nuchal line (m) ■
  Temporal crest (m') ★ ■
Jugular foramen (q) ●
Petrooccipital fissure (q') ●

(Paramedian section ●)

Cranial cavity

Rostral cran. fossa (r) ●
Middle cran. fossa (u) ●
  Hypophysial fossa (v) ●
  Piriform fossa (w) ●
Caudal cran. fossa (x) ●
Pontine impression (y) ●
Medullary impression (z) ●

Neurocranial bones

II. Parietal bone ★ ■

III. Interparietal bone ■

IV. Temporal bone ★ ■

a. Petrous part (6) ■ ●
Mastoid process (7) ■
Internal acoustic meatus
  Internal acoustic pore (8) ●
Facial canal (9) ●
  Stylomastoid foramen (10) ■
  Styloid process (10') ■
  Petrotympanic fissure (12) ■
Cerebellar fossa (13) ●

b. Tympanic part (15) ★
External acoustic meatus
  External acoustic pore (16) ★ ■
Tympanic bulla (17) ■
Muscular process (17") ■ ●

c. Squamous part (18) ★
Zygomatic process (19) ★ ■
Mandibular fossa (20) ■
  Articular surface (21) ■
  Retroarticular process (22) ■

V. Ethmoid Bone ●

Cribriform plate (23) ●
Crista galli (24) ●
Ethmoid labyrinth (25) ●
Ethmoturbinates
  Ectoturbinates (not shown)
  Endoturbinates (27) ●
    Dorsal nasal concha (28) ●
    Middle nasal concha (29) ●

VI. Occipital bone ■ ●

Squamous part (30) ■ ●
  External occipital protuberance (31) ■ ●
  Internal occipital protuberance (31') ●
Lateral part (32) ■ ●
  Occipital condyle (33) ■ ●
  Condylar canal (34) ■ ●
  Hypoglossal nerve canal (35) ■ ●
  Jugular and paracondylar process (36) ★ ■ ●
Basilar part (37) ●
  Foramen magnum (38) ■ ●
  Muscular tubercle (40) ■ ●

VII. Sphenoid bone ■ ●

Basisphenoid bone
Body (41) ■ ●
  Sella turcica (42) ●
Wing [Ala] (43) ■ ●
  Groove for ophthalmic and maxillary nn. (44') ●
  Foramen orbitorotundum (44") p. 31 ★
  Oval foramen (45) ★ ■ ●
  Pterygoid crest (46) ★ ■

Presphenoid bone
Body (50) ■ ●
Wing [Ala] (51) ■
  Orbitosphenoid crest (51') ●
  Optic canal (52) ★ ●

Face

Facial bones

Sphenopalatine foramen (E) ■ ●

XII. Incisive bone ■ ●

Body of incisive bone (66) ★ ■ ●
Alveolar process (67) ★ ■ ●
Palatine process (68) ★ ■ ●
Nasal process (69) ★ ■ ●

XIII. Palatine bone ■ ●

Perpendicular plate (70) ■ ●
Horizontal plate (71) ■ ●

XIV. Pterygoid bone ■ ●

Hamulus (72) ■ ●

XV. Vomer ●

XVI. Ventral nasal concha ●

XVII. Mandible ◆

Mandibular canal
  Mandibular foramen (74) ◆
  Mental foramen (75) ◆
Body of the mandible (76) ◆
  Diastema (J) ◆
  Ventral border (77) ◆
  Vascular groove (77') ◆
  Alveolar border (78) ◆
  Mylohyoid line (79) ◆
Ramus of the mandible (80) ◆
  Angle of the mandible (81) ◆
  Masseteric fossa (83) ◆
  Pterygoid fossa (84) ◆
  Condylar process (85) ◆
    Head of mandible (86) ◆
    Neck of mandible (87) ◆
Mandibular notch (88) ◆
Coronoid process (89) ◆

XVII. Mandible ◆

33

3. SKULL WITH PARANASAL SINUSES AND HORNS

a) The **PARANASAL SINUSES** (see also p. 45) may be studied from prepared skulls, but many of the clinically important septa are not solid bone; they are completed by membranes that do not survive maceration. The paranasal sinuses develop by evagination of the nasal mucosa into the spongy bone (diploë, b, p. 33)● between the **external** and **internal plates** (a, c)● of the cranial and facial bones. Therefore each sinus is lined by respiratory epithelium and, except for the lacrimal and palatine sinuses, which are diverticula of the maxillary sinus, each has a direct opening to the nasal cavity. Unfortunately, when inflammation occurs, the mucous membrane swells and closes the aperture, blocking normal drainage of the sinus. This condition may require surgical drainage.

The paranasal Sinuses of the Ox

Group I	Group II
Maxillary	Frontal
Lacrimal	Caudal
Palatine	Rostral
Conchal	Medial
Dorsal	Intermediate
Ventral	Lateral
	Sphenoid
	Ethmoid cells
	Middle conchal sinus

I. **The first group of sinuses** open into the middle nasal meatus (p. 45, 6)

1. The **maxillary sinus (7)** occupies the maxilla and extends back under the orbit into the thin-walled **lacrimal bulla (E)** and into the zygomatic bone, thereby surrounding the orbit rostrally and ventrally. The **nasomaxillary opening** is high on the medial wall just ventral to the **lacrimal canal (D)** and midway between the orbit and the facial tuber. It opens into the middle nasal meatus.

The maxillary sinus communicates with the **lacrimal sinus (5)** and through the **maxillopalatine opening (F)** over the **infraorbital canal (G)** with the **palatine sinus (10)**. See also p. 45, j.

There is a large opening in the bony wall between the ventral nasal meatus and the palatine sinus, but this is closed in life by the apposition of their mucous membranes.

2. Also opening into the middle nasal meatus is the **dorsal conchal sinus (6)** in the caudal part of the dorsal concha, and

3. the **ventral conchal sinus** in the caudal part of the ventral concha (XVI) p. 33●. See also p. 45.

II. **The second group of sinuses** open into ethmoidal meatuses in the caudal end of the nasal cavity.

1. The **frontal sinuses** are variable in size and number. In the newborn calf, they occupy only the frontal bone rostrodorsal to the brain. *In the aged ox the caudal frontal sinus is very extensive, invading also the parietal, interparietal, occipital, and temporal bones.* Left and right frontal sinuses are separated by a **median septum (B)**. The **caudal frontal sinus (1)** is bounded rostrally by an **oblique transverse septum (B')** that runs from the middle of the orbit caudomedially to join the median septum in the transverse plane of the caudal margin of the orbit. The caudal boundary is the occipital bone and the lateral boundary is the **temporal line (k)***. There is an extension into the zygomatic process. The **supraorbital canal (C)**, conducting the frontal vein, passes through the caudal frontal sinus in a plate of bone that appears to be a septum, but is always perforated. The caudal frontal sinus has three clinically important diverticula: the **nuchal (H), cornual (J),** and **postorbital (K) diverticula**. The caudal frontal sinus has only one aperture: at its rostral extremity there is a small outlet to an ethmoid meatus. *There is no frontomaxillary opening in any domestic animal except the Equidae.* The **rostral frontal sinuses (2, 3, 4)** lie between the rostral half of the orbit and the median plane. Each has an opening at its rostral end to an ethmoid meatus. A part of the **dorsal nasal concha (6)** projects caudally between two of the rostral frontal sinuses. The lateral rostral frontal sinus is separated by a thin septum from the lacrimal sinus.

2. The **sphenoid sinus (8)**, when present, opens into an ethmoid meatus.

3. The **ethmoid cells (9)** in the medial wall of the orbit, and

4. The **sinus of the middle concha** (p. 45, g) open into ethmoid meatuses.

b) The **HORNS (CORNUA)** project from the caudolateral angle of the frontal bone in both sexes, (except for hornless breeds, which have only a knob-like thickening of the bone.) Round, and tapering conically to a small apex, their form is not only species and breed specific, but is also quite variable individually. In the cow they are slender and long—in the bull, thick and short, and in the steer also thick, but longer. We recognize a **base**, a **body**, and an **apex**. The osseous core of the horn is the cornual process of the frontal bone (p. 31, 3'), which until shortly before birth is a rounded thickening. This elongates after birth to become a massive bony cone, and beginning at six months is pneumatized from the caudal frontal sinus. This is clinically important in deep wounds of the horns and in dehorning methods.

The bony process, like the distal part of the digit, is covered by greatly modified skin.

I. The subcutis is absent and the periosteum is fused with the dermis.

II. The **dermis** bears distinct papillae, which become longer on the base and especially toward the body, and lie step-wise over each other parallel to the surface. On the apex they are large free vertical tapering papillae. The dermis forms the positive die on which the living epidermis is molded.

III. The **epidermis of the horn** produces from its living cells the cornified horn sheath (stratum corneum) as **horn tubules** corresponding to the dermal papillae. The tubules are bound together by intertubular horn. **Longitudinal growth** of the horns occurs under the previously formed conical horn sheath through the production of a new cone of horn by the living epidermal cells, pushing the horny substance toward the apex. This can be seen on a longitudinal section. The horn consists of a stack of cones, each produced during a growth period, the horn sheath becoming thicker toward the apex. Radial growth pressure inside the rigid sheath compresses and flattens the tubules so that they are not recognizable in the body. On the apex of the cornual process additional tubular horn is formed over the free papillae. Growth is mainly longitudinal; growth in diameter is of lesser importance.

The formation of horn substance is steady in the bull; therefore the horns appear smooth on the surface. In the cow, growth is periodical and variable in rate, causing superficial rings and grooves. The **rings** are the product of regular, and the **grooves** the product of irregular horn formation, which is explained primarily by repeated pregnancies, but also by nutritional deficiencies and possibly diseases.

On the base of the horn at the transition from the skin to the horn sheath there is an epidermal zone called the **epikeras** that is comparable to the periople of the equine hoof.

The **blood supply** of the horns comes from the cornual aa. and vv. from the supf. temporal a. and v.

The **innervation** is supplied by the cornual br. of the zygomaticotemporal br. (see p. 40) and also the supraorbital and infratrochlear nn., all from the ophthalmic n.

The **lymph** is drained to the parotid ln.

Paranasal Sinuses and Horns

(dorsal)

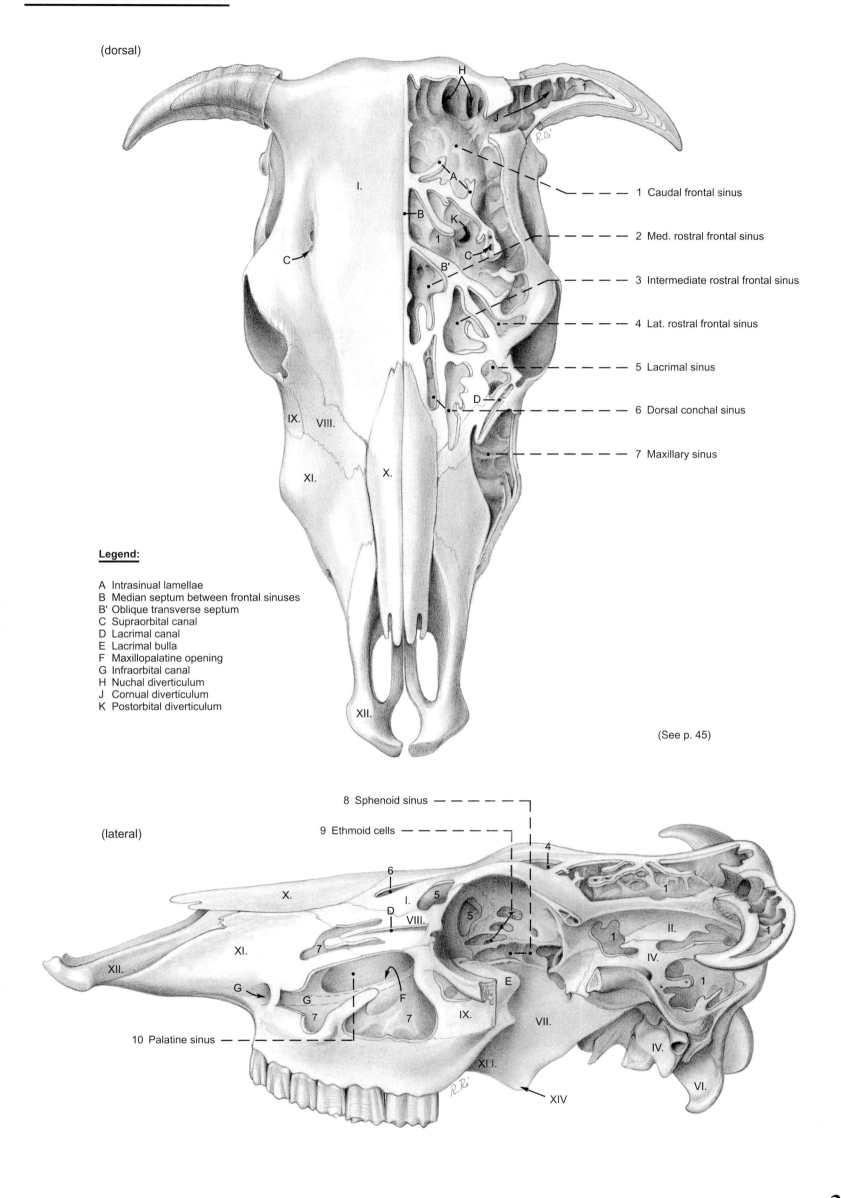

1 Caudal frontal sinus

2 Med. rostral frontal sinus

3 Intermediate rostral frontal sinus

4 Lat. rostral frontal sinus

5 Lacrimal sinus

6 Dorsal conchal sinus

7 Maxillary sinus

Legend:

A Intrasinual lamellae
B Median septum between frontal sinuses
B' Oblique transverse septum
C Supraorbital canal
D Lacrimal canal
E Lacrimal bulla
F Maxillopalatine opening
G Infraorbital canal
H Nuchal diverticulum
J Cornual diverticulum
K Postorbital diverticulum

(See p. 45)

8 Sphenoid sinus

9 Ethmoid cells

(lateral)

10 Palatine sinus

The Roman numerals refer to the bones of the skull on pp. 31 and 33.

4. SUPERFICIAL VEINS OF THE HEAD, FACIAL N. (VII), AND FACIAL MUSCLES

> To demonstrate the superficial veins and nerves, the head is split in the median plane and the skin is removed, except for a narrow strip of skin around the horn, eye, nose, and mouth, noting the cutaneus faciei (A) and the frontalis, which is spread superficially over the frontal region. The parotidoauricularis and zygomaticoauricularis are transected and reflected to expose the parotid gland. The dorsal part of the gland above the maxillary v. is removed piecemeal, sparing the vessels and nerves in the gland, and the large parotid lymph node ventral to the temporo-mandibular joint.

a) The **SUPERFICIAL VEINS** (refer to p. 37) are drained by the **external jugular v. (k)** whose main branches, the linguofacial and maxillary vv., cross the lateral surface of the mandibular gland. The **linguo-facial v. (16)**, after giving off the **lingual v.**, is continued as the **facial v. (8)**. The lingual v. gives off the sublingual v. as in the dog. The sternomandibularis (F) must be reflected to see the facial v. where it crosses the ventral border of the mandible in the vascular groove with the **facial a. (f)**, **ventr. buccal br. (33)** of the facial n., **parotid br. (h)** of the buccal n. (V3),* and **parotid duct (j)**. On the lateral surface of the mandible the **supf. and deep vv. of the lower lip (28)** are given off. From the caudal side of the facial v. at this level, the **deep facial v. (27)** passes deep to the masseter to the **deep facial plexus** (text fig. b) and to the orbit. The facial vessels continue dorsally, supplying **deep and superficial vessels of the upper lip (21)**. The vein supplies the **lat. nasal v. (9)** and **dorsal nasal v. (7)**, and is continued by the **v. of the angle of the eye (6)**. The latter *passes dorsomedial to the orbit and becomes the frontal v., which courses in the supraorbital groove (p. 31, 1') to the supraorbital foramen.*

Caudal to the angle of the mandible, medial to the parotid gl., the **maxillary v. (15)** gives off the **caud. auricular v. (14)** and the **ventral masseteric v. (34)**. (The occipital v. comes from the int. jugular v.) Before the maxillary v. turns deep to the ramus of the mandible it gives rise to the large **supf. temporal v. (31)**, which gives off the *short* **transverse facial v. (30)**, the **rostral auricular v. (18)**, and the **cornual v. (17)**, and turns rostrally into the orbit to become the **dorsal ext. ophthalmic v. (19)**.

b) The **FACIAL N. (VII)** as it leaves the stylomastoid foramen, gives off the **caud. auricular n.** and **internal auricular br.**, *which does not give off the cutaneous brr. that go to the base and inner surface of the auricle in the horse and dog; these are supplied exclusively by the auricular branch of the vagus n.* Dorsally, the facial n. gives off the **auriculopalpebral n. (29)**, which divides into the rostral auricular brr. and the zygomatic br. The latter runs forward on the surface of the zygomatic arch to the eyelids and ends in palpebral brr. In the parotid gland the facial n. divides into dorsal and ventral buccal brr. The **dorsal buccal br. (32)** emerges at the ventral

end of the parotid ln. under the parotid gland. It is joined by a large branch of the sensory auriculotemporal n. (V3, g) and courses toward the upper lip, supplying facial muscles and cutaneous sensation. The **ventral buccal br. (33)** is more slender than the dorsal br. *It follows the caudal and ventral borders of the masseter (unlike that of the horse) to the vascular groove, whence it runs along the ventral border of the buccinator and depressor labii inferioris to the lower lip. The cervical br. (Ramus colli) is absent in the ox.*

c) The **FACIAL MUSCLES** include lip and cheek muscles, the muscles of the eyelids and nose, and ear muscles. The **levator nasolabialis (5)** is a broad thin muscle originating from the frontal bone *and the frontalis. Between its superficial and deep layers pass the* **levator labii superioris (22)** and **caninus (23)**. These two muscles and the **depressor labii superioris (24)** originate close together from the facial tuber. The levator labii superioris covers the ventral part of the infraorbital foramen, which is nevertheless palpable. The **depressor labii inferioris (25)** originates deep to the masseter from the caudal part of the alveolar border of the mandible. The **zygomaticus (11)** originates from the masseteric fascia ventral to the orbit and runs obliquely across the masseter and buccinator to the **orbicularis oris (10)** at the corner of the mouth. The **buccinator (26)** forms the muscular layer of the cheek. The **molar part** is covered by the masseter and the depressor labii inferioris. The **buccal part** is a thin layer of mostly vertical fibers.

The muscles of the eyelids are the **orbicularis oculi (4)**, **frontalis (1)**, **levator palpebrae superioris** (see p. 41, 13), and **malaris (20)**. *The frontalis* (not present in the horse) *takes over the function of the absent retractor anguli oculi lat., and augments the action of the levator palpebrae superioris.* Of the ear muscles, the **parotidoauricularis (13)** extends on the surface of the parotid gland from the ventral part of the parotid fascia to the intertragic notch. The **zygomaticoauricularis (12)** begins on the zygomatic arch and runs back to end at the intertragic notch. The **cervicoscutularis (2)** originates from the lig. nuchae and the skull behind the intercornual protuberance. *The short* **interscutularis (3)** *comes from the cornual process and the temporal line, and has no connection with the contralateral muscle.*

Arteries and Veins of the Head

Legend: (Numbers differ from those in text.)

1 Common carotid a.
2 External carotid a.
3 Occipital a.
4 Linguofacial tr. and v.
5 Lingual a. and v.
6 Submental a. and v.
7 Sublingual a. and v.
8 Facial a. and v.
9 Supf. and deep
   inf. labial a. and v.
10 Superior labial a., supf.
   and deep sup. labial vv.
11 Rostral lat. nasal a.
   and lat. nasal v.
12 Dors. nasal a. and v.
13 Arterial br. and
   v. of angle of eye
14 Ventr. masseteric br. and v.
15 Caud. auricular a. and v.
16 Supf. temporal a. and v.
17 Rostr. auricular a. and v.
18 Transverse facial a. and v.
19 Cornual a. and v.
19' Inf. and sup. palpebral aa.
20 Maxillary a. and v.
21 Inferior alveolar a. and v.
22 Mental a. and v.
23 Ext. ophth. a.,
   dors. ext. ophth. v.

24 Supraorbital a. and v.
25 Malar a. and v.
26 A. of angle of eye
27 Infraorbital a. and v.
28 Ext. jugular v.
29 Buccal v.
30 Deep facial v.
31 Frontal v.

a Pterygoid plexus
b Deep facial plexus
c Ophthalmic plexus

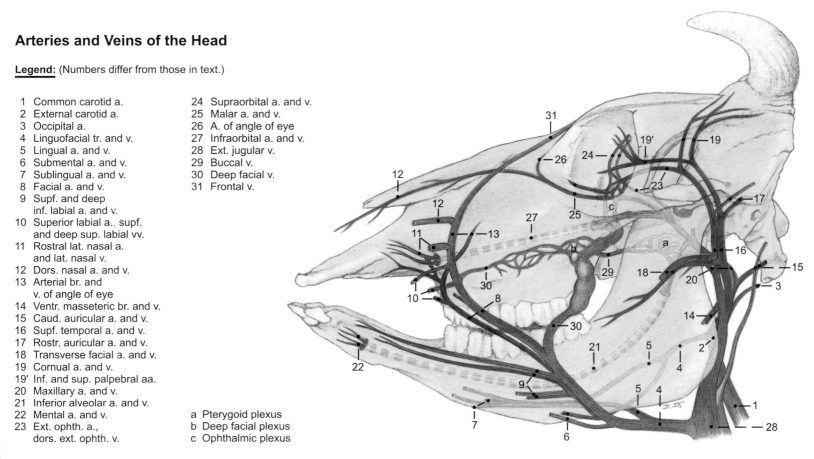

* V = Trigeminal n., V1 = Ophthalmic n. V2 = Maxillary n. V3 = Mandibular n.

Arteries and Veins of the head, Facial n. and Facial muscles

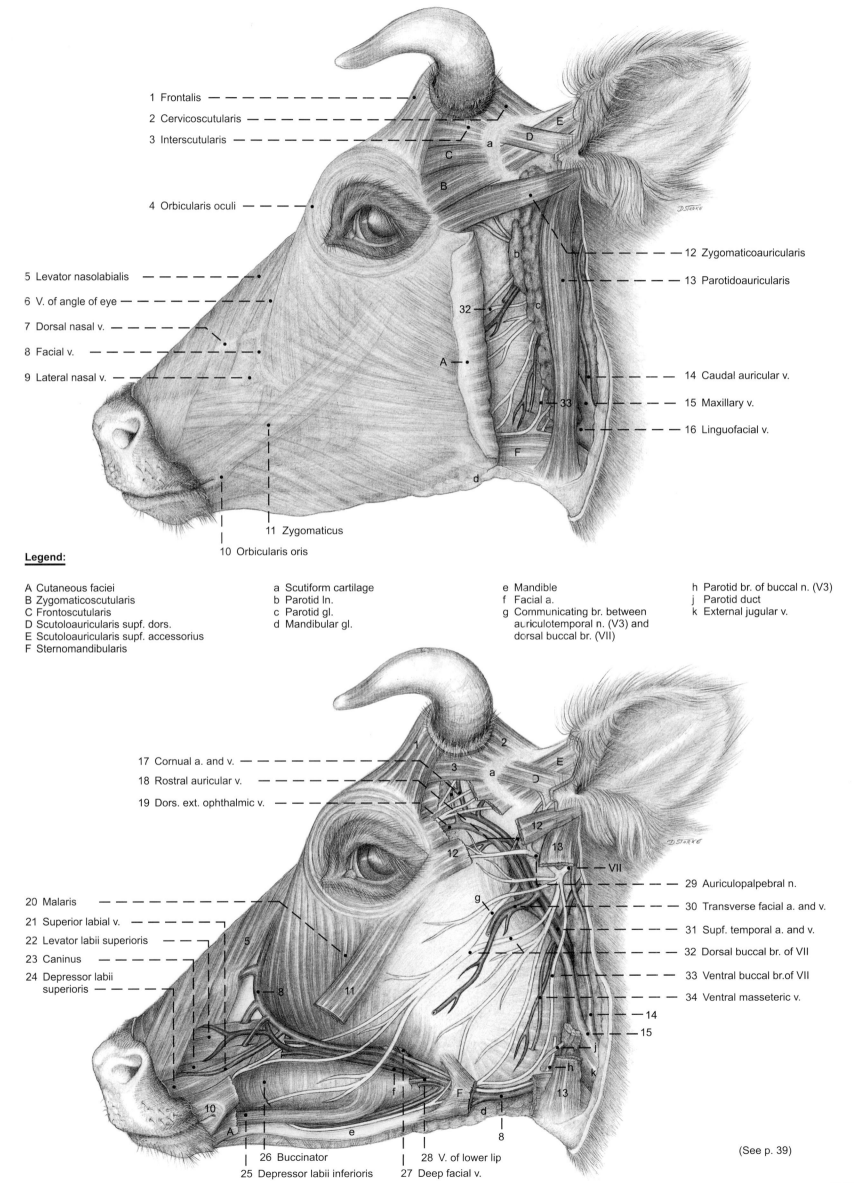

1 Frontalis

2 Cervicoscutularis

3 Interscutularis

4 Orbicularis oculi

5 Levator nasolabialis

6 V. of angle of eye

7 Dorsal nasal v.

8 Facial v.

9 Lateral nasal v.

12 Zygomaticoauricularis

13 Parotidoauricularis

14 Caudal auricular v.

15 Maxillary v.

16 Linguofacial v.

11 Zygomaticus

10 Orbicularis oris

Legend:

A Cutaneous faciei
B Zygomaticoscutularis
C Frontoscutularis
D Scutoloauricularis supf. dors.
E Scutoloauricularis supf. accessorius
F Sternomandibularis

a Scutiform cartilage
b Parotid ln.
c Parotid gl.
d Mandibular gl.

e Mandible
f Facial a.
g Communicating br. between auriculotemporal n. (V3) and dorsal buccal br. (VII)

h Parotid br. of buccal n. (V3)
j Parotid duct
k External jugular v.

17 Cornual a. and v.

18 Rostral auricular v.

19 Dors. ext. ophthalmic v.

20 Malaris

21 Superior labial v.

22 Levator labii superioris

23 Caninus

24 Depressor labii superioris

29 Auriculopalpebral n.

30 Transverse facial a. and v.

31 Supf. temporal a. and v.

32 Dorsal buccal br. of VII

33 Ventral buccal br. of VII

34 Ventral masseteric v.

26 Buccinator

25 Depressor labii inferioris

28 V. of lower lip

27 Deep facial v.

(See p. 39)

37

5. TRIGEMINAL N. (V3 AND V2), MASTICATORY MM., SALIVARY GLL., AND LYMPHATIC SYSTEM

For the dissection of the temporalis and masseter the covering facial muscles and superficial nerves and vessels are removed. The masseter is removed in layers, showing its tough tendinous laminae, its almost horizontal and oblique fiber directions and its innervation by the masseteric n. (V3) passing through the mandibular notch. Medial to the masseter is the large **deep facial venous plexus (2)**. To remove the zygomatic arch three sagittal cuts are made: I. at the temporomandib. joint, II. through the zygomatic bone rostral to its frontal and temporal processes, and III. through the zygomatic process of the frontal bone. In the course of disarticulation of the temporomandib. joint the temporalis is separated from its termination on the coronoid proc., whereby its innervation from the deep temporal nn. is demonstrated. The mandible is sawed through rostral to the first cheek tooth. After severing all structures attached to the medial surface of the mandible, the temporomandib. joint is disarticulated by strong lateral displacement of the mandible while the joint capsule is cut. The fibrocartilaginous **articular disc** compensates for the incongruence of the articular surfaces.

a) The **TRIGEMINAL N. (V)** of the ox exhibits no marked differences in its branches from that of the dog and horse.

I. The **mandibular n. (V3)** is sensory to the teeth, oral mucosa, and skin of the lower jaw, as well as the tongue, parotid gl., and part of the ear. Unlike the other divisions of the trigeminal n. (V1 and V2) it also has somatic motor components. These are in the following branches: the **masticatory n. (20)** divides into the **deep temporal nn. (18)** and **masseteric n. (19)** which innervate the corresponding muscles. Branches to the pterygoids, tensor tympani, and tensor veli palatini have corresponding names. The inferior alveolar n. gives off, before entering the mandibular foramen, the **mylohyoid n. (29)** for the muscle of that name and for the rostral belly of the digastricus, and sends cutaneous branches to the rostral part of the intermandibular region. The following branches of the mandibular n. have no somatic motor components: The *many-branched* **buccal n. (4)** conducts sensory fibers and receives parasympathetic fibers from the glossopharyngeal n. (IX) via the *large oval* otic ganglion to the oral mucosa and the buccal salivary glands. *Its* **parotid br. (16)**, *which occurs only in ruminants, turns around the rostral border of the masseter and runs back to the parotid gland close to the duct.* The **auriculotemporal n. (26)** turns caudally to the ear, skin of the temporal region, and parotid gland, supplying sensory branches and parasympathetic innervation (from IX via the otic ganglion). The nerve then turns rostrally and joins the dorsal buccal br. of VII as the **communicating br. with the facial n. (1)** thereby supplying sensation to the skin of the cheek. The **lingual n. (30)** is sensory to the sublingual mucosa and tongue. From the **chorda tympani (VII —27)** it receives taste fibers for the rostral 2/3 of the tongue, and parasympathetic fibers for the sublingual and mandibular glands. Its **sublingual n. (33)** runs as in the dog but not as in the horse, on the lat. surface of the sublingual gll. to the floor of the mouth. The sensory **inferior alveolar n. (28)** passes through the **mandibular foramen** to the mandibular canal. It supplies the lower teeth and after emerging from the mental foramen as the **mental n. (5)** it supplies the skin and mucosa of the lower lip and chin.

II. The **maxillary n. (V2—21)** is sensory and contains parasympathetic components from VII via the pterygopalatine ganglion. It gives off the zygomatic n. and the pterygopalatine n. with the major palatine, minor palatine, and caudal nasal nn. Its rostral continuation is the **infraorbital n. (6)** which gives off sensory brr. in the infraorbital canal for the upper teeth, and after emerging from the foramen divides into numerous branches for the dorsum nasi, nostril, planum nasolabiale, upper lip, and the nasal vestibule. (For the ophthalmic n., V1, see p. 40.)

b) The **MASTICATORY MM. INCLUDING THE SUPERFICIAL INTERMANDIBULAR MM.** are innervated by the mandibular n. (V3). The caudal belly of the digastricus is innervated by the facial n. (VII). Of the **external masticatory mm.**, as in the horse, the **masseter (13)** *is larger than the* **temporalis (17)**, and, covered by a glistening aponeurosis, presents a superficial layer with almost horizontal muscle fibers, and a deep layer with caudoventral fiber direction. The **internal masticatory mm.**: the **medial pterygoid (22)** and the **lateral pterygoid (22)**, are clearly separate. The **superficial intermandibular mm.** are the mylohyoideus (25) digastricus (31). *There is no occipitomandibularis in the ox. The digastricus, which does not perforate the stylohyoideus, terminates rostral to the vascular groove on the medial surface of the ventral border of the mandible. Right and left digastrici are connected ventral to the lingual process of the basihyoid by transverse muscle fibers.*

c) The **LARGE SALIVARY GLANDS** are the parotid, mandibular, monostomatic sublingual, and polystomatic sublingual gll.

I. The **parotid gland (14, p. 37, c)** is elongated and thick. It lies along the caudal border of the masseter from the zygomatic arch to the angle of the mandible. Numerous excretory ducts converge to the **parotid duct (15)** at the ventral end of the gland. *The duct runs with the facial vessels from medial to lateral through the vascular groove in the ventral border of the mandible,* ascends in the groove along the rostral border of the masseter, and enters the oral vestibule opposite the fifth upper cheek tooth (M2). The deep surface of the gland is related to the maxillary and linguofacial vv., the end of the ext. carotid a., the mandibular gl., and the parotid ln. The facial n. with the origin of its buccal branches is enveloped by the parotid gland.

II. The **mandibular gland (9)** is curved, lying medial to the angle of the mandible and extending from the paracondylar process to the basihyoid. *Its enlarged bulbous end is palpable in the intermandibular region, where it is in contact with the contralateral gland.* The deep surface is related to the lat. retropharyngeal ln., common carotid a., pharynx, and larynx. The **mandibular duct (32)** leaves the middle of the concave border of the gland and courses deep to the mylohyoideus and dorsal to the monostomatic sublingual gl. to the sublingual caruncle on the floor of the oral cavity rostral to the frenulum of the tongue.

III. The **monostomatic sublingual gl. (24)** is about 10 cm long. Its **major sublingual duct** ends near the mandibular duct under the sublingual caruncle.

IV. The **polystomatic sublingual gl. (23)** extends in a chain of lobules from the palatoglossal arch to the incisive part of the mandible. The microscopic sublingual ducts open under the tongue on each side of a row of conical papillae extending caudally from the sublingual caruncle .

The **small salivary glands:**

The **buccal gll.** are developed best in the ox.

The superficial layer of the **dorsal buccal gll. (3)** is on the surface of the buccinator. The deep layer is covered by the muscle. They extend from the angle of the mouth to the facial tuber and are covered caudally by the masseter. *The* **middle buccal gll. (7)** *are found in ruminants between two layers of the buccinator and dorsal to the vein of the lower lip.* The **ventral buccal gll. (8)** lie on the mandible from the angle of the mouth to the rostral border of the masseter. They are ventral to the vein of the lower lip and covered, except the caudal part, by the buccinator. Small salivary gll. are present throughout the oral mucosa. Total secretion of saliva in the ox is about 50 liters in 24 hours.*

d) The **LYMPHATIC SYSTEM.** *Ruminant lymph nodes differ from those of the horse; they are usually single large nodes rather than groups of small nodes. All of the following nodes are routinely incised in meat inspection.* The **parotid ln. (12)** lies between the rostral border of the parotid gl. and the masseter, ventral to the temporomandibular joint. It is palpable in the live animal. The **mandibular ln. (10)** lies ventral to the mandible, halfway between the rostral border of the masseter and the angle of the mandible, in contact with the facial vein. It is covered laterally by the sternomandibularis and the facial cutaneous m., but is palpable in the live animal; it is lateral to the bulbous ventral end of the mandibular gl., which is in contact with the contralateral gl. and should not be mistaken for the mandibular ln.

The **medial retropharyngeal ln.** is in the fat between the caudodorsal wall of the pharynx, through which it can be palpated, and the longus capitis. Its lateral surface is related to the large (1.5 x 0.5 cm) **cranial cervical ganglion** and cranial nn. IX to XII.

The **lateral retropharyngeal ln. (11)** receives all of the lymph from the other lymph nodes of the head and is drained by the tracheal trunk. It lies in the fossa between the wing of the atlas and the mandible, covered laterally by the mandibular gland.

* Somers, 1957

Mandibular n. (V3), Maxillary n. (V2), and Salivary glands

Legend:

a Mandible
b Levator labii superioris
c Caninus
d Depressor labii superioris
e Buccinator
f Facial vein
g Vein of lower lip
h Sternomandibularis

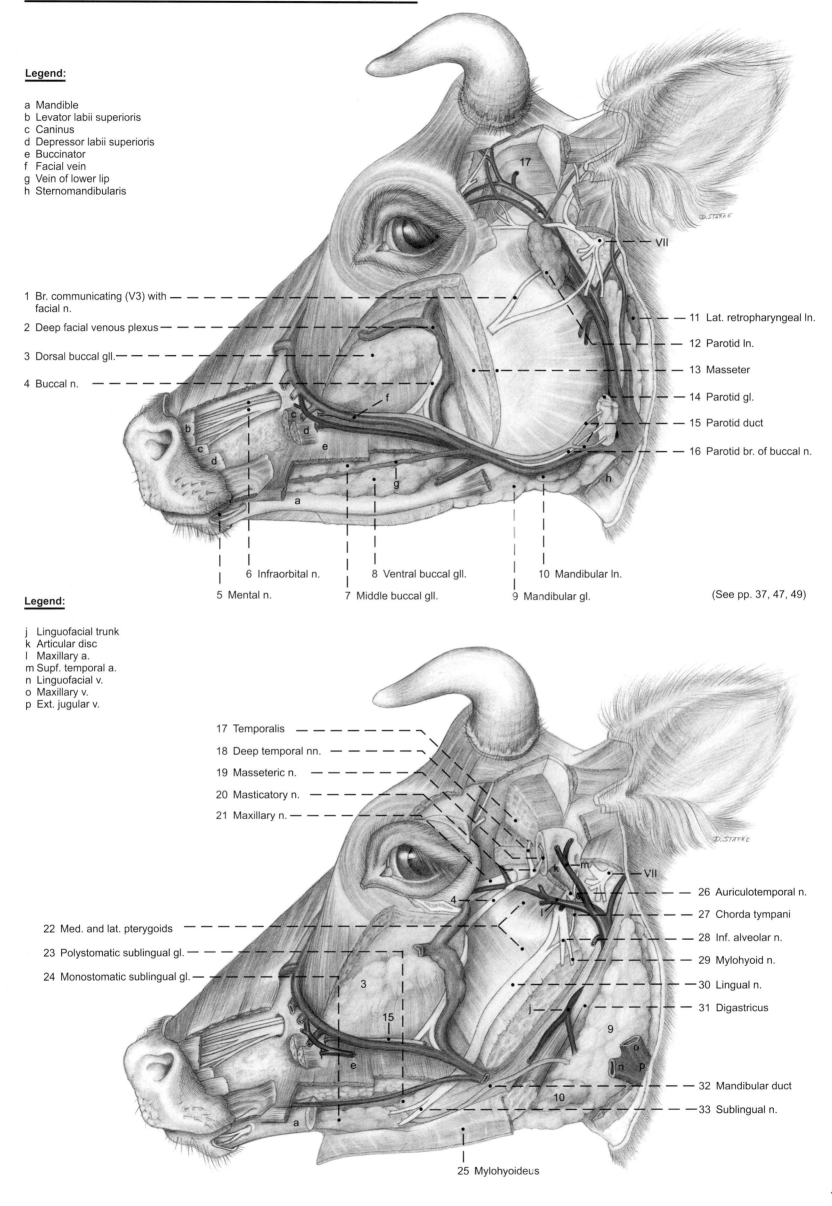

1 Br. communicating (V3) with facial n.
2 Deep facial venous plexus
3 Dorsal buccal gll.
4 Buccal n.

11 Lat. retropharyngeal ln.
12 Parotid ln.
13 Masseter
14 Parotid gl.
15 Parotid duct
16 Parotid br. of buccal n.

VII

6 Infraorbital n.
5 Mental n.
7 Middle buccal gll.
8 Ventral buccal gll.
9 Mandibular gl.
10 Mandibular ln.

(See pp. 37, 47, 49)

Legend:

j Linguofacial trunk
k Articular disc
l Maxillary a.
m Supf. temporal a.
n Linguofacial v.
o Maxillary v.
p Ext. jugular v.

17 Temporalis
18 Deep temporal nn.
19 Masseteric n.
20 Masticatory n.
21 Maxillary n.

22 Med. and lat. pterygoids
23 Polystomatic sublingual gl.
24 Monostomatic sublingual gl.

VII

26 Auriculotemporal n.
27 Chorda tympani
28 Inf. alveolar n.
29 Mylohyoid n.
30 Lingual n.
31 Digastricus

32 Mandibular duct
33 Sublingual n.

25 Mylohyoideus

39

6. ACCESSORY ORGANS OF THE EYE

The **ACCESSORY ORGANS** include the eyelids and conjunctiva, the lacrimal apparatus, and the cone of striated bulbar muscles with their fasciae and nerves. They will be described in the order in which they are exposed (see also the text figure and p. 43).

I. The **upper and lower eyelids** (palpebra superior, **A**, and **inferior**, **B**) consist of an outer layer of haired skin, a middle fibromuscular layer, and the palpebral conjunctiva. The fibrous part of the middle layer is attached to the osseous orbital margin and increases in density toward the free border to form the **tarsus**, which contains the **tarsal glands**.

The **eyelashes (cilia, D)** *of the lower lid are fewer and shorter than those of the upper lid, but they are present in the ox.*

The striated muscles are: the strong **orbicularis oculi (C)**, and in the upper eyelid, the termination of the **levator palpebrae superioris (13)** *and fibers of the* **frontalis**. The upper and lower **tarsal mm.** are parts of the smooth muscle system of the orbit, which retracts the eyelids and protrudes the eyeball under sympathetic stimulation. The **palpebral conjunctiva (10)** is continuous at the **fornix (11)** with the **bulbar conjunctiva (12)**, which ends at the **limbus of the cornea.**

The **third eyelid (8)** consists of a fold of conjunctiva in the medial angle, enclosing the T-shaped outer end of the **cartilage of the third eyelid.**

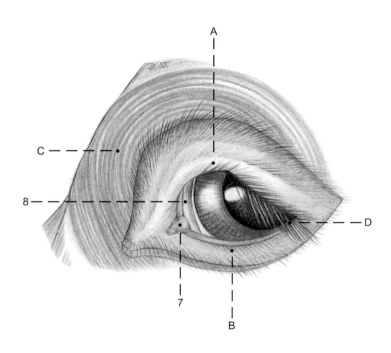

The deep part of the cartilage is surrounded by the **gland of the third eyelid,** *larger than in the horse,* extending about 5 cm straight back into the fat medial to the eyeball and discharging tears through orifices on the bulbar side of the third lid.

II. The **lacrimal apparatus.** The **lacrimal gl. (9)** lies in the dorsolateral quadrant of the orbit, with the *broad dorsal part* under the root of the zygomatic proc., and a *long thin tail* which extends around the lateral margin of the orbit.

The lacrimal ducts pass from the ventral end of the gland to orifices in the lateral fornix. The gland of the third eyelid is the largest accessory lacrimal gland. The tears collect around the **lacrimal caruncle (7)** in the **lacrimal lake** in the medial angle anterior to the third eyelid. They are drained through the **upper (5)** and **lower (6) lacrimal puncta** and **lacrimal canaliculi (4)** which join at the **lacrimal sac (3).** This is drained by the **nasolacrimal duct (2)** to the **nasolacrimal orifice (1)** *concealed on the medioventral surface of the alar fold.*

III. The **bulbar muscles** are surrounded by the **periorbita** which, in the osseous part of the orbit, is the periosteum, containing the **trochlea (19),** but caudolaterally where the bony orbit is deficient in domestic mammals, the periorbita alone forms the wall of the orbit. It is a tough, fibrous, partially elastic membrane stretched from the lateral margin of the orbit to the **pterygoid crest.** The lacrimal gland and the levator palpebrae superioris are covered only by the periorbita. The remaining structures are also enveloped in the **deep orbital fasciae:** the **fasciae of the muscles** and the **bulbar fascia (vagina bulbi).**

The **ophthalmic n. (V 1)** (see p. 53) divides while still in the for. orbitorotundum into the following three nerves:

1. The usually double **lacrimal n.** runs along the lateral surface of the lateral rectus and gives off branches to the lacrimal gl. and the upper eyelid. *The two strands of the lacrimal n. then unite and the* **zygomaticotemporal br.** *so formed* perforates the periorbita and turns caudally under the zygomatic proc. of the frontal bone to the temporal region, where it sends twigs to the skin *and continues ventral to the temporal line as the* **cornual branch** *to the skin on the cornual process.*

2. The **frontal n.** *gives rise to the* **nerve to the frontal sinuses,** *which perforates the wall of the orbit.* The frontal n. then passes around the dorsal margin of the orbit (unlike that of the horse) and becomes the **supraorbital n.** to the frontal region.

3. The **nasociliary n.** gives off the **long ciliary nn.,** which penetrate the sclera and supply sensation to the vascular tunic (see p. 42) and cornea; the **ethmoidal n.,** with sensory and autonomic fibers to the caudal nasal mucosa; and the **infratrochlear n.** The last turns around the mediodorsal margin of the orbit to the skin of the medial angle of the eye and the frontal region.

Almost all of the striated bulbar muscles: **dorsal (16), medial (14),** and **ventral (17) recti; ventral oblique (20), levator palpebrae sup. (13),** and **retractor bulbi (21),** except its lateral part, are innervated by the **oculomotor n. (III).**

Only the **dorsal oblique (18)** is innervated by the **trochlear n. (IV).**

The **lateral rectus (15)** and the **lateral part of the retractor bulbi (21)** are served by the **abducent n. (VI).**

The bulbar muscles originate around the optic canal, with the exception of the ventral oblique, which comes from a fossa on the medial wall of the orbit just above the lacrimal bulla. With the exception of the levator palpebrae sup. all of the bulbar muscles terminate on the sclera.

Lacrimal apparatus

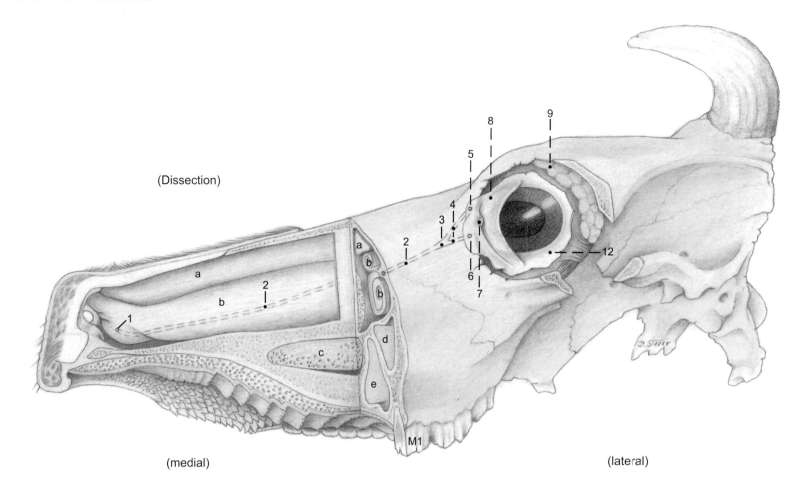

(Dissection)

(medial)   (lateral)

(See pp. 45, 47)

Legend:

1 Nasolacrimal orifice
2 Nasolacrimal duct
3 Lacrimal sac
4 Lacrimal canaliculi
5 Superior lacrimal punctum
6 Inferior lacrimal punctum
7 Lacrimal caruncle
8 Third eyelid
9 Lacrimal gland

Legend:

a Dorsal nasal concha
b Ventral nasal concha
c Venous plexus
d Maxillary sinus
e Palatine sinus

Bulbar muscles (Left eye)

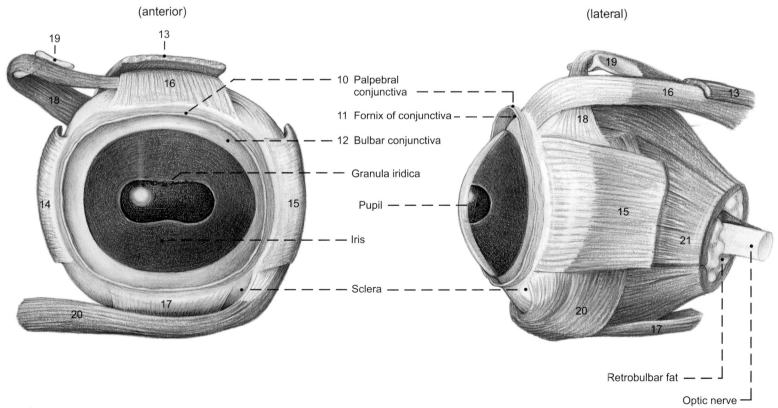

(anterior)   (lateral)

10 Palpebral conjunctiva
11 Fornix of conjunctiva
12 Bulbar conjunctiva
Granula iridica
Pupil
Iris
Sclera
Retrobulbar fat
Optic nerve

Legend:

13 Levator palpebrae superioris
14 Medial rectus
15 Lateral rectus
16 Dorsal rectus
17 Ventral rectus
18 Dorsal oblique
19 Trochlea
20 Ventral oblique
21 Retractor bulbi

7. THE EYEBALL (BULBUS OCULI)

The eyeball of the ox is smaller than that of the horse, and is not flattened so much anteroposteriorly. For orientation, the pupil and the **optic nerve** are taken as reference points. The pupil is at the anterior pole, and *the optic n. is below and slightly lateral to the posterior pole.* Like other ungulates, the ox has a transversely elliptical **pupil (5)**. When it dilates, it becomes round. The black projections (**granula iridica, 5**) on the upper and lower margins of the pupil are vascular appendages covered by pigmented epithelium from the back of the iris. Those on the lower margin are small. On eyeballs sectioned on the equator and meridionally, one can study the external (fibrous) tunic, the middle (vascular) tunic, and the internal tunic (retina).

I. The **fibrous tunic** comprises the **sclera (1)**, enclosing the greater part of the bulb in its dense white connective tissue, and the transparent **cornea (3)**. These parts join at the **corneal limbus (2)**.

II. The **vascular tunic** consists of the choroid, ciliary body, and iris.

The **choroid (15)** is highly vascular and pigmented. In its posterior part, just above the optic disc, is the blue-green, reflective **tapetum lucidum (16)**, *a fibrous structure of roughly semicircular outline with a horizontal base.*

The **ciliary body**, containing the weak **ciliary m. (J)**, is the anterior continuation of the choroid. Its most prominent feature is the **ciliary crown (corona ciliaris, 10)**, composed of vascular, radial **ciliary processes (10)**, from which the **zonular fibers (9)** extend to the equator of the lens. Posterior to the ciliary processes is the **ciliary ring (orbiculus ciliaris, 11)**, a zone bearing minute **ciliary folds (11)**. It is narrower medially than elsewhere. The posterior epithelium is the pars ciliaris retinae.

Between the ciliary body and the pupil is the **iris (4)** with the **sphincter (G)** and **dilator (H) mm.** of the pupil, The bovine iris is dark because of the heavy pigmentation of the posterior epithelium (pars iridica retinae).

III. The **retina** lines the entire vascular coat, so that each part of the vascular coat has a double inner layer derived from the two-layered ectodermal optic cup of the embryo. The greater part of the retina is the **optical part (12)**, extending from the **optic disc (20)** to the ciliary body at the **ora serrata (13)**. It contains the visual elements in its **nervous layer** and has an outer **pigmented layer**, which adheres to the vascular tunic when the nervous layer is detached. The outer layer is free of pigment over the tapetum.

The **blind part (pars ceca, 14)** of the retina lines the iris and ciliary body. In the **iridial part** the outer layer contributes the sphincter and dilator mm., and the inner layer is pigmented; in the **ciliary part**, the outer layer is pigmented.

At the **optic disc (20)** the nerve fibers of the retina exit through the **area cribrosa** of the sclera, acquire a myelin sheath, but no neurolemma, and form the **optic n. (17)**, which is morphologically a tract of the brain, covered by a thin **internal sheath (18)** corresponding to the pia mater and arachnoidea, and a thick **external sheath (19)** corresponding to the dura mater.

IV. The **lens (6)** is surrounded by the elastic **lens capsule (j)**, which is connected to the ciliary body by the zonular fibers. Under the capsule, the anterior surface of the lens is covered by the lens epithelium. Toward the **equator (k)** the epithelial cells elongate to form the lens fibers—the substance of the lens. The fibers, held together by an amorphous cement, meet on the anterior and posterior surfaces of the lens in three sutures (radii lentis), which are joined to form a Y (the lens star), best seen in the fresh state.

V. Inside the eyeball the anterior and posterior chambers lie before the lens and the vitreous body lies behind it. The **anterior chamber (7)** is between the cornea and iris. It communicates freely through the pupil with the **posterior chamber (8)** which is between the iris and the lens with its zonula. Viewed from the anterior chamber the circular **pectinate ligament (h)** is seen in the **iridocorneal angle (g)**, attaching the iris by delicate radial trabeculae to the **scleral ring** at the corneal limbus. Between these trabeculae are the **spaces of the iridocorneal angle (of Fontana)**, through which the **aqueous humor** drains to the circular **venous plexus of the sclera (42)**.

The **vitreous chamber (22)** lies between the lens and the retina, and is filled by the vitreous body. Its stroma is a network that holds in its meshes a cell-free jelly, the water content of which determines the intraocular pressure.

VI. The **blood supply** of the eye comes from the int. and ext. ophthalmic aa. and the malar a. The small **int. ophthalmic a. (24)** *comes from the rostral epidural rete mirabile (see p. 50),* accompanies the optic n., and anastomoses with the ext. ophthalmic a. and the post. ciliary aa. The **ext. ophthalmic a. (23)**, from the maxillary a., *forms the* **ophthalmic rete mirabile** *deep in the orbit on the ventral surface of the dorsal rectus.* The **supraorbital a.** arises from the rete, gives off in the orbit the **ext. ethmoidal a.** and **ant. conjunctival aa.**, and enters the supraorbital canal, supplying the frontal sinus and emerging to supply the frontalis m. and skin. Also arising from the rete are the **muscular brr. (28)** and the **lacrimal a.** The muscular brr. supply the eye muscles and give off **ant. ciliary aa. (33)** and **posterior conjunctival aa. (35)**. The **ext. ophthalmic a.** divides into two **long post. ciliary aa. (25, 26)**, which give off **short post. ciliary aa. (27)** near the eyeball, and continue to the equator of the eyeball before they enter the sclera. In the ciliary region of the iris they form the **major arterial circle of the iris (36)**. Near the bulbar end of the optic n. the long post. ciliary aa. supply small **choroidoretinal aa. (31)**, which accompany the optic n. and supply the *four* **retinal arteries** *seen with the ophthalmoscope in the fundus of the eye. Accompanied by the corresonding veins, they appear near the center of the disc and spread out over the interior of the retina in a pattern characteristic of the ox, with the largest vessels directed dorsally.* The venous blood of the eyeball is drained through the **vorticose vv. (38–41)**, **ciliary vv. (27–33)**, and the **choroidoretinal vv. (31)** to the intraorbital ophthalmic venous plexus.

Organic of vision

Right eye

(medial)

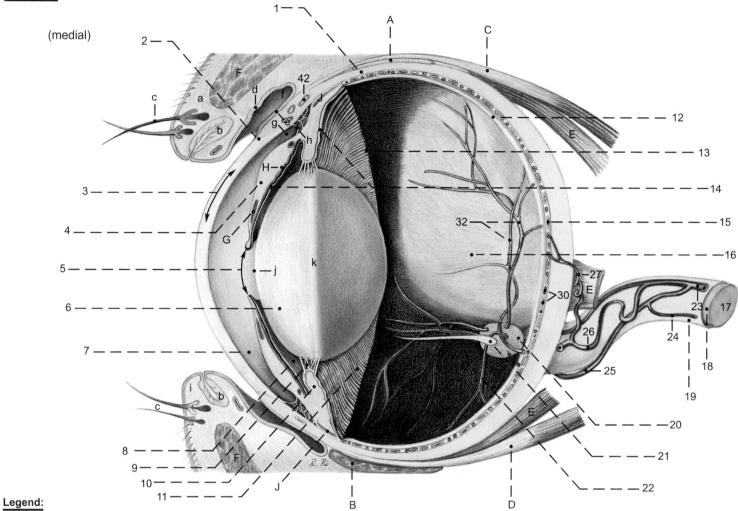

R. Rü

Left eye

(lateral)

(See pp. 40, 41)

D. Starke

Legend:

Fibrous tunic:
1 Sclera
2 Limbus of cornea
3 Cornea
4 Iris
5 Pupil with granula iridica

6 Lens
7 Anterior chamber
8 Posterior chamber
9 Zonular fibers
Ciliary body:
10 Ciliary crown and ciliary processes
11 Ciliary ring (orbiculus ciliaris) and ciliary folds

Retina:
12 Optical part of retina
13 Ora serrata
14 Blind part of retina (pars ceca)
15 Choroid
16 Tapetum lucidum

17 Optic n.
18 Internal sheath of optic n.
19 External sheath of optic n.
20 Optic disc
21 Hyaloid process
22 Vitreous chamber

8. NOSE AND NASAL CAVITIES, ORAL CAVITY AND TONGUE

> The nasal septum is removed to expose the nasal cavity.

a) NOSE.

I. *The end of the nose and the upper lip are covered by hairless skin—the* **planum nasolabiale (22)**, *where the skin is marked by minute grooves and raised areas with the openings of* **serous nasolabial glands**. *Incision reveals a thick layer of glandular tissue.* The **nostril (23)** *is rounded medioventrally and extends dorsolaterally as the* **alar groove (24)** *between the lateral border of the nostril and the* **wing of the nose (ala nasi, 24)**. *The wing is med. in the horse, dorsomed. in ruminants, and lat. in man and dog. In the ox it is held up by the rostral part of the* **dorsal lat. nasal cartilage (26)**. *The alar cartilage and nasal diverticulum of the horse are absent in the ox. The ventrolateral border of the nostril is supported by the* **lateral accessory nasal cartilage (27)**, *attached to the dorsal lateral nasal cartilage. In addition, a* **medial accessory nasal cartilage (25)** *and a* **ventral lateral nasal cartilage (28)** *are present.*

II. Each **nasal cavity** begins with the **vestibule (12)**, a narrow zone of hairless skin and stratified squamous epithelium. The rest of the nasal cavity is lined by respiratory epithelium, except the olfactory region in the caudal part. The **dorsal concha (5)** is between the **dorsal (4)** and **middle (6)** meatuses. The caudal part of the middle meatus is divided into dorsal and ventral channels by the **middle concha (2)**. The **ventral concha (7)** is between the middle and **ventral (8)** meatuses. The **common meatus (3)** is next to the nasal septum and connects the other three meatuses. *Because the vomer is not attached to the caudal half of the hard palate, the right and left ventral meatuses communicate caudal to the plane of the second cheek tooth.* The ventral concha is continued rostrally by the **alar fold (11)** to the wing of the nose. *The* **nasolacrimal orifice (10)** *is just caudal to the mucocutaneous border, concealed on the medioventral surface of the alar fold, but in the live ox the wing can be drawn dorsolaterally to cannulate the nasolacrimal duct.* The **basal fold (13)** extends from the floor of the ventral meatus to the alar fold. The ventral meatus is the only one through which a stomach tube can be passed. The dorsal nasal concha is connected to the nostril by the **straight fold (9)**. **Cavernous venous plexuses (29)** are present in the three nasal folds, in the conchae, and on the sides of the vomer and ventral border of the **nasal septum**. *In aged cattle the rostral end of the nasal septum is ossified.* A nasal concha is the whole shell-like structure, including the inner and outer mucous membranes, the submucosa containing cavernous venous plexuses, and the middle lamina, or os conchae, of thin, partly cribriform, bone. The caudal part of the nasal cavity, lined by olfactory epithelium, contains the **ethmoid conchae (1)**, which include the **middle concha (2)**. The bones of the ethmoid conchae are called turbinates. The caudal part of the ventral concha encloses a single cavity—the **ventral conchal sinus (h)**. *The rostral part forms* **dorsal and ventral scrolls (7)** *which enclose several smaller cavities (h')*. *The dorsal concha forms a single* **dorsal conchal sinus (f)**.

The **incisive duct** runs rostroventrally from the floor of the nasal cavity through the palatine fissure *to open into the mouth at the incisive papilla just caudal to the dental pad (a)*.

The **vomeronasal organ** lies on the floor of the nasal cavity lateral to the nasal septum. Its duct opens into the incisive duct within the hard palate, and its caudal end is rostral to the first cheek tooth.

The lateral nasal gland is absent in the ox. (See the paranasal sinuses, p. 34.)

b) ORAL CAVITY.

The **lips** *are not so mobile and selective as in the horse; they accept nails and pieces of fence wire that cause traumatic reticulitis. Near the angle of the mouth the cornified* **labial papillae (b)** *become long and sharp and directed caudally like the* **buccal papillae (b)** *inside the cheek. Together they serve to retain the cud during the wide lateral jaw movements of rumination.* The **oral vestibule (14)** is the space between the teeth and the lips and cheeks. The **oral cavity proper (17)** is enclosed by the teeth and **dental pad (a)** (see also p. 32), except at the diastema and at the palatoglossal arches, where it opens into the pharynx. On the rostral two-thirds of the **hard palate (c, d, 16)** are the transverse **palatine ridges (16)** *whose raised caudal borders bear a row of minute caudally directed spines*. The **palatine venous plexus (c)** is thickest between the premolars and just rostral to them. Attached to the **floor of the oral cavity** (see text figure) is the broad, *double* **frenulum of the tongue (B)**. Rostrolateral to the the frenulum is the large, flat **sublingual caruncle (A)**, which conceals the orifices of the ducts of the mandibular gl. and the monostomatic sublingual gl. Caudal to the caruncle on each side is a row of conical papillae. Med. and lat. to the papillae are the minute orifices of the polystomatic sublingual gll. (p. 38).

c) TONGUE.

The **dorsal surface (dorsum linguae)** *is divided by the transverse* **lingual fossa (18)** *into a flat apical part and a high, rounded* **torus linguae (19)**. *The tip (apex, 15) of the tongue is pointed.* The apical half of the tongue is covered on the dorsum and margin by fine, *sharp* **filiform papillae (D)** *directed backward and adapted to the use of the tongue as an organ of prehension in grazing*. Scattered among the filiform papillae are round **fungiform papillae (C)**, which bear taste buds, as do the **vallate papillae (F)**. The latter form an irregular double row of about twelve on each side of the caudal part of the torus, which is covered by large **conical and lentiform papillae (E)**. *Foliate papillae are absent.* The palatoglossal arches (lat. to G) are attached to the sides of the **root of the tongue (21)**. On the root and on both sides of the **median glossoepiglottic fold** are many small orifices of the crypts of the **lingual tonsil (H)** and its glands.

Tongue

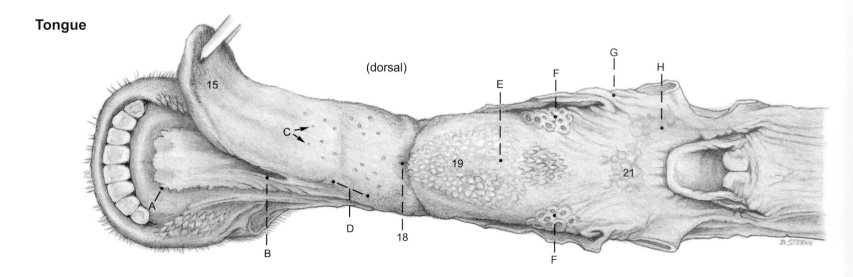

Nasal cavity, Oral cavity, and External nose

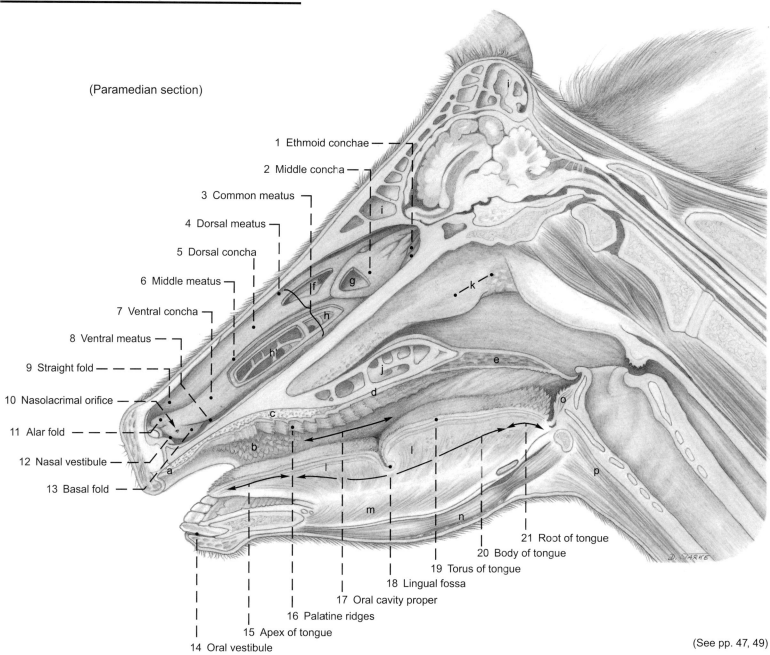

(Paramedian section)

1 Ethmoid conchae
2 Middle concha
3 Common meatus
4 Dorsal meatus
5 Dorsal concha
6 Middle meatus
7 Ventral concha
8 Ventral meatus
9 Straight fold
10 Nasolacrimal orifice
11 Alar fold
12 Nasal vestibule
13 Basal fold

14 Oral vestibule
15 Apex of tongue
16 Palatine ridges
17 Oral cavity proper
18 Lingual fossa
19 Torus of tongue
20 Body of tongue
21 Root of tongue

(See pp. 47, 49)

Legend:

a Dental pad
b Labial and buccal papillae
  (See also text figure)
c Palatine venous plexus
d Hard palate

e Soft palate
f Dorsal conchal sinus
g Middle conchal sinus
h Ventral conchal sinus

h' Bulla and cells of
   ventral concha
i Frontal sinus
j Palatine sinus
k Pharyngeal septum and
  pharyngeal tonsil

l Proper lingual muscle
m Genioglossis
n Geniohyoideus
o Hyoepiglotticus
p Sternohyoideus

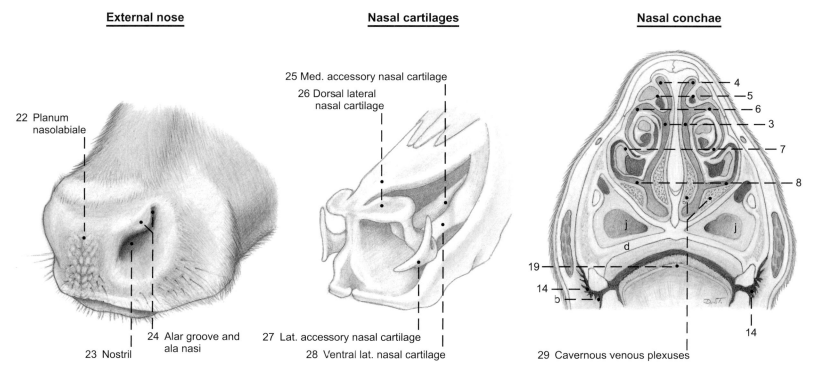

External nose

22 Planum
   nasolabiale

23 Nostril
24 Alar groove and
   ala nasi

Nasal cartilages

25 Med. accessory nasal cartilage
26 Dorsal lateral
   nasal cartilage

27 Lat. accessory nasal cartilage
28 Ventral lat. nasal cartilage

Nasal conchae

4
5
6
3
7
8

19
14
b

14

29 Cavernous venous plexuses

45

9. PHARYNX AND LARYNX

Dissection and study are carried out from the medial cut surface as well as the lateral side. Laterally, the pterygoids, digastricus, stylohyoideus, and occipitohyoideus are removed, as well as the remnants of the mandibular and parotid glands.

a) The cavity of the **PHARYNX** consists of three parts: the oropharynx, laryngopharynx, and nasopharynx. The **oropharynx (pars oralis, B)** communicates with the oral cavity through the **isthmus of the fauces**, which is bounded dorsally by the soft palate (velum palatinum), ventrally by the tongue, and laterally by the **palatoglossal arches** (p. 44, text fig.). The oropharynx extends to the base of the epiglottis, and its lateral wall contains the palatine tonsil (4, 14). The **laryngopharynx (pars laryngea, D)** lies below the **intrapharyngeal ostium**, which is surrounded by the free border of the **soft palate (3)** (raised by forceps) and the right and left **palatopharyngeal arches**. The arches meet on the caudal wall over the arytenoid cartilages. When the animal is breathing, the larynx projects through the ostium into the nasopharynx, and the cavity of the laryngopharynx is obliterated, except for the lateral **piriform recesses**, which conduct saliva around the larynx to the esophagus without the necessity of swallowing. In swallowing, the intrapharyngeal ostium and the larynx are closed, and the function of the laryngopharynx changes from **respiratory** to **digestive**. The caudal part of the laryngopharynx (D) joins the **esophagus** over the cricoid lamina without visible demarcation. The **nasopharynx (pars nasalis, A)** extends from the **choanae (p. 31, F)** to the intrapharyngeal ostium, and is separated from the oropharynx by the **soft palate (3)**. The choanae are divided dorsally by the crest of the vomer, covered by mucosa with a thick submucosal cavernous venous plexus. *Caudal to the vomer in ruminants, the membranous* **pharyngeal septum (2)** *divides the dorsal part of the nasopharynx lengthwise, and extends to the caudodorsal wall, where it contains the pharyngeal tonsil (p. 45, k).* On the wall of the nasopharynx lateral to the tonsil, is a slit—the **pharyngeal orifice of the auditory tube (1)**, leading to the middle ear.

I.   The **pharyngeal muscles** are identified from the lateral surface, sparing the arteries and the pharyngeal branches of cranial nerves IX and X, which innervate the muscles and the mucosa. (See p. 49.)

Muscles of the soft palate: The **tensor veli palatini (11)**, has a superficial part originating from the muscular process of the temporal bone and terminating in a tendon that passes around the hamulus of the pterygoid bone. The deep part originates on the pterygoid bone and works in the opposite direction to open the auditory tube by pulling on its cartilage.* The **levator veli palatini (12)** also originates from the muscular process. With the contralateral muscle it forms a sling in the soft palate. The **palatinus** (not illustrated) comes from the choanal border of the *palatine bones and runs through the median line of the soft palate.** The **palatopharyngeus** (p. 49, e) forms a thin band in the palatopharyngeal arch and acts as a constrictor of the intrapharyngeal ostium. It may also be classed with the:

Rostral pharyngeal constrictors: The **pterygopharyngeus (13)**, comes from the hamulus of the pterygoid bone and passes caudally lateral to the levator. The **rostral stylopharyngeus** (not illustrated) lies on the lateral wall of the pharynx rostral to the stylohyoid bone. It is inconstant in most species, *but constant in ruminants.* It arises from the medial surface of the distal half of the bone and terminates with the pterygopharyngeus.

Middle pharyngeal constrictor: The **hyopharyngeus (16)** originates mainly from the thyrohyoid, but also from the keratohyoid and the ventral end of the stylohyoid.

Caudal pharyngeal constrictors: The **thyropharyngeus (17)** comes from the oblique line on the thyroid cartilage. The **cricopharyngeus (18)** comes from the lateral surface of the cricoid. All pharyngeal constrictors terminate on the pharyngeal raphe.

The only **dilator of the pharynx** is the **caudal stylopharyngeus (15)**, originating from the proximal half of the stylohyoid, it passes between the rostral and middle constrictors, and *in the ox, terminates mainly on the dorsal border of the thyroid cartilage, so that it draws the larynx upward and forward.* Another part turns around the rostral border of the hyopharyngeus to terminate on the lateral pharyngeal wall and act as a dilator of the pharynx.

II.   The **pharyngeal lymphatic ring** consists of the palatine, pharyngeal, lingual, and tubal tonsils, and the tonsil of the soft palate.

The **palatine tonsil (14)** *is concealed outside the mucosa of the lateral wall of the oropharynx. Only the orifice of the central* **tonsillar sinus (4)**, *into which the crypts of the follicles open, is visible.* The sides of the **pharyngeal tonsil** (see p. 45) are marked by long ridges and grooves, in which the openings of mucous glands can be seen. The **lingual tonsil** has been described (p. 44). The **tubal tonsil**, in the lateral wall of the pharyngeal orifice of the auditory tube, is flat and nonfollicular. The **tonsil of the soft palate**, on the oral side, consists of some lymphatic tissue and a few follicles. On the medial surface, the paired **medial retropharyngeal lnn. (p. 49, a)**, important clinically and in meat inspection, lie in the fat between the caudal wall of the pharynx and the longus capitis (f).

III. The **auditory tube** connects the middle ear with the nasopharynx. The tubal cartilage, *unlike that of the horse, does not extend into the mucosal flap that closes the pharyngeal orifice. The latter is in a transverse plane just rostral to the temporomandibular joint, and at the level of the base of the ear.* The tube is medial to the tensor veli palatini. *Of the domestic mammals, only the Equidae have a diverticulum of the tube (guttural pouch).*

b)   The **LARYNX** (see also text fig.) *Because there are no laryngeal ventricles or vestibular folds, the wall of the the* **laryngeal vestibule (E)** *is smooth. The vestibular lig. of the horse is represented by a flat, fan-shaped sheet of fibers.*

The **vocal fold (F)** *is only a low ridge* containing the **vocal ligament (5)**. The **glottis (F)** is composed of the vocal folds, arytenoid cartilages, and the **glottic cleft (rima glottidis)**. Behind the glottis is the **infraglottic cavity (G)**.

I.   The **cartilages of the larynx** show the following species differences in the ox: The **epiglottic cartilage (H)** *is broad and rounded.* The corniculate, vocal, and muscular processes of the **arytenoid cartilages (J)** resemble those of the dog and horse, *but there is no cuneiform process.* The **thyroid cartilage (K)** *has a* **rostral notch (K')**, *absent in other species, and the caudal notch is not palpable in the live animal.* The **laryngeal prominence (K")** *a landmark, is not at the rostral end of the cartilage, as is the human "Adam's apple", but two-thirds of the way toward the caudal end. The lamina of the* **cricoid cartilage (L)** *is short.*

(dorsal)

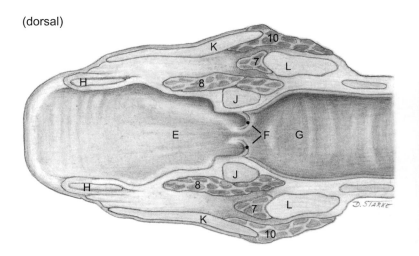

II.   The **LARYNGEAL MUSCLES** act like those of the dog and horse. The **cricoarytenoideus dorsalis (9)** is the primary dilator of the glottis. *Because there is no lateral ventricle, the ventricularis and vocalis are combined in the* **thyroarytenoideus (8)**. Other constrictors of the glottis are the **cricoarytenoideus lateralis (7)**, **cricothyroideus (10)**, and **arytenoideus transversus (6)**.

The **innervation of the larynx** by the cranial and recurrent laryngeal nn. from the vagus n. corresponds to that of the horse and dog.

* Himmelreich, 1964

Pharynx and Larynx

(Paramedian section)

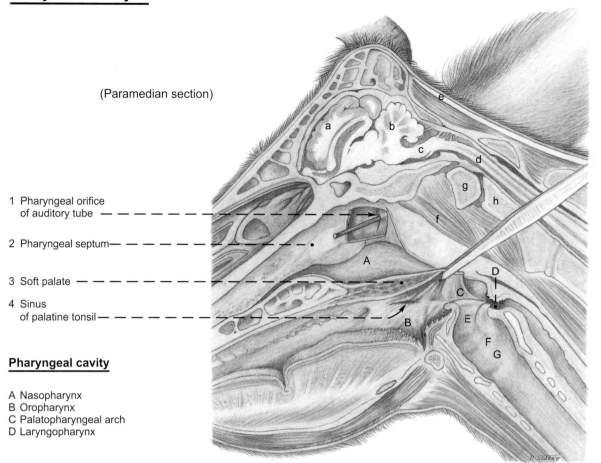

1 Pharyngeal orifice of auditory tube

2 Pharyngeal septum

3 Soft palate

4 Sinus of palatine tonsil

Pharyngeal cavity

A Nasopharynx
B Oropharynx
C Palatopharyngeal arch
D Laryngopharynx

Legend:

(Brain, see p. 51)

a Cerebrum
b Cerebellum
c Medulla oblongata
d Medulla spinalis (Spinal cord)
e Lig. nuchae
f Longus capitis
g Atlas
h Axis

Laryngeal cavity

E Laryngeal vestibule
F Glottis and vocal fold
G Infraglottic cavity

(medial)

Cricoarytenoid lig.

5 Vocal lig.

Laryngeal cartilages

H Epiglottic
J Arytenoid
K Thyroid
K' Rostral notch
K" Laryngeal prominence
L Cricoid

(lateral)

6 Arytenoideus transversus
7 Cricoarytenoideus lat.
8 Thyroarytenoideus
9 Cricoarytenoideus dors.
10 Cricothyroideus

(lateral)

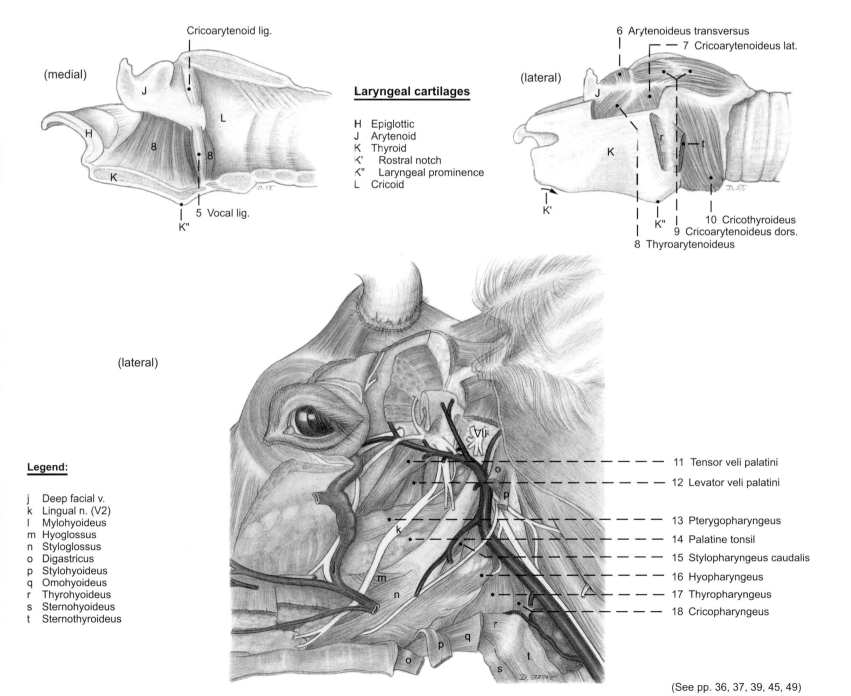

Legend:

j Deep facial v.
k Lingual n. (V2)
l Mylohyoideus
m Hyoglossus
n Styloglossus
o Digastricus
p Stylohyoideus
q Omohyoideus
r Thyrohyoideus
s Sternohyoideus
t Sternothyroideus

11 Tensor veli palatini
12 Levator veli palatini
13 Pterygopharyngeus
14 Palatine tonsil
15 Stylopharyngeus caudalis
16 Hyopharyngeus
17 Thyropharyngeus
18 Cricopharyngeus

(See pp. 36, 37, 39, 45, 49)

10. ARTERIES OF THE HEAD AND HEAD-NECK JUNCTION, THE CRANIAL NN. OF THE VAGUS GROUP (IX–XI), AND THE HYPOGLOSSAL N. (XII)

> For the demonstration of these aa. and nn.: laterally the dorsocaudal third of the stylohyoid bone, and medially the rectus capitis ventralis and longus capitis are removed.

a) The **ARTERIES OF THE HEAD** show species-specific characteristics different from the dog and horse (for veins and arteries of the head, see text fig. p. 36).

The **common carotid a.** (16, see also p. 61) reaches the head-neck junction accompanied dorsally by the vagosympathetic trunk, and ventrally by the recurrent laryngeal n. Here it gives off the **sternomastoid brr.** (15). At the thyroid gl. it gives off, as in the horse, the *inconstant* **caud. thyroid a.** and the **cran. thyroid a.** (17). The latter gives rise to the **caud. laryngeal br.** which accompanies the caud. laryngeal n. The **cran. laryngeal a.** with its laryngeal and pharyngeal brr. *comes either directly from the common carotid a.* or, as in the horse, from the cran. thyroid a. *Shortly before its termination the common carotid a. gives off the ascending pharyngeal a. for the soft palate, tonsils, and pharynx.*

The common carotid a. is continued by its largest terminal br., the external carotid a., whose origin is marked by the origin of the **occipital a.** (9) *because the smaller terminal br., the internal carotid a., undergoes atrophy of its extracranial part in the ox. By three months after birth it is completely closed.*

The **external carotid a.** (11), as it turns dorsally, gives off the **linguofacial trunk** (4) rostroventrally. This divides into the facial and lingual aa. The **lingual a.** (5) runs medial to the mandible along the stylohyoid bone, gives off the sublingual a., and passes medial to the hyoglossus into the tongue. The **facial a.** (6) also runs first medial to the mandible, and then turns at the vascular groove, *covered by the sternomandibularis*, onto the lateral surface at the rostral border of the masseter. After giving off the **caudal auricular a.** (8) caudodorsally, the **masseteric br.** (2) rostroventrally, and the **supf. temporal a.** (7) dorsally, the external carotid is continued by the **maxillary a.** (1) directed rostrodorsally toward the base of the skull.

b) The **THYROID GL.** (18) consists of *two flat lobulated irregularly triangular lobes* connected by a *parenchymatous* isthmus. The lobes are lateral to the trachea, esophagus, and cricoid cartilage, and the isthmus passes ventral to the trachea at the first or second cartilage. *In old cattle the isthmus may be reduced to a fibrous band.*

c) The **PARATHYROID GLL.** The **external parathyroid gl.** is 6–10 mm long and reddish-brown. *It is always cranial to the thyroid gl., usually dorsomedial to the common carotid a., about 3 cm caudal to the origin of the occipital a.* It may be on the caudal border of the mandibular gl. The **internal parathyroid gl.** is 1–4 mm long, and brown. *It is on the tracheal surface of the lobe of the thyroid gl., near the craniodorsal border, embedded in the parenchyma.*

d) The **ESOPHAGUS** (23, see also p. 60) in the cranial third of the neck, is dorsal to the trachea; between the third and sixth vertebrae it lies on the left side of the trachea; and at the thoracic inlet it is in a left dorsolateral position.

e) The **TRACHEA** (24, see also p. 60) *of the ox changes the shape of its cross section in life and after death* mainly by the state of contraction of the trachealis muscle attached to the inside of the tracheal cartilages. *It is relatively small (4 x 5 cm).*

f) **CRANIAL NERVES OF THE VAGUS GROUP (IX–XI)** emerge through the jugular foramen, as in the horse and dog.

I. The **glossopharyngeal n. (IX, 3)** innervates mainly the tongue with its large **lingual br.** Before it divides into dorsal and ventral brr., the lingual br. in the ox *bears a lateropharyngeal ganglion* medial and rostroventral to the stylohyoid. The **pharyngeal br.** supplies several branches to the pharynx.

II. The **vagus n. (X, 20)** has the widest distribution of all the cranial nn. Its nuclei of origin are in the nucleus ambiguus of the medulla oblongata for the motor fibers and in the parasympathetic nucleus of the vagus for the parasympathetic fibers. The sensory nuclei are in the nucleus of the solitary tract and in the nucleus of the spinal tract of C. N. V (see pp. 54, 55). The pseudounipolar nerve cells of the afferent fibers are in the proximal ganglion and in the distal ganglion of the vagus, which is very small in the ox, and lies near the jugular foramen. The vagus, after leaving the skull, first gives off the **pharyngeal brr.** (21), whose cranial brr. join those of C. N. IX in the pharyngeal plexus, supplying pharyngeal muscles and mucosa. The caudal continuation innervates the thyropharyngeus and cricopharyngeus and becomes the **esophageal br.** This is motor to the cran. part of the cervical esophagus, and joins the caud. laryngeal n. The **cranial laryngeal n.** (13) originates from the vagus caudal to the pharyngeal brr., and runs cranioventrally, crossing lateral to the pharyngeal brr. Its **external br.** usually joins the pharyngeal br., then separates again to innervate the cricothyroideus. The **internal br.** of the cran. laryngeal n. enters the larynx through the thyroid fissure and innervates the mucosa. *It then courses caudally inside the thyroid lamina and emerges caudal to the larynx to join the esophageal br.* or the **caudal laryngeal n.** (19) which comes from the recurrent laryngeal n. In the thorax the vagus gives off the **recurrent laryngeal n.**, which, on the right side, turns dorsally around the caudal surface of the subclavian a. and runs cranially between the common carotid a. and the trachea. On the left side, the recurrent n. turns medially around the aorta and the lig. arteriosum, passes medial to the great arteries, and runs cranially between the esophagus and trachea. Both nerves terminate as the **caudal laryngeal nerves** which pass deep to the cricopharyngeus to innervate all of the laryngeal muscles except the cricothyroideus.

After giving off the recurrent laryngeal n., the vagus still carries parasympathetic and visceral afferent fibers serving the heart, lungs, and abdominal organs as far as the descending colon. The visceral afferents greatly predominate (see pp. 65, 73).

III. The **accessory n. (XI, 10)** divides at the level of the atlas into a **dorsal br.** to the cleidooccipitalis and trapezius, and a **ventral br.** to the cleidomastoideus and sternocephalicus (see p. 60).

g) The **HYPOGLOSSAL N. (XII, 12)** emerges through the hypoglossal canals. It innervates the **proper (intrinsic) muscle of the tongue** (f) and the following extrinsic muscles: styloglossus, hyoglossus, and genioglossus. The **geniohyoideus** (h) and **thyrohyoideus** (see p. 47) are also supplied by the hypoglossal n. with a variable contribution from the first cervical n. via the ansa cervicalis.

h) From the **SYMPATHETIC TRUNK** of the autonomic system, fibers pass in the region of the thoracic inlet through the cervicothoracic ganglion (p. 65) and middle cervical ganglion and then in the **vagosympathetic trunk** (14) to the head. Here in the **cran. cervical ganglion** (22), large in the ox, the fibers synapse with ganglion cells whose postganglionic sympathetic fibers run in perivascular (mainly periarterial) plexuses in the adventitia of the large vessels of the head to their distribution in glands and internal eye muscles.

Arteries of the head and Cranial nn. IX, X, XI, XII

(lateral)

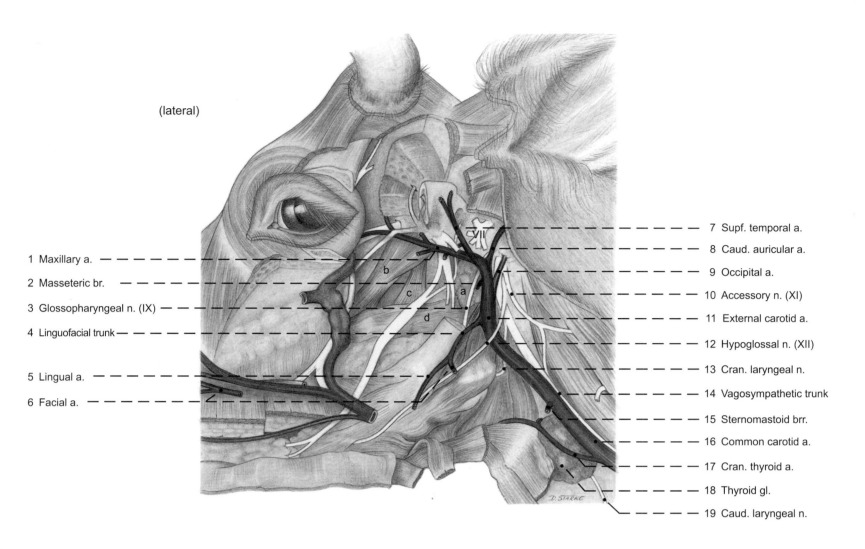

1 Maxillary a.
2 Masseteric br.
3 Glossopharyngeal n. (IX)
4 Linguofacial trunk
5 Lingual a.
6 Facial a.

7 Supf. temporal a.
8 Caud. auricular a.
9 Occipital a.
10 Accessory n. (XI)
11 External carotid a.
12 Hypoglossal n. (XII)
13 Cran. laryngeal n.
14 Vagosympathetic trunk
15 Sternomastoid brr.
16 Common carotid a.
17 Cran. thyroid a.
18 Thyroid gl.
19 Caud. laryngeal n.

Legend:

a Med. retropharyngeal ln.
b Tensor veli palatini
c Levator veli palatini
d Pterygopharyngeus
e Palatopharyngeus
f Proper lingual m.
g Genioglossus
h Geniohyoideus
i Sternohyoideus
j Hyoepiglotticus

(medial)

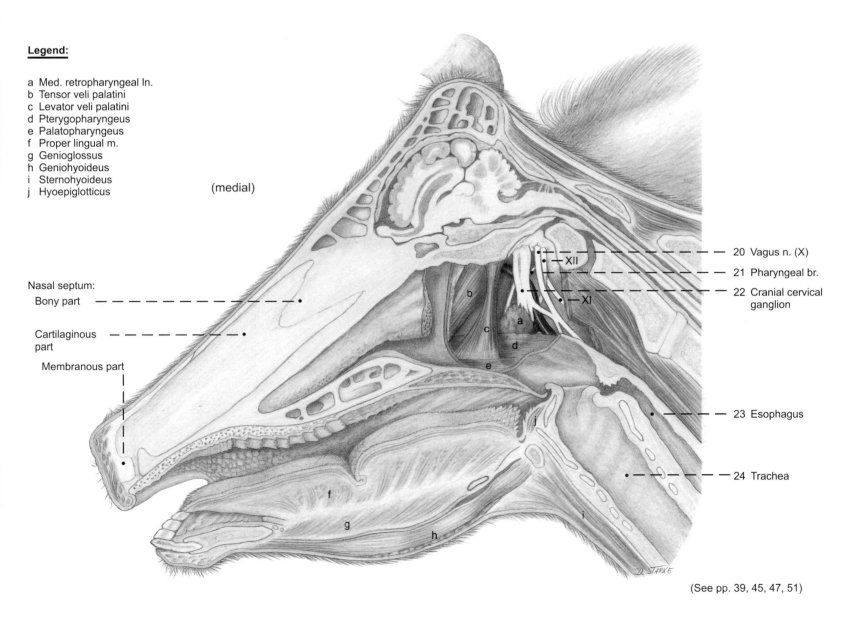

Nasal septum:

Bony part

Cartilaginous part

Membranous part

20 Vagus n. (X)
21 Pharyngeal br.
22 Cranial cervical ganglion
23 Esophagus
24 Trachea

(See pp. 39, 45, 47, 51)

49

CHAPTER 4: CENTRAL NERVOUS SYSTEM AND CRANIAL NERVES

1. THE BRAIN

To remove the half-brain from the bisected head, the cut end of the spinal cord is first lifted from the dura mater, cutting the attachments of the denticulate lig. and the cervical nn. Then the brain is detached by identifying and cutting the cranial nn. in caudorostral order, midway between the brain and the dura. The roots of the **hypoglossal n. (XII)** emerge from the ventrolateral groove, lateral to the **decussation of the pyramids**, and exit through the dura, and to the hypoglossal canals. The nerves of the vagus group (IX, X, XI) emerge from the lateral funiculus of the medulla oblongata. The **accessory n. (XI)** has a long **spinal root**, which begins at the fifth cervical segment and runs up to unite with the small **cranial root**. The **glossopharyngeal (IX)** and **vagus (X) nerves** originate by a continuous series of rootlets and pass out through the jugular foramen with the accessory n. The **vestibulocochlear (VIII)** and **facial (VII) nerves** also arise close together from the medulla, between the cerebellum and the trapezoid body, with VIII dorsolateral to VII, and run dorsolaterally to the internal acoustic meatus. The small **abducent n. (VI)** passes out through the trapezoid body at the lateral edge of the pyramid, and enters a hole in the dura on the floor of the cranium in the transverse plane of the internal acoustic meatus. The large **trigeminal n. (V)** comes from the end of the pons just rostral to the facial n. and runs rostroventrally to the largest aperture in the dura. Nn. IV and III come from the midbrain (13, 14). The **trochlear n. (IV)**, the only one to emerge from the dorsal surface of the brain stem, arises behind the caudal colliculus, decussates with the contralateral nerve, and passes around the lateral surface of the midbrain, on or in the free border of the tentorium cerebelli, to the floor of the cranium. The larger **oculomotor n. (III)** arises from the crus cerebri, caudolateral to the hypophysis, which should be carefully dissected out of the Sella turcica (p. 31, 42) while maintaining its connection with the brain. The internal carotid a. will be cut between the rete mirabile and the arterial circle of the cerebrum. Nerves III, IV, VI, and the ophthalmic and maxillary nerves join outside the dura and leave the cranium through the orbitoround for. in ruminants and swine. The **optic n. (II)** is cut distal to the optic chiasm. The optic tract connects the chiasm to the diencephalon. To free the cerebral hemisphere, the median dorsal fold of the dura (falx cerebri) is removed and preserved for study of the enclosed sagittal sinus, and the membranous tentorium cerebelli is cut at its dorsal attachment. (There is no osseous tentorium in ruminants.) The half-brain is lifted out of the dura by inserting scalpel handles between the cerebrum and the dura dorsally and between the olfactory bulb and the ethmoidal fossa, severing the **olfactory nn. (I)**.

a) The **BRAIN** is relatively small. Because species-specific differences are of minor significance among domestic mammals, reference to a general textbook description is advised. Only a few features of the bovine brain will be mentioned here; greater importance will be given to the illustrations.

I. The dorsal part of the **rhombencephalon**, the **cerebellum (17)**, is much more complex and irregular than in man, and the **vermis (H)** is not very prominent.

II. The **midbrain (mesencephalon)** exhibits four dorsal eminences, the **rostral** and **caudal colliculi**. The caudal pair is smaller. On the ventral surface is the **cerebral crus**.

III. The **diencephalon** is connected through its **hypothalamus (9)** with the **infundibulum (10)** of the **hypophysis (11)**. Caudal to the infundibulum is the **mammillary body (12)**. The **pineal gl. (8)** projects dorsocaudally from the diencephalon.

IV. The greatest part of the **telencephalon (cerebrum)** is the **hemisphere (F)**. It consists of the **cortex (A)** and the **white matter (B)**. It is markedly convoluted on the surface, bearing **gyri (folds)** and **sulci (grooves)**. The herbivora have additional variable and inconstant sulci which make the brain more complex than the brains of carnivores. On the **rhinencephalon (3)** the **olfactory bulb** is smaller than in the dog and horse. It is continuous caudally with the **olfactory peduncle**, which branches into **lateral and medial olfactory tracts**.

b) The **VENTRICULAR SYSTEM**. In the roof of the **fourth ventricle (h)** the **caudal medullary velum (j)** is invaginated by a **choroid plexus**. The **third ventricle (a)** is in the median plane; it encircles the interthalamic adhesion (7), and with its **choroid plexus (a')**, extends over the pineal gl. as the **suprapineal recess (d)**. The third ventricle also extends into the pineal gl. The **cerebral aqueduct (g)** connects the third and fourth ventricles. Rostrally, the third ventricle communicates on each side through an **interventricular foramen (f)** with a **lateral ventricle**, which contains a **choroid plexus** continuous with that of the third ventricle. A long process of the lateral ventricle extends into the olfactory bulb.

Section of cerebrum (dorsal)

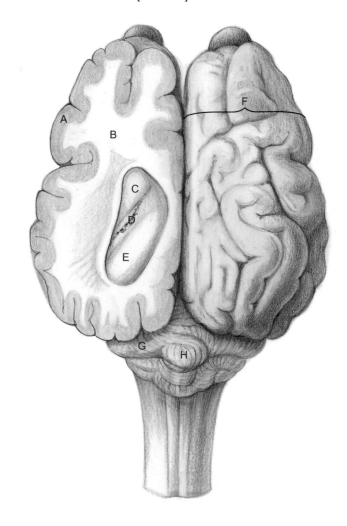

Legend:

A Cerebral cortex [Gray matter]
B White matter
C Head of caudate nucleus
D Choroid plexus of lateral ventricle
E Hippocampus
F Cerebral hemisphere
G Cerebellar hemisphere
H Vermis

Brain [Encephalon] and Cranial Nerves

Base of brain (ventral)

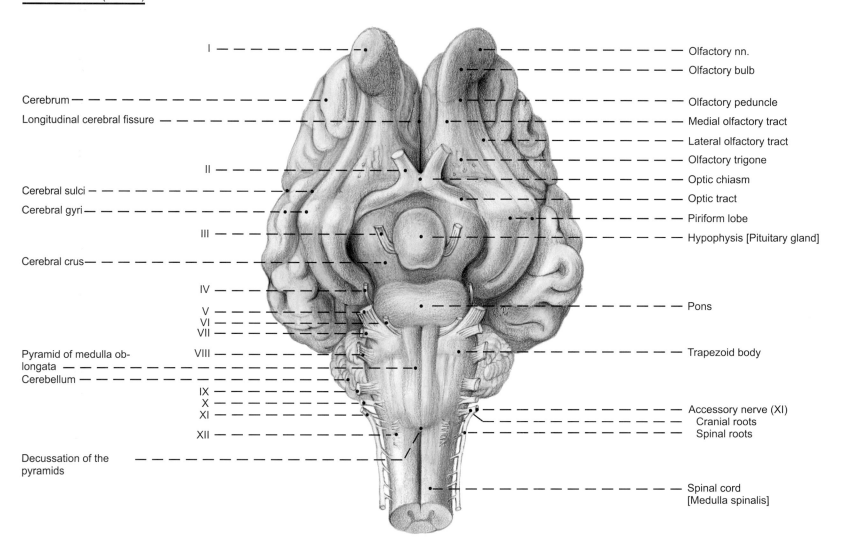

I — Olfactory nn.
— Olfactory bulb
Cerebrum — — Olfactory peduncle
Longitudinal cerebral fissure — — Medial olfactory tract
— Lateral olfactory tract
II — — Olfactory trigone
Cerebral sulci — — Optic chiasm
Cerebral gyri — — Optic tract
— Piriform lobe
III — — Hypophysis [Pituitary gland]
Cerebral crus —
IV —
V — — Pons
VI —
VII —
Pyramid of medulla ob- VIII — — Trapezoid body
longata
Cerebellum —
IX —
X — — Accessory nerve (XI)
XI — — Cranial roots
— Spinal roots
XII —
Decussation of the
pyramids — Spinal cord
[Medulla spinalis]

Median section of the brain

Legend:

a   Third ventricle
a'   Choroid plexus of third ventricle
b   Optic recess
c   Infundibular recess
d   Suprapineal recess
e   Pineal recess
f   Interventricular foramen
g   Cerebral aqueduct
h   Fourth ventricle
i   Rostral medullary velum
j   Caudal medullary velum

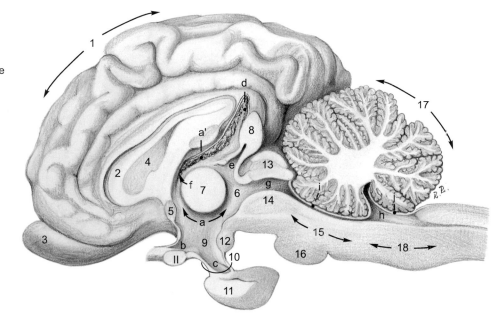

Cerebrum:	Diencephalon:	Mesencephalon [Midbrain]:	Rhombencephalon:
1 Hemisphere	6 Thalamus	Tectum	15 Metencephalon
2 Corpus callosum	7 Interthalamic adhesion	13 Lamina tecti	16 Pons
3 Rhinencephalon	[Intermediate mass]	[Rostral and caudal colliculi]	17 Cerebellum
4 Septum pellucidum	8 Epiphysis [Pineal gland]	14 Tegmentum	18 Myelencephalon
5 Rostral commissure	9 Hypothalamus		[Medulla oblongata]
	10 Infundibulum		
	11 Hypophysis [Pituitary gl.]		
	12 Mamillary body		

2. CRANIAL NERVES I–V

NERVE	PAGE	NAME/FIBER FUNCTION	DISTRIBUTION	REMARKS
I	50	**Olfactory nn. (special sensory)**	Olfactory region in caud. nasal cavity	1st neuron in olfactory mucosa, synapse in olfactory bulb
II	42, 50	**Optic n. (special sensory)**	Optical part of retina	Evagination of diencephalon
III	40, 50	**Oculomotor n. (m., psy.)***		Orig. mesencephalon, exits by for. orbitorotundum
(1)		• Dorsal br. (m.)	Dors. rectus, levator palpebrae superioris, retractor bulbi	
(2)		• Ventr. br. (m., psy.)	Med. and ventr. recti, ventral oblique	Psy. neurons synapse in ciliary gangl. and pass in ciliary nn. to eyeball
IV	40, 50	**Trochlear n. (m.)**	Dorsal oblique	Orig. mesencephalon, exits skull by for. orbitorotundum
V	38, 50	**Trigeminal n.**		Orig. rhombencephalon and mesencephalon. Nerve of 1st pharyngeal arch
V1	40	• Ophtalmic n. (s.)	Dorsum nasi, ethmoid bone, lacrimal gl., upper eyelid	Exits skull by foramen orbitorotundum
(3)	40	•• Nasociliary n. (s.)		
(4)	40	••• Ethmoid n. (s.)	Dorsal nasal mucosa	Enters nasal cavity through ethmoid for. and cribriform plate
(5)	40	••• Infratrochlear n. (s.)	Conjunctiva, 3rd lid, lacrimal caruncle, skin of med. angle of eye	Crosses dors. margin of orbit below trochlea; may reach cornual process
(6)	40	••• Long ciliary nn. (s., psy.)	Iris and cornea, ciliary muscle	Psy. fibers from ciliary ganglion
(7)	40	•• Lacrimal n. (s., psy., sy.)	Lacrimal gl., skin and conjunctiva of lat. angle of eye	Thin lat. and med. brr., which, after junction with r. communicans from zygomatic n., join to form zygomaticotemporal br.
(8)	40	••• Zygomaticotemporal br.	Skin of temporal region	
(9)	40	•••• Cornual br.	Cornual dermis	Dehorning anesthesia!
(10)	40	•• Frontal n. (s.)	Skin of frontal region and upper eyelid	Ends as supraorbital n. in skin of frontal region
V2	38	• Maxillary n. (s.)		Exits skull from for. orbitorotundum
(11)		•• Zygomatic n. (s., psy.)		Communicating br. with lacrimal n. (V1)
(12)		••• Zygomaticofacial br. (s.)	Lower eyelid	Exits orbit at lat. angle of eye
(13)		•• Pterygopalatine n. (s., psy.)		Psy. fibers from pterygopalatine ganglion
(14)		••• Major palatine n. (s., psy.)	Mucosa and gll. of the hard palate	Goes through caudal palatine for., palatine canal, and major palatine for.
(15)		••• Minor palatine nn. (s., psy.)	Soft palate with its glands	Exit palatine canal through minor palatine foramina
(16)		••• Caud. nasal n. (s.)	Ventr. parts of nasal cavity, palate	Enters nasal cavity through sphenopalatine for.
(17)	38	•• Infraorbital n. (s.)	Skin of dorsum nasi, nares, and upper lip	Traverses maxillary for. and infraorbital canal and for.
V3	38	• Mandibular n. (s., m.)		Exits skull by oval foramen
(18)	38	•• Masticatory n. (m.)		
(19)	38	••• Deep temporal nn. (m.)	Temporalis	
(20)	38	••• Masseteric n. (m.)	Masseter	Goes through mandibular notch
(21)		•• Med. and lat. pterygoid nn. (m.)	Med. and lat. pterygoid mm.	The otic gangl. (s., psy.) at root of buccal n., is large in the ox
(22)		•• Tensor tympani n. (m.)	Tensor tympani	Enters tympanic cavity
(23)		•• Tensor veli palatini n.	Tensor veli palatini	
(24)	38	•• Auriculotemporal n. (s., psy., sy.)	Skin of auricle and temporal region, Parotid gl.	Turns around the neck of the mandible, psy. fibers from otic ganglion
(25)	38	••• Communicating brr. with facial n. (s.)		Connection with dors. buccal br. (VII)
(26)	38	•• Buccal n. (s. psy.)	Mucosa of cheek and buccal gll.	Psy. fibers from otic gangl.
(27)	38	••• Parotid br. (psy.)	Parotid gl.	Follows parotid duct backward through vascular groove
(28)	38	•• Lingual n. (taste, s., psy.)	Sensory to floor of mouth and tongue, taste from rostral 2/3 of tongue	Receives taste, s., and psy. fibers from chorda tympani (VII). (Psy. fibers synapse in mandibular ganglion.)
(29)	38	••• Sublingual n. (s., psy.)	Mucosa of rostral floor of mouth	Carries psy. fibers to mandibular and sublingual gll.
(30)	38	•• Inferior alveolar n. (s.)	Inferior teeth and gingiva	Traverses mandibular foramen and canal
(31)	38	••• Mylohyoid n. (m.)	Mylohyoid, rostral belly of digastricus	
(32)	38	••• Mental n. (s.)	Skin and mucosa of chin and lower lip	Leaves the mandib. canal at the mental foramen

* Fiber function: s. = sensory, m. = motor and proprioceptive, sy. = sympathetic, psy. = parasympathetic

Cranial nerves

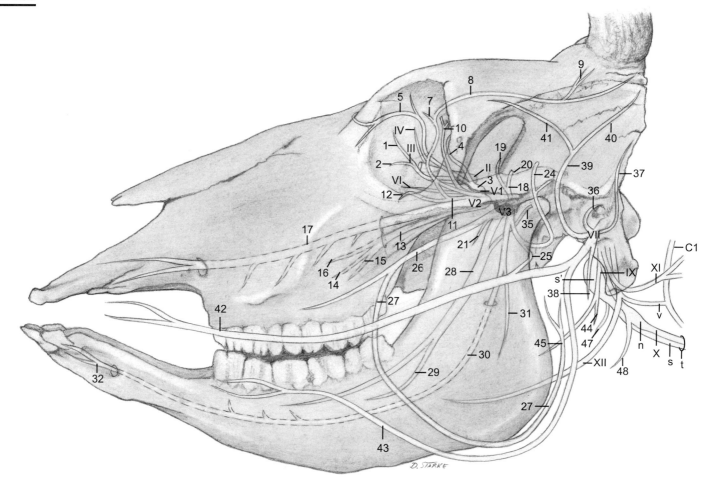

Legend:

A Cribriform plate
B Optic canal
C Ethmoid foramen
D For. orbitorotundum
E Oval foramen
F Stylomastoid for.
G Int. acoustic meatus
H Foramen magnum
J Jugular foramen
K Hypoglossal canal

L Lacrimal gl.
M Nasal gll.
N Palatine gll. (soft palate)
N' Palatine gll. (hard palate)
O Buccal gll.
P Monostomatic sublingual gl.
P' Polystomatic sublingual gl.
Q Mandibular gl.
R Parotid gl.

a Olfactory region
b Retina
c Fungiform papillae
d Ciliary ganglion
d' Short ciliary nn.
e Pterygopalatine gangl.
e' Orbital brr.
e" N. of pterygoid canal
   (major and deep petrosal nn.)
f Mandibular ganglion
g Trigeminal ganglion
h Otic ganglion

h' Minor petrosal n.
j Vallate papillae
k Geniculate ganglion
l Proximal ganglia
m Distal gangl. (petrosal)
m' Tympanic n.
n Distal gangl (nodose)
o Carotid glomus
p Carotid sinus
q Vestibular n.
q' Sup. vestibular gangl.
q" Inf. vestibular gangl.
r Cochlear n.

r' Spiral gangl. of cochlea
s Sympathetic trunk
s' Cranial cervical gangl.
t Vagosympathetic trunk
u Spinal root of accessory n.
v Ansa cervicalis

● Special sensory neuron
● Sensory neuron
● Parasympathetic neuron
◉ Sympathetic neuron
● Motor neuron

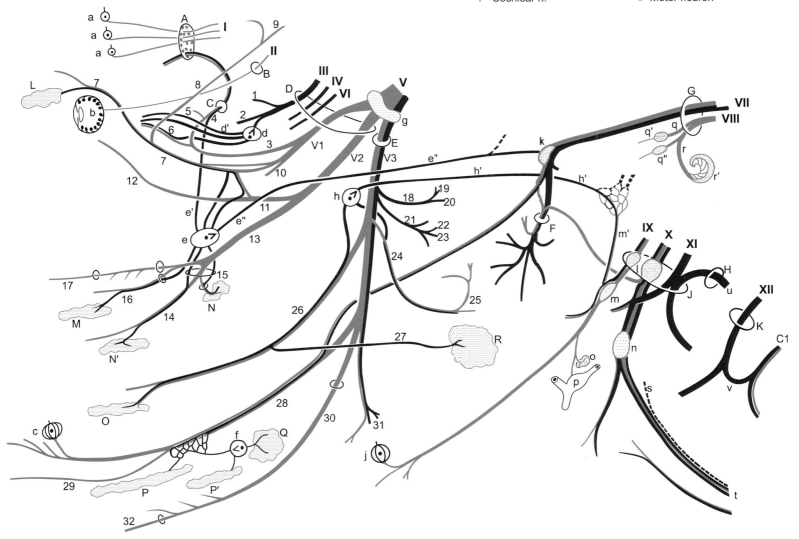

3. CRANIAL NERVES VI–XII

NERVE	PAGE	NAME/FIBER FUNCTION	DISTRIBUTION	REMARKS
VI	40, 50	**Abducent n. (m.)**	Lat. rectus, lat. part of retractor bulbi	Orig.: Rhombencephalon; exits skull at for. orbitorotundum
VII	36, 50	**Facial n. (intermediofacial n.) (taste, m., psy.)***	Mm. of face and ear, lacrimal and salivary gll.	Goes through int. acoustic meatus into facial canal and leaves through stylomastoid for.; nerve of 2nd pharyngeal arch
(33)		• Major petrosal n. (psy.)	Gll. of nose and palate, and lacrimal gll.	Joins the deep petrosal n. (sy.) to form the n. of the pterygoid canal, which goes to pterygopalatine ganglion
(34)		• N. to stapedius (m.)	Stapedius	
(35)	38	• Chorda tympani (taste, psy.)	Mandibular and sublingual gll., rostral 2/3 of tongue, taste	Leaves petrous temporal bone through petrotympanic fissure and joins lingual n. (V3)
(36)	36	• Int. auricular br. (s.)	Int. surface of auricle	Passes through auricular cartilage
(37)	36	• Caud. auricular n. (m.)	Auricular mm.	Communicates with the dors. brr. of first 2 cervical nn.
(38)		• Digastric br. (m.)	Caud. belly of digastricus	
		• Parotid plexus (psy.)	Parotid gl.	Impulses from auriculopalpebral n. (V3)
(39)	36	• Auriculopalpebral n. (m.)		Communicates with auriculotemporal n. (V3)
(40)		•• Rostral auricular brr. (m.)	Rostral auricular mm.	
(41)		•• Zygomatic br. (m.)	Orbicularis oculi, levator anguli oculi med., frontalis	Ends with palpebral brr.
(42)	36	• Dorsal buccal br. (m.)	Mm. of upper lip, planum nasale, and nostril	Communicating br. (s.) with auriculotemporal n. (V3)
(43)	36	• Ventral buccal br. (m.)	Buccinator, depressor labii inferioris	Passes through vascular groove with facial a. and v.
VIII	50	**Vestibulocochlear n. (special sensory)**		Orig.: Medulla oblongata; enters int. acoustic pore
		• Cochlear n. (hearing)	Spiral organ of the cochlea	1st neuron: in spiral gangl. of cochlea; 2nd neuron: in rhombencephalon
		• Vestibular n. (equilibrium)	Ampullae of semicircular ducts, maculae of utriculus and sacculus	1st neuron: in vestibular gangl.; 2nd neuron in rhombencephalon
IX	48, 50	**Glossopharyngeal n. (taste, s., m. psy.)**	Mucosa of tongue and pharynx, tonsils, tympanic cavity	Orig.: medulla oblongata; exits skull through jugular for. Nerve of 3rd pharyngeal arch; 1st n. of vagus group
(44)	48	• Pharyngeal br. (s., m.)	Pharyngeal mucosa, caud. stylopharyngeus	Forms pharyngeal plexus with pharyngeal brr. of vagus (X)
(45)		• Lingual br. (taste, s., psy.)	Mucosa of soft palate and root of tongue with its taste buds	Before it divides into dorsal and ventr. brr. this n. bears the lateropharyngeal ganglion
X	48, 50	**Vagus n. (s., m., psy.)**	Viscera of the head, neck, thorax, and abdomen	Orig.: medulla oblongata; exits skull from jugular foramen; n. of 4th pharyngeal arch; *2nd n. of vagus group*
(46)		• Auricular br. (s.)	Skin of ext. acoustic meatus	Enters the facial canal and joins the facial n. (VII)
(47)	48	• Pharyngeal brr. (s., m.)	Pharyngeal mm. and mucosa	Caud. contribution to pharyngeal plexus, ends as esophageal br.
(48)	48	• Cran. laryngeal n. (s., m.)		Branches off from distal ganglion and crosses lat. to pharyngeal br.
(49)	48	•• External br. (m.)	Cricothyroideus	Joins pharyngeal brr.
(50)	48	•• Internal br. (s.)	Laryngeal mucosa rostral to the rima glottidis	Passes through the thyroid fissure
	48, 60	• Recurrent laryngeal n. (s., m., psy.)	Branches to cardiac plexus, trachea, and esophagus	Separates from the vagus in the thorax and turns cranially
	48	•• Caud. laryngeal n. (s., m.)	All laryngeal mm. except cricothyroid, laryngeal mucosa caud. to rima glottidis	
XI	48, 50	**Accessory n. (m.)**		Exits skull through jugular for.; 3rd n. of vagus group
(51)		• Cran. root: int. br. (m.)		Orig.: medulla oblongata, joins vagus n. and gives it motor fibers
(52)		• Spinal root: ext. br. (m.)		Orig. cervical spinal cord
	48	•• Dorsal br. (m.)	Trapezius and cleidooccipitalis	
	48	•• Ventral br. (m.)	Cleidomastoideus and sternocephalicus	
XII	48, 50	**Hypoglossal n. (m.)**	Proper lingual m., genio-, stylo-, and hyoglossus; together with ventr. br. of 1st cervical n.: genio- and thyrohyoideus	Orig.: Medulla oblongata, leaves the skull via hypoglossal canal, forms the ansa cervicalis with 1st cervical n.

* Fiber function: s. = sensory, m. = motor and proprioceptive, sy. = sympathetic, psy. = parasympathetic

Cranial nerves

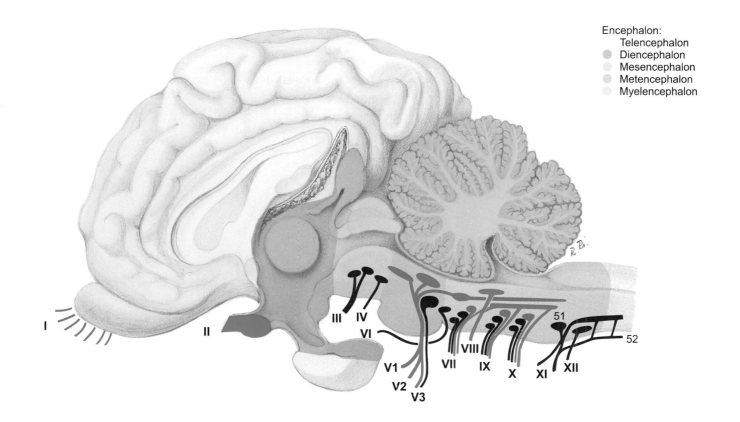

Encephalon:
Telencephalon
● Diencephalon
● Mesencephalon
● Metencephalon
● Myelencephalon

I II III IV VI V1 V2 V3 VII VIII IX X XI XII 51 52

Legend:

A	Cribriform plate	L	Lacrimal gl.
B	Optic canal	M	Nasal gll.
C	Ethmoid foramen	N	Palatine gll. (soft palate)
D	For. orbitorotundum	N'	Palatine gll. (hard palate)
E	Oval foramen	O	Buccal gll.
F	Stylomastoid for.	P	Monostomatic sublingual gl.
G	Int. acoustic meatus	P'	Polystomatic sublingual gl.
H	Foramen magnum	Q	Mandibular gl.
J	Jugular foramen	R	Parotid gl.
K	Hypoglossal canal		

a Olfactory region
b Retina
c Fungiform papillae
d Ciliary ganglion
d' Short ciliary nn.
e Pterygopalatine gangl.
e' Orbital brr.
e" N. of pterygoid canal (major and deep petrosal nn.)
f Mandibular ganglion
g Trigeminal ganglion
h Otic ganglion

h' Minor petrosal n.
j Vallate papillae
k Geniculate ganglion
l Proximal ganglia
m Distal gangl. (petrosal)
m' Tympanic n.
n Distal gangl. (nodose)
o Carotid glomus
p Carotid sinus
q Vestibular n.
q' Sup. vestibular gangl.
q" Inf. vestibular gangl.
r Cochlear n.

r' Spiral gangl. of cochlea
s Sympathetic trunk
s' Cranial cervical gangl.
t Vagosympathetic trunk
u Spinal root of accessory n.
v Ansa cervicalis

● Special sensory neuron
● Sensory neuron
● Parasympathetic neuron
◍ Sympathetic neuron
● Motor neuron

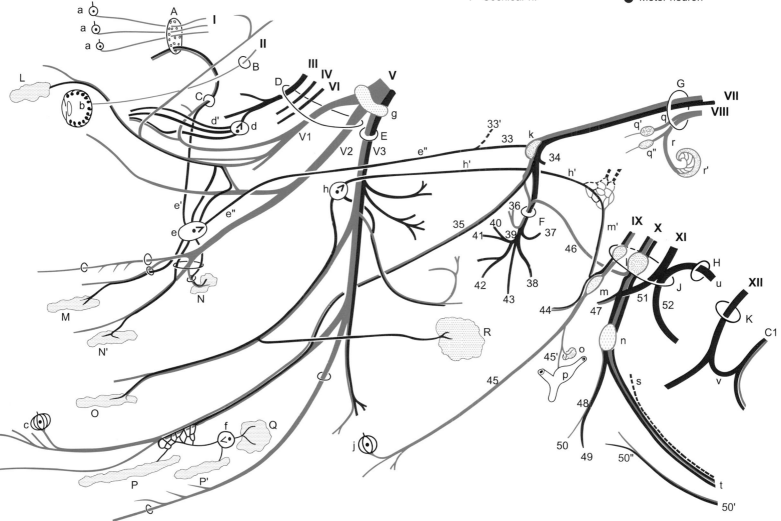

55

4. SPINAL CORD AND AUTONOMIC NERVOUS SYSTEM

> Demonstration specimens are provided for the study of the spinal cord. The arches of the vertebrae and portions of the meninges have been removed to show the dorsal surface of the cord. Transverse sections are studied to see the distribution of gray and white matter, the course of the central canal, and the positions of the fiber tracts.

The following statements concern only a few specific characteristics of the ox. For the rest, the generally applicable textbook descriptions and the detailed illustrations in the neurological literature may be consulted.

a) The **SPINAL CORD (MEDULLA SPINALIS)** is surrounded by the meninges in the vertebral canal. In animals it has a greater biological importance than in man, and in the ox its mass is almost as great as that of the brain. The spinal cord presents a **cervical enlargement** and a **lumbar enlargement**. The central canal is predominantly transversely oval, as in the horse. The cord ends as the **conus medullaris (16)**, containing the sacral and caudal segments. This extends in the two-month-old calf through vert. S3, and at ten months, through vert. S2*, but in the adult the conus extends only into vert. S1. The difference is caused by the so-called "ascent of the cord," really by the continued growth of the vertebral column after the growth of the cord has slowed. This results in a longer course of the spinal nerves within the vertebral canal before they reach their intervertebral foramina, forming the **cauda equina (18)**, which is composed of the conus medullaris, the **terminal filament (17)** of connective tissue, and the sacral and caudal nerves. The clinical importance is in the danger of injury to the cord by lumbosacral puncture. The space between the spine of vert. L6 and the sacral crest overlies the intervertebral disc and the cranial part of the body of vert. S1. In the mature ox, although the sacral segments of the cord are all in vert. L6, the caudal segments, the last lumbar nerve, the sacral nerves, and some caudal nerves are vulnerable. Epidural anesthesia is performed in the ox by injection between the first and second caudal vertebrae, and lumbosacral puncture is restricted to diagnostic withdrawal of cerebrospinal fluid.

b) **THE AUTONOMIC NERVOUS SYSTEM** includes the sympathetic part, the paraympathetic part, and the intramural intestinal plexuses.

The efferent nerve fibers:

I. The **sympathetic part** consists mainly of **efferents** with pre- and postsynaptic neurons, and also contains **afferents** with only one neuron. It is also called the thoracolumbar nervous system because the nerve cell bodies of the efferents are in the lateral horns of the corresponding segments of the spinal cord. However, the **sympathetic trunk (12)** extends farther caudally, to the first caudal vertebra, where the paired ganglia unite in the ganglion impar. The thoracolumbar body parts and organs are supplied by **relatively short** (nearly transverse) **communicating brr.** to the ganglia of the sympathetic trunk.

1. The **thoracic organs** are supplied by **postsynaptic unmyelinated neurons** that come from the **cervicothoracic ggl. (5)** or from the **ansa subclavia (4)** or from the **middle cervical ggl. (3)** and go, e.g. as cardiac nn. or pulmonary nn., to the corresponding organs. They form with branches of the vagus n. (e.g. cardiac brr. or pulmonary brr.) autonomic plexuses for the thoracic organs (e.g. **cardiac plexus, 7**).

2. The **abdominal organs** are mainly supplied through the **major splanchnic n. (13)**, which leaves the sympathetic trunk at the level of vert. T 10, and passes over the lumbocostal arch of the diaphragm to the **celiac ggl.** and **cran. mesenteric ggl. (14)**. In addition, the minor splanchnic nn. and the lumbar splanchnic nn. from the lumbar sympathetic trunk go to the **solar plexus** or to the **caud. mesenteric ggl. (15)**. The **myelinated presynaptic first neurons** come mainly without synapse through the ggll. of the sympathetic trunk,

and most of the neurons synapse first in the following **prevertebral ggll.: celiac ggl. (14), cran. (14), and caud. (15) mesenteric ggll.** The **unmyelinated postsynaptic second neurons** reach the areas they supply through periarterial plexuses of the visceral aa., e.g. those of the intestinal wall.

The communicating brr. to the somatic thoracic and lumbar nn. (white communicating brr.) synapse in the **ggll. of the sympathetic trunk (12)**, and the second neurons (gray communicating brr.) conduct sympathetic impulses to those nn. The **body parts and organs** (Nos. 3–6) cranial or caudal to the thoracolumbar body segments are supplied by **relatively long** (longitudinal) **nerves.**

3. The **head** is supplied by efferent sympathetic neurons from the **cervicothoracic ggl.** that pass through the ansa subclavia and the middle cervical ggl. and the **vagosympathetic trunk (2)** to the **cran. cervical ggl. (1)**. This ggl. at the level of the base of the skull is the last synaptic transfer station. From here only postsynaptic unmyelinated neurons, as perivascular plexuses, reach, with blood vessels of the same name, their areas of innervation in the head (e.g. int. carotid plexus, maxillary plexus).

4. The **neck** is supplied by the **vertebral n. (11)**. It leaves the **cervicothoracic ggl.** and passes through the foramina transversaria of the cervical vertebrae as far as the third. It gives gray rami communicantes to the 2nd to 6th cervical nn.

5. The **pelvic cavity** receives sympathetic neurons over two different pathways. The dorsal path goes through the lumbar and sacral sympathetic trunk and into the **sacral splanchnic nn.** which run together with the **pelvic n. (10)** to the **pelvic plexus (9)**. The ventral path goes from the lumbar sympathetic trunk through the **lumbar splanchnic nn. (15)** to the **caud. mesenteric ggl. (15)** and over the **hypogastric n. (18)** to the mixed autonomic pelvic plexus. Here at the pelvic inlet, on the lateral wall of the rectum, is the transfer to the postsynaptic neurons which supply the pelvic organs and the descending colon.

6. The **limbs** are supplied by postganglionic unmyelinated neurons. From the **cervicothoracic ggl.** at the cran. end of the thoracic sympathetic trunk, they reach the thoracic limb, and from the caud. end of the lumbar sympathetic trunk they reach the pelvic limb. They first pass through the brachial plexus or lumbosacral plexus in the somatic nn., and more distally enter the adventitia of blood vessels.

II. The **parasympathetic part** to which **cranial nn. III, VII, IX, and X** and the **pelvic n. (10)** belong, supplies with its efferents the glands and smooth muscle cells in e.g. the gut, and also in the eye and in the salivary and lacrimal gll. The efferents are connected through two neurons in series to carry the impulse from the CNS to the target organ. In the vagus, the presynaptic axon is very long, extending from the CNS to the synapse with the second neuron in the target organ. Vagal fibers extend as far as the transverse colon. For the origin and distribution of the vagus, see pp. 48, 54, and 72.

The afferent nerve fibers:

The **sympathetic** and **parasympathetic nn.** contain afferents of sensory neurons that measure the contraction or distention of hollow organs and transmit pain. The vagus at the diaphragm contains more than 80 % afferent fibers. The cell bodies of the sympathetic afferents lie in the spinal ganglia, and those of the vagus are in the proximal (jugular) and distal (nodose) ganglia near the base of the skull (see p. 48).

* Weber, 1942

Spinal cord and Autonomic nervous system

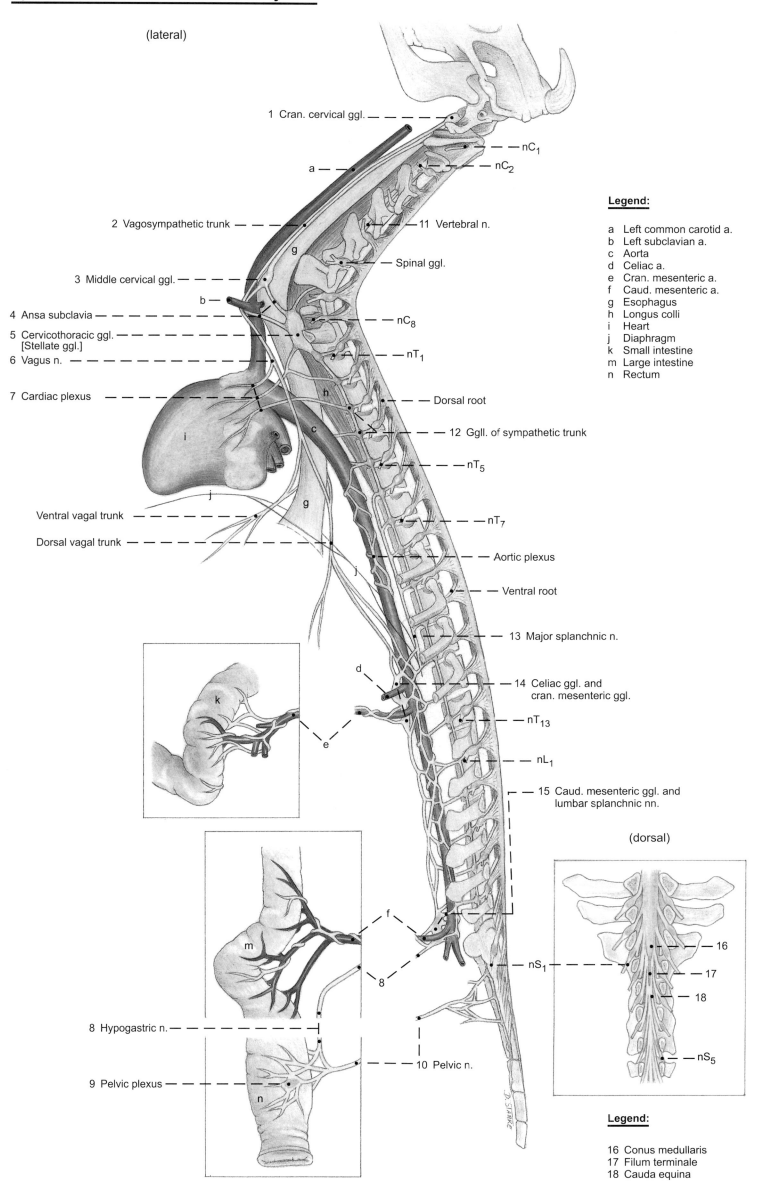

(lateral)

1 Cran. cervical ggl.

— nC$_1$

a

— nC$_2$

2 Vagosympathetic trunk

11 Vertebral n.

g

Spinal ggl.

3 Middle cervical ggl.

b

4 Ansa subclavia

— nC$_8$

5 Cervicothoracic ggl.
[Stellate ggl.]

6 Vagus n.

— nT$_1$

7 Cardiac plexus

h

Dorsal root

i

c

12 Ggll. of sympathetic trunk

— nT$_5$

j

Ventral vagal trunk

g

— nT$_7$

Dorsal vagal trunk

Aortic plexus

j

Ventral root

13 Major splanchnic n.

d

14 Celiac ggl. and
cran. mesenteric ggl.

k

— nT$_{13}$

e

— nL$_1$

15 Caud. mesenteric ggl. and
lumbar splanchnic nn.

(dorsal)

f

m

— 16

8

nS$_1$

— 17

— 18

8 Hypogastric n.

10 Pelvic n.

9 Pelvic plexus

n

— nS$_5$

Legend:

a Left common carotid a.
b Left subclavian a.
c Aorta
d Celiac a.
e Cran. mesenteric a.
f Caud. mesenteric a.
g Esophagus
h Longus colli
i Heart
j Diaphragm
k Small intestine
m Large intestine
n Rectum

Legend:

16 Conus medullaris
17 Filum terminale
18 Cauda equina

57

CHAPTER 5: VERTEBRAL COLUMN, THORACIC SKELETON, AND NECK

1. VERTEBRAL COLUMN, LIGAMENTUM NUCHAE, RIBS, AND STERNUM

> Review the basic parts of the bones on individual bones and mounted skeletons, and study the special features in the ox mentioned below.

a) The **VERTEBRAL COLUMN** is composed of seven cervical vertebrae, thirteen (12–14) thoracic vertebrae, six (7) lumbar vertebrae, five sacral vertebrae, and eighteen to twenty (16–21) caudal vertebrae.

The vertebrae are joined by fibrocartilaginous intervertebral discs, and surround the **vertebral canal (7)**. The basic parts: **body (1)**, **arch (8)**, and **processes** are developed differently according to function.

I. The cervical vertebrae (C1–C7) are generally shorter than in the horse. The **spinous process (12)** is longer than in the horse, and inclined cranially. Only on the seventh is it almost vertical, and *on the third and fourth cervical vertebrae the free end is split*. On the first, the spinous process is represented by a tubercle (29'). The *massive* **transverse process (13)** of the third to the fifth bears a cranial **ventral tubercle (13')** and a caudal **dorsal tubercle (13")** as in the dog and horse. On the sixth cervical vertebra the ventral tubercle is replaced by a sagittal quadrilateral plate, the **ventral lamina (13')**. The **cranial (16)** and **caudal (17)** articular processes are *very small* compared to those of the horse. The **atlas (C1)** *lacks a transverse foramen (15)*; the **dorsal arch** bears a large **dorsal tubercle (29')**; and the **ventral arch**, a large **ventral tubercle (30')**, *which is sometimes bifid*. The **axis (C2)** is *shorter than in the horse*; its **dens (32)** is *semicylindrical*; the spinous process (12) is a high and straight crest, but not split caudally as it is in the horse. The **lateral vertebral foramen (31')**, absent in the dog, is *very large*.

II. The **thoracic vertebrae (T1–T13)** have relatively long bodies compared to the dog and horse. The **spinous process (12)** of the first to the fifth thoracic vertebra is broad with sharp cranial and caudal borders, and provided on the free end with a cartilaginous cap until about the third year. These ossify by the eighth year. The **withers (interscapular region)** is *not as high as in the horse*. The seventh to eleventh thoracic spines are strongly inclined caudally. *The spine is vertical on the last thoracic (anticlinal) vertebra. In most thoracic vertebrae the caudal vertebral notch (11) is closed by a bridge of bone to form a* **lateral vertebral foramen (11')**. The **mamillary processes (20)** are not very prominent; on the last two thoracic vertebrae they merge with the **cranial articular processes (16)**.

Costovertebral articulations

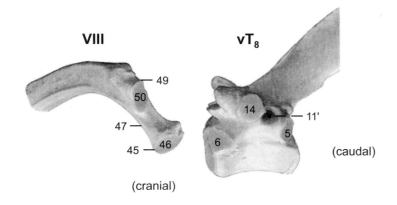

VIII — 49, 50, 47, 45, 46 (cranial)

vT$_8$ — 14, 11', 6, 5 (caudal)

III. The lumbar vertebrae (L1–L6) have a *long body* and a *flat arch* with an *almost square, cranially and caudally extended*, **spinous process (12)**. The horizontal **transverse processes (13)** are *curved cranially* and separated by wide spaces. The cranial lumbar vertebrae often have *lateral vertebral foramina* as in the thoracic vertebrae. The mamillary processes are always fused with the cranial articular processes.

IV. The sacral vertebrae (S1–S5) are completely fused to form the **sacrum** after 3–4 years. Depending on breed, the sacrum is more or less arched dorsally. Ventrally it has a distinct groove for the median sacral artery. The spinous processes are fused to form a **median sacral crest (35)** (as in the dog, but unlike the horse) with an occasional interruption between the fourth and fifth vertebrae. The **sacral promontory (38)** is the cranial ventral prominence of the first sacral vertebra. It is palpable per rectum. The *auricular surfaces of the alae face caudodorsally*. The fused articular processes form a ridge, the **intermediate sacral crest (37)**, *which bridges over the narrow* **dorsal sacral foramina (39)**, *and lies medial to the last sacral foramen. This is very large and not divided into dorsal (39) and ventral (40) foramina because the last two transverse processes are not completely fused.*

V. The caudal [coccygeal] vertebrae (Cd1+) and their processes are significantly larger and better developed than in the horse. The progressively narrowing **vertebral canal (7)** *extends to the fifth caudal vertebra*. The paired **hemal processes (21)** (present as in the dog, unlike the horse) *may be closed to form* **hemal arches (22)** *from the second to the fifth caudal vertebra.*

b) Of the thirteen **RIBS**, eight are **sternal ribs (41)** and five are **asternal (42)**. They increase in length to the tenth rib and, especially in the middle of the thorax, they are *flat toward the sternal end with sharp caudal borders, and wider than in the dog and horse*, whereby the intercostal spaces become narrower. The **head (45)** and the **tubercle (49)** are well developed and separated by a long **neck (47)**. The **knee [genu costae, 53]** *is at the costochondral junction*.

c) The body of the **STERNUM**, formed by five **sternebrae (56)**, *is slightly arched dorsally and flattened dorsoventrally. The triangular* **manubrium sterni (54)** *is raised craniodorsally and has no manubrial cartilage. It is attached to the body of the sternum by a true joint.* The **xiphoid process (57)** is smaller than in the horse. A sternal crest is absent, as in the dog.

d) The elastic **NUCHAL LIGAMENT** is generally better developed than in the dog and horse. It consists of a paired **funiculus (A)** and a **lamina (B)**, which is paired in the cranial part and unpaired in the caudal part.

The funiculus is divided into right and left halves attached to the external occipital protuberance. They extend, without attachment to the cervical vertebrae, to the withers, and become gradually wider to form the sagittally positioned, flat, wide parts *lateral to the first to fifth thoracic spinous processes, but not capping them. The wide parts gradually become narrower and unite to form the* **supraspinous ligament (C)**, which extends to the sacrum. It is elastic cranially, but becomes collagenous in the midlumbar region. The lamina arises with its cranial paired part from spinous processes C2–C4 and fuses with the funiculus. The caudal unpaired part, *also elastic*, which in the horse is thin and contains few elastic fibers, arises from vertebrae C5–C7 and terminates on the first thoracic spinous process under the wide parts of the funiculus. A **supraspinous bursa** may be present between the first few thoracic spines and the wide parts of the funiculus.

Vertebral column, Thoracic skeleton, and Nuchal ligament

Vertebral column and Bones of the thorax

Cervical vertebrae (C1–C7)
Thoracic vertebrae (T1–T13, 14)
Lumbar vertebrae (L1–L6)
Sacral vertebrae (S1–S5)
Caudal [Coccygeal] vertebrae (Cd1–Cd16, 21)
Body of vertebra (1)
  Ventral crest (2)
  Cranial end (3)
  Caudal end (4)
  Caud. costal fovea (5)
  Cran. costal fovea (6)
Vertebral canal (7)
Vertebral arch (8)
Intervertebral foramen (9):
  Cran. vertebral notch (10)
  Caud. vertebral notch (11)
  Lat. vertebral foramen (11')
Spinous process (12)
Transverse process (13)
  Ventral tubercle (C3–C5) (13') [Ventral lamina C6]
  Dorsal tubercle (C3–C5) (13")
  Costal fovea (T1–T13) (14)
  Transverse foramen (C2–C6) (15)
Cran. articular process (16)
Caud. articular process (17)
Costal process (18)
  [Transverse proc.] (L1–L6)
  [Ventr. tubercle] (C3–C5)]
Mamillary process (T+Cd) (20)
Hemal process (Cd2–Cd15) (21)
Hemal arch (Cd4 + Cd5) (22)
Interarcuate space:
  Lumbosacral (23)
  Sacrocaudal (24)

Atlas [C1]

Lateral mass
  Transverse proc. [Wing of atlas, Ala] (26)
    Alar foramen (27')
    Lat. vertebral foramen (28)
Dorsal arch (29)
  Dorsal tubercle (29')
Ventral arch (30)
  Ventral tubercle (30')

Axis [C2]

Lat. vertebral foramen (31')
Dens (32)

Sacrum [S1–S5]

Wing [Ala] of sacrum (33)
Median sacral crest (35)
Lat. sacral crest (36)
Intermediate sacral crest (37)
Promontory (38)
Dorsal sacral foramen (39)
Ventral sacral foramen (40)

Ribs [Costae]

Sternal ribs (41)
Asternal ribs (42)
Costal bone [Os costale] (44)
  Head of rib (45)
    Artic. surface of head (46)
  Neck of rib (47)
  Body of rib (48)
  Costal tubercle (49)
    Artic. surf. of tubercle (50)
  Angle of rib (51)
Costal cartilage (52)
Knee of rib [Genu costae] (53)

Sternum

Manubrium (54)
Body of sternum (55)
  Sternebrae (56)
Xiphoid process (57)

Legend:

Nuchal ligament:
A Funiculus nuchae
B Lamina nuchae
C Supraspinous lig.

C1 (caudodorsal)

C2 (lateral)

C6

C7

T13

L5 + L6

S1–S5

Cd1

Cd5

(lateral)

(dorsolateral)

(ventral)

(caudal)

2. NECK AND CUTANEOUS MUSCLES

A dorsomedian skin incision is made from the skull to the level of the last rib, and laterally along the last rib to its costochondral junction. A skin incision from the cranial end of the first incision is directed ventrally behind the base of the ear and across the angle of the mandible to the ventromedian line. The skin is reflected ventrally, sparing the cutaneous muscles, ext. jugular v., and cutaneous nerves, and continuing to the ventromedian line of the neck, on the lateral surface of the limb to the level of the sternum, and to a line extending from the axilla to the last costochondral junction. This flap of skin is removed. Note the dewlap [Palear], a breed-variable ventromedian fold of skin on the neck and presternal region.

a) Of the CUTANEOUS MUSCLES, the *cutaneus colli is thin and often impossible to demonstrate*. It originates from the ventro-median cervical fascia. The **cutaneus trunci** resembles that of the horse; whereas the cranially attached **cutaneus omobrachialis**, absent in the dog, is *thinner* than in the horse, and *occasionally unconnected to the cutaneus trunci*. For the preputial muscles, see p.66.

b) The **SUPERFICIAL SHOULDER GIRDLE MUSCLES (TRUNK—THORACIC LIMB MUSCLES):**

The **trapezius** with its **cervical part (11)** and **thoracic part (11')** is *significantly better developed than in the horse*. This fan-shaped muscle originates from the funicular nuchal lig. and supraspinous lig. between the atlas and the 12th (10th) thoracic vertebra and ends on the spine of the scapula. The cervical part is connected ventrally to the **omotransversarius (8)**, which, as in the dog, extends between the acromion and the transverse process of the atlas (axis), where it is fused with the tendon of the splenius. The **brachiocephalicus** consists of the **cleidobrachialis** (clavicular part of deltoideus, p. 4) and the **cleidocephalicus**. The two parts of the latter in the ox are the cleido-occipitalis and the cleidomastoideus. The **cleido-occipitalis (7),** *and the cleidomastoideus, originate from the clavicular intersection—an indistinct line of connective tissue across the brachiocephalicus cranial to the shoulder joint. The cleido-occipitalis is joined to the cleidomastoideus as far as the middle of the neck, separates from it, adjoins the ventrocranial border of the trapezius, and ends on the funicular nuchal lig. and occipital bone.* The **cleidomastoideus (6)** *lies ventral to the cleidooccipitalis, is partially covered by it, and ends as a thin muscle with a slender tendon on the mastoid process and the tendon of the longus capitis.* The **sternocephalicus** consists of the sternomastoideus and sternomandibularis.

The **sternomastoideus mm. (4)** originate from the the manubrium sterni only, are fused in the caudal third of the neck, and terminate in common with the cleidomastoideus. The **sternomandibularis (5)** originates laterally from the manubrium and from the first rib; and, crossing the sternomastoideus, runs ventral to the jugular groove and ends with a thin tendon on the rostral border of the masseter and aponeurotically on the mandible and the depressor labii inferioris. The sternomastoideus and cleidomastoideus are homologous to the human sternocleidomastoideus.

The **latissimus dorsi (12)** arises from the thoracolumbar fascia and from the 11th and 12th ribs. The fibers run cranioventrally to a common termination with the teres major and an aponeurotic connection *with the coracobrachialis and deep pectoral as well as the long head of the triceps.*

Of the **superficial pectoral muscles**, the flat **transverse pectoral (25')** originates from the sternum and ends on the medial deep fascia of the forearm. The **descending pectoral (25)** is a thick muscle originating from the manubrium and ending with the brachiocephalicus on the crest of the humerus. It is *not as visible under the skin as in the horse.*

c) **JUGULAR GROOVE AND LATERAL PECTORAL GROOVE:** The **jugular groove** is bounded dorsally by the cleidomastoideus, ventrally by the **sternomandibularis**, and, in the cranial half of the neck, medially by the sternomastoideus. The **ext. jugular vein (3)** lies in the groove. At the junction of the head and neck it bifurcates, giving rise to the **maxillary (2)** and **linguofacial (1) veins**. At the thoracic inlet it gives off a dorsal branch, the **superficial cervical vein (21)**; and gives off the **cephalic vein (10)** to the lateral pectoral groove between the brachiocephalicus and the descending pectoral muscle.

3. DEEP SHOULDER GIRDLE MUSCLES, VISCERA AND CONDUCTING STRUCTURES OF THE NECK

The superficial shoulder girdle muscles and the sternomastoideus and sternomandibularis are transected near their attachments on the limb and sternum and removed, leaving short stumps. The accessory n. (c) and the roots of the phrenic nerve (C5 to C7, q) must be spared in the dissection.

a) **DEEP SHOULDER GIRDLE MUSCLES:** The **rhomboideus** consists of the **rhomboideus cervicis (28)** and **thoracis (28')** *but no rhomboideus capitis, unlike the dog*. These are covered by the trapezius, originate from the funicular nuchal lig. and supraspinous lig. between C2 and T7 (T8), and terminate on the medial surface of the scapular cartilage. The **deep pectoral (26 and p. 5, t)** is a strong unified muscle which ends primarily on the major and minor tubercles. *A branch of the tendon fuses with the latissimus dorsi and ends on the tendon of origin of the coracobrachialis.* The **subclavius (26')**, absent in the dog, is *not well developed. It extends from the first costal cartilage to the deep surface of the clavicular intersection.* The **serratus ventralis** extends from the 2nd (3rd) cervical vertebra to the 9th rib, and is *clearly divided* into **serratus ventralis cervicis (27)** and **thoracis**. The **serratus ventralis thoracis (27')** arises by distinct muscle slips and is interspersed with strong tendinous layers. It is *attached not only to the facies serrata of the scapula, but penetrates with a thick broad tendon between the parts of the subscapularis to end in the subscapular fossa.*

b) **LONG HYOID MUSCLES:** The **sternohyoideus (14)**, **sternothyroideus (15)**, and omohyoideus do not belong to the shoulder girdle muscles, but are long muscles of the hyoid bone and thyroid cartilage. The first two resemble those of the horse, *but do not have a tendinous intersection; they are, however, connected by a tendinous band in the middle of the neck.* The **omohyoideus (13)** is *thin and does not come from the shoulder, but from the deep cervical fascia, and thereby indirectly from the transverse processes of the 3rd and 4th cervical vertebrae. In the angle between the sternomastoideus and sternomandibularis, and crossed laterally by the external jugular vein, it passes medially under the mandibular gland to end with the sternohyoideus on the basihyoid.*

c) **VISCERA AND CONDUCTING STRUCTURES OF THE NECK:** In the middle of the space for the viscera and conducting structures is the **trachea (19)**. *In life the tracheal cartilages are arched to give it a vertical oval section, but after death it has a tear-drop shape.* Dorsolateral to the trachea is the **common carotid artery (16)**, with the **vagosympathetic trunk (17)**, The latter is accompanied by the small **int. jugular v**. *This may be absent.* The **esophagus (18)** is dorsal in the first third of the neck; in the other two thirds it is on the left side of the trachea and at the thoracic inlet it is dorsolateral. The *left* **recurrent n. (18)** *accompanies the esophagus ventrally; the right recurrent n. accompanies the trachea dorsolaterally.*

d) **LYMPHATIC SYSTEM AND THYMUS:** The **superficial cervical lymph node (9)** *lies in the groove cranial to the supraspinatus, covered by the omotransversarius and cleido-occipitalis.* It receives lymph from the neck, thoracic limb, and thoracic wall back to the 12th rib. *Its efferent lymphatics go to the tracheal trunk; on the left, also to the thoracic duct.* The **cranial deep cervical lnn. (22)** lie near the thyroid gland; the **middle deep cervical lnn. (23)**, in the middle third of the neck on the right of the trachea and on the left of the esophagus. The **caudal deep cervical lnn. (24)** are placed around the trachea near the first rib. They receive lymph from the cervical viscera, ventral cervical muscles and preceding lymph nodes of the head, neck, and thoracic limb. (See the table of lymph nodes.) Some of their efferents have the same termination as those of the superficial cervical ln.; others end in the cran. vena cava. The **thymus (20)** is fully developed only in the fetus. It consists of an *unpaired left thoracic part* (may be maintained to six years of age), a V-shaped paired cervical part with the unpaired apex directed toward the thoracic cavity, and a paired cranial part (already retrogressed at birth).

Regions of the neck and chest

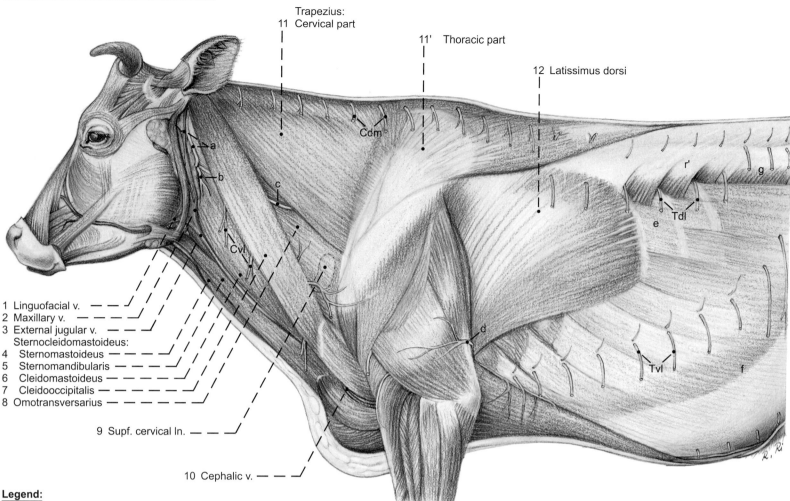

Trapezius:
11 Cervical part
11' Thoracic part
12 Latissimus dorsi

1 Linguofacial v.
2 Maxillary v.
3 External jugular v.
Sternocleidomastoideus:
4 Sternomastoideus
5 Sternomandibularis
6 Cleidomastoideus
7 Cleidooccipitalis
8 Omotransversarius

9 Supf. cervical ln.

10 Cephalic v.

Legend:

a Great auricular n. and
  caud. auricular v.
b Transverse n. of the neck
c Accessory n.
d Intercostobrachial n.
e External intercostal mm.
f External oblique abd. m.

g Internal oblique abd. m.
h Longus capitis
i Intertransversarius longus
j Ventral cervical
  intertransversarii
k Splenius
l Semispinalis capitis

m Spinalis et semispinalis
  thoracis et cervicis
Longissimus:
n Longissimus capitis et atlantis
n' Longissimus cervicis
n' Longissimus thoracis
n''' Longissimus lumborum

Iliocostalis:
o Iliocostalis cervicis
o' Iliocostalis thoracis
o" Iliocostalis lumborum
Scalenus:
p Scalenus dorsalis
p' Scalenus ventralis

q C6 root of phrenic n.
r Serratus dors. cranialis
r' Serratus dors. caudalis
s Brachial plexus
t Cran. pectoral nn.
u Caud. pectoral nn.
v Long thoracic n.
w Lat. thoracic n.

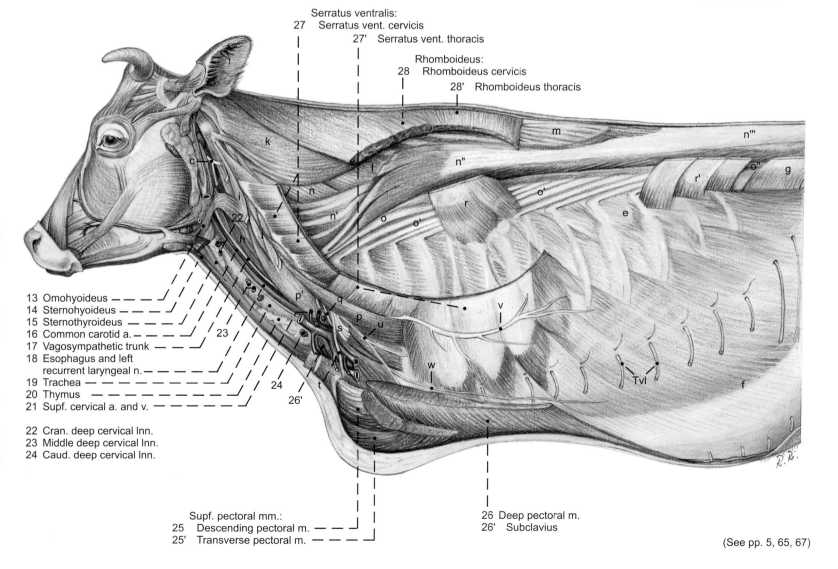

Serratus ventralis:
27 Serratus vent. cervicis
27' Serratus vent. thoracis

Rhomboideus:
28 Rhomboideus cervicis
28' Rhomboideus thoracis

13 Omohyoideus
14 Sternohyoideus
15 Sternothyroideus
16 Common carotid a.
17 Vagosympathetic trunk
18 Esophagus and left
   recurrent laryngeal n.
19 Trachea
20 Thymus
21 Supf. cervical a. and v.

22 Cran. deep cervical lnn.
23 Middle deep cervical lnn.
24 Caud. deep cervical lnn.

Supf. pectoral mm.:
25 Descending pectoral m.
25' Transverse pectoral m.

26 Deep pectoral m.
26' Subclavius

(See pp. 5, 65, 67)

61

Cdm = Med. dors. cut. brr. of cervical nn. Tdl = Dorsolat. cut. brr. of thoracic nn. Tvl = Ventrolat. cut. brr. of thoracic nn.

CHAPTER 6: THORACIC CAVITY
1. RESPIRATORY MUSCLES AND THORACIC CAVITY WITH LUNGS

The deep shoulder girdle muscles and the vessels and nerves of the limb, with attention to their roots, are cut as close as possible to the thoracic wall, and the limb is removed. **The diaphragmatic line of pleural reflection**, where the costal pleura is reflected as the diaphragmatic pleura, is clinically important as the caudoventral boundary of the pleural cavity. In the dorsal end of the 11th intercostal space, a small opening is made through the intercostal muscles into the pleural cavity; then the caudoventral limits of the **costodiaphragmatic recess (7)** are probed and marked on the ribs as the intercostal muscles are removed. The line extends from the knee of the 7th or 8th rib, through the middle of the 11th, to the angle of the 13th rib at the lateral border of the muscles of the back. The **basal border of the lung** is also marked on the ribs. After study of the **lung field**, the ribs, with the exception of the 3rd, 6th, and 13th, are cut above the line of pleural reflection and removed, sparing the diaphragm and noting the slips of origin of the ext. oblique abdominal muscle.

a) The **RESPIRATORY MUSCLES** (see appendix on myology) belong partly to the muscles of the back and partly to those of the thorax. They function as **expiratory muscles** in the contraction of the thorax or as **inspiratory muscles** in the expansion of it. The obligate respiratory muscles are aided by the auxiliary respiratory muscles. The **diaphragm** is the primary respiratory muscle and the partition between the thoracic and abdominal cavities.

The **line of diaphragmatic attachment** *rises steeply, running across the ribs from the knee of the 8th, across the 11th rib below its middle to the vertebral end of the 13th rib.* In ruminants the two **costal parts (3)** of the diaphragm *are clearly separated from the 13–15 cm wide* **sternal part** *(not illustrated) by clefts between muscle fibers.* The **lumbar part (2)** resembles that of the horse in its relation to the aortic hiatus and esophageal hiatus, but *sends muscle fiber bundles from the* **right and left crura**, *sometimes with fibrocartilaginous inlays, to the* **foramen venae cavae (5)**. This lies on the right in a relatively large **tendinous center (4)**, which on inspiration is at the level of the 7th rib.

b) The **THORACIC CAVITY** is protected by the bony thoracic cage [thorax] and extends from the especially narrow cranial thoracic aperture [thoracic inlet] to the diaphragm. It contains the two **pleural cavities** of unequal size. The pleural sacs project into the thoracic inlet as the **cupulae pleurae (15)**. The left one does not extend beyond the first rib. The right **one** projects 4–5 cm cranial to the first rib. The **parietal pleura** includes the **costal pleura (6)**, **diaphragmatic pleura (8)**, and the **mediastinal pleura (16)**, where right and left pleural sacs adjoin and where they cover the **pericardium** as **pericardial pleura (18)**. The **visceral pleura** covers the lungs as the **pulmonary pleura**, which is connected to the mediastinal pleura by the short pulmonary ligament. This is present only in the caudal area. The **mediastinal recess (9)** is a diverticulum of the right pleural cavity containing the accessory lobe of the right lung.

The **costodiaphragmatic recess (7)** is the potential space between the **basal border of the lung** and the **diaphragmatic line of pleural reflection**. The latter runs slightly craniodorsal to the line of diaphragmatic attachment, dipping ventrally at every intercostal space.

c) The **MEDIASTINUM** *is thicker than in the horse*. The heart occupies the **middle mediastinum** and divides the rest of the mediastinum into **cranial (16)**, **caudal**, **dorsal**, and **ventral parts**. The mediastinum is composed of the two mediastinal pleural layers and the fibrous substantia propria between them. It encloses the usual organs and structures: the esophagus, trachea, blood and lymph vessels, lymph nodes, nerves, and the pericardium. *The* **cranial mediastinum** *is pushed against the left thoracic wall in the first and second intercostal spaces, ventral to the great vessels, by the cranial lobe of the right lung. The* **caudal mediastinum**, *containing the left phrenic nerve, is attached to the left side of the the diaphragm.* Together with a fold on the right, the **plica venae cavae (h)**, they enclose the **mediastinal recess (9)**, containing the accessory lobe of the right lung. *Perforations of the mediastinum, allowing communication between right and left pleural cavities, as described in the dog and horse, do not occur in the ox.*

d) The **LUNGS** are *accessible for percussion and auscultation in a cranial and a caudal lung field*. The total area is relatively small.

The **cranial lung field** is of lesser significance for clinical examination. It lies cranial to the thoracic limb in the first three intercostal spaces. The **caudal lung field** is bounded cranially by the tricipital line and dorsally by the muscles of the back. The **basal border** as determined by percussion or auscultation is 3–4 cm above the actual border of the lung, which is too thin for clinical examination. It is *almost straight in contrast to the curvature in the dog and horse*. It intersects the cranial border at the knee of the 6th rib. In the 7th intercostal space it intersects the dorsal plane through the shoulder joint. In the 11th space it meets the dorsal border.

The **right lung** *is considerably larger than the* **left lung**. The interlobar and intralobar fissures are distinctly marked so that both the **right** and **left cranial lobes** are divided into **cranial (19)** and **caudal (20) parts**, unlike the dog and horse. In addition to the **caudal lobe (30)** of both lungs, the right lung has an **accessory lobe (29)**, as in all domestic mammals, and a **middle lobe (23)**, absent in the horse. *In addition, the right cranial lobe has a special* **tracheal bronchus (22)** *that comes from the trachea cranial to the* **bifurcation (26)**. *Also, the bovine lung has a distinctly visible lobular structure outlined by an increase in the amount of connective tissue.*

e) The **LYMPHATIC SYSTEM** is not only clinically important (as in the dog and especially in the horse), but also of great practical interest in meat inspection; therefore a knowledge of it is indispensable. (See the appendix on the lymphatic system.) *Lymph nodes routinely examined in meat inspection are*: the **left (24)**, **middle (27)**, and **cranial (21) tracheobronchial lnn.**, *the latter lying cranial to the origin of the tracheal bronchus*; and the small, inconstant **right tracheobronchial lnn. (25)**, called the supervisor's node. Routinely palpated for enlargement are the **pulmonary lnn. (28)** concealed in the lung near the main bronchi. Also routinely examined are the **cranial (14)**, **middle (12)**, and **caudal (13) mediastinal lnn.** The latter consist of a group of small nodes between the esophagus and aorta and *one 15–25 cm long ln.* that extends dorsal to the esophagus to the diaphragm and drains a large area on both sides of the latter. Finally, included in the routine examination are the **thoracic aortic lnn. (11)** dorsal to the aorta and medial to the sympathetic trunk.

In special cases the following are examined: the **intercostal lnn. (10)** lateral to the sympathetic trunk, and the **cranial sternal ln. (17)** dorsal to the manubrium sterni and ventral to the internal thoracic vessels.

The caudal sternal lnn. and the *phrenic ln. on the thoracic side of the foramen venae cavae are unimportant for meat inspection.*

Most of the lymphatic drainage passes through the mediastinal lnn. and the terminal part of the tracheal duct, as well as the **thoracic duct (1)**, *which does not go through the aortic hiatus, but through the right crus of the diaphragm. At T5 it crosses to the left side of the esophagus and trachea. It may be enlarged to form an ampulla before it opens into the bijugular trunk.*

Right thoracic cavity and Lungs

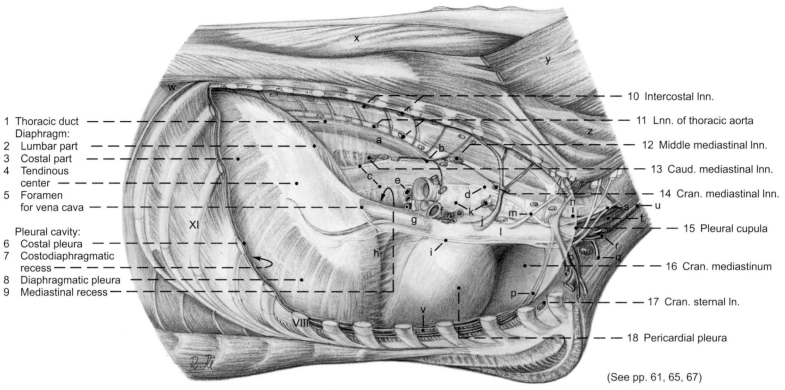

1 Thoracic duct
Diaphragm:
2 Lumbar part
3 Costal part
4 Tendinous
   center
5 Foramen
   for vena cava

Pleural cavity:
6 Costal pleura
7 Costodiaphragmatic
   recess
8 Diaphragmatic pleura
9 Mediastinal recess

10 Intercostal lnn.
11 Lnn. of thoracic aorta
12 Middle mediastinal lnn.
13 Caud. mediastinal lnn.
14 Cran. mediastinal lnn.
15 Pleural cupula
16 Cran. mediastinum
17 Cran. sternal ln.
18 Pericardial pleura

(See pp. 61, 65, 67)

Legend:

A Main bronchus
B Lobar bronchus
C Segmental bronchus
a Thoracic aorta
b Bronchoesophagial a.
c Dors. and vent. vagal trunks

d Right vagus n.
e Pulmonary vv.
f Pulmonary a.
g Caud. vena cava
h Plica venae cavae
i Phrenic n.

j Right azygos v.
k Trachea and tracheal bronchus
l Cran. vena cava
m Costocervical v.
n Right recurrent laryngeal n.
o Right subclavian a. and v.

p Internal thoracic a. and v.
q Cephalic v.
r Supf. cervical a. and v.
s Vagosympathetic trunk
t Common carotid a. and
   internal jugular v.
u External jugular v.

v Transverse thoracic m.
w Retractor costae
x Spinalis et semispinalis
   cervicis et capitis
y Semispinalis capitis
z Longissimus cervicis

Lungs and Bronchial Inn.

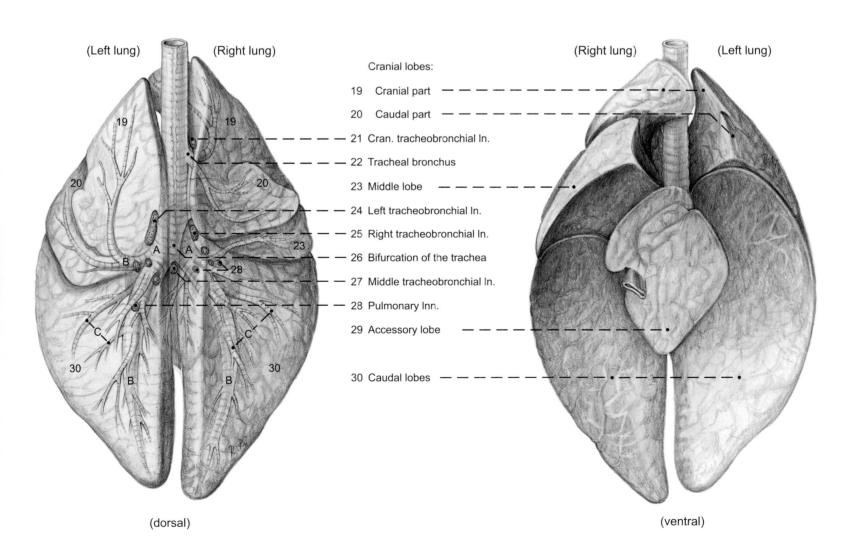

(Left lung)   (Right lung)

Cranial lobes:

19 Cranial part
20 Caudal part
21 Cran. tracheobronchial ln.
22 Tracheal bronchus
23 Middle lobe
24 Left tracheobronchial ln.
25 Right tracheobronchial ln.
26 Bifurcation of the trachea
27 Middle tracheobronchial ln.
28 Pulmonary lnn.
29 Accessory lobe
30 Caudal lobes

(Right lung)   (Left lung)

(dorsal)   (ventral)

The surface of the heart is studied in situ; the internal relations are studied on isolated hearts. The visible blood vessels and nerves are identified.

a) The **HEART (COR)** is relatively small in comparison to that of the horse. Its weight varies between 0.4 and 0.5 percent of the body weight. Its absolute weight in cows averages 2.4 kg and in bulls 2.6 kg.

The **heart is located** between the planes of the 3rd and 5th intercostal spaces in the ventral half of the thoracic cavity. The inclination of the **cardiac axis** is relatively steep, with the **base** of the heart directed craniodorsally. The **apex (x)** of the heart is directed caudoventrally, but does not reach the sternum. The greater part of the heart lies on the left of the median plane and brings the pericardium into contact with the left thoracic wall in the 3rd and 4th intercostal spaces. Its **left ventricular border (w)** presses the pericardium into contact with the left side of the diaphragm close to the median plane, and *this is clinically significant because of the proximity of the reticulum, with its penetrating hardware*. The **heart field**, clinically important for auscultation and percussion, is an outline of the heart projected on the left thoracic wall from the 3rd to the 5th intercostal space. On the surface of the heart in addition to the **paraconal (16)** and **subsinuosal (18)** interventricular grooves, *there is an* **intermediate groove** *on the left ventricular border that does not reach the apex*. Also species-specific are the distinctly *dentate margins of the auricles*, which overhang the base of the heart, but are smaller than those of the horse. The *friable white structural fat (suet)* that can make up as much as 24 percent of the weight of the heart lies in four interconnected lobes *on the right and left atria between the great vessels and in the coronary grooves.*

The **pericardium** is attached by two divergent **sternopericardiac ligaments (14)** to the sternum at the level of the notches for the 6th costal cartilages.

Of the **coronary arteries**, the **left coronary a. (15)** is *substantially larger (left coronary supply type as in the dog, but unlike the horse and pig.)* It gives off the **paraconal interventricular branch (16)** in the groove of the same name, as well as the **circumflex branch (17)** which runs around the caudal surface of the heart in the coronary groove, and ends as the **subsinuosal interventricular branch (18)** in the groove of the same name. The small **right coronary a. (19)** takes a circumflex course in the **coronary groove** between the right atrium and ventricle.

The **heart bones** are remarkable features of the **heart skeleton**—the fibrous rings around and between the valves. *The large, 3–6 cm, three-pronged right heart bone (g) and the small, 2 cm, left heart bone (g') are in the aortic ring.*

b) The remaining **BLOOD VESSELS** show greater differences from the dog than from the horse.

The first branch of the **aortic arch**, as in the horse, is the **brachiocephalic trunk (13)**, the common trunk of the vessels to cranial parts of the thorax, to the thoracic limbs, and to the head and neck. It gives off first the left subclavian a., then the right subclavian a., and continues as the **bicarotid trunk** for the **left (4)** and **right** (see p. 63) **common carotid aa.** The **left (6)** and **right** (see p. 63) **subclavian aa.** give off cranially the **costocervical trunk (3)** for vessels to the vertebrae, spinal cord, and brain (**vertebral a. 2**); to the neck (**deep cervical a., 2** and **dorsal scapular a., 1**); and to the ribs (supreme intercostal a., which can also originate from the subclavian a. or the aorta). Dorsocranially the subclavian gives off the **superficial cervical a. (5)**, and caudally, the **internal thoracic a. (7)**, which is the last branch before the subclavian turns around the first rib and becomes the axillary a. The **thoracic aorta (8)** gives off dorsal intercostal aa. and on the right, dorsal to the base of the heart, the **bronchoesophageal a.**, whose **bronchial (12)** and **esophageal (11)** branches may originate as separate arteries from the aorta or an intercostal a. The tracheal bronchus is supplied by its own branch, either from the aorta or from the bronchial branch.

The **veins** show a distribution similar to that of the arteries. A **right azygos v.**, (see p. 63), present in the dog and horse, *is only rarely developed as far as the last thoracic vertebra in the ox, and may be absent caudal to the 5th dorsal intercostal v.* The **left azygos v. (10)** *is always present. It drains into the coronary sinus of the right atrium. It does not occur in the dog and horse.*

c) The **NERVES** in the thoracic cavity are the same as in the dog and horse. The **greater splanchnic n.** *takes origin from the* **sympathetic trunk (9)** *at the 6th to 10th ganglia*, unlike the dog and horse, *and separates from the trunk just before they pass over the diaphragm in the lumbocostal arch.*

Section through the Base of the Heart

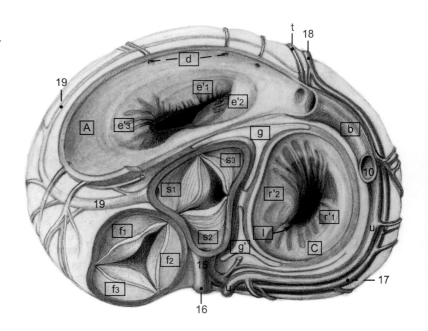

A Right atrium	**C** Left atrium
a Sinus of venae cavae	Pulmonary vv.
b Coronary sinus	(See p. 65 p)
c Pectinate mm.	
d Veins of right heart	

g Right heart bone	
g' Left heart bone	
h Fossa ovalis	
i Epicardium	
j Myocardium	
k Endocardium	

B Right ventricle	**D** Left ventricle
e Right atrioventricular valve [Tricuspid valve]	r Left atrioventricular valve [Mitral valve]
e'1 Parietal cusp	r'1 Parietal cusp
e'2 Septal cusp	r'2 Septal cusp
e'3 Angular cusp	r"1 Subauricular papillary m.
e"1 Small papillary mm.	r"2 Subatrial papillary m.
e"2 Great papillary m.	s Aortic valve
e"3 Subarterial papillary m.	s1 Right semilunar valvule
f Pulmonary valve	s2 Left semilunar valvule
f1 Right semilunar valvule	s3 Septal semilunar valvule
f2 Left semilunar valvule	
f3 Intermediate semilunar valvule	

l Atrioventricular orifice	
m Interventricular septum	
n Septomarginal trabeculae	
o Trabeculae carneae	
p Tendinous cords	

* The letters in this legend are framed in the heart illustrations (pp. 64, 65).

Left Thoracic cavity and Heart

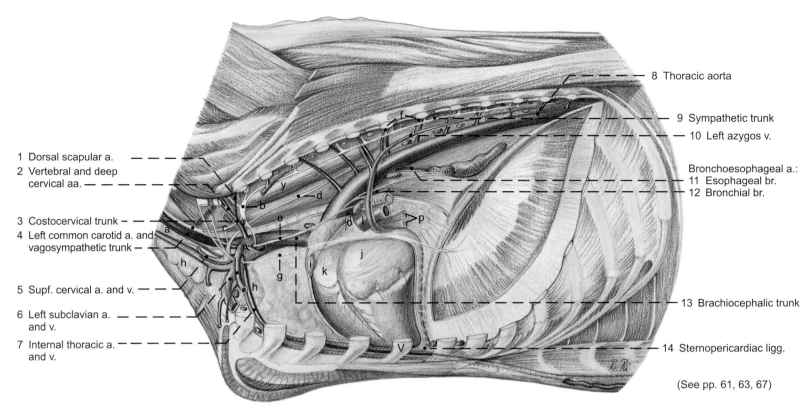

1 Dorsal scapular a.
2 Vertebral and deep cervical aa.
3 Costocervical trunk
4 Left common carotid a. and vagosympathetic trunk
5 Supf. cervical a. and v.
6 Left subclavian a. and v.
7 Internal thoracic a. and v.

8 Thoracic aorta
9 Sympathetic trunk
10 Left azygos v.
Bronchoesophageal a.:
11 Esophageal br.
12 Bronchial br.

13 Brachiocephalic trunk

14 Sternopericardiac ligg.

(See pp. 61, 63, 67)

Legend: (Lnn. see p. 63)

a Trachea and int. jugular v.
b Cervicothoracic ganglion
c Middle cervical ganglion
d Thoracic duct
e Vagus n.

f Intercostal aa. and vv.
g Left phrenic n.
h Thymus
i Right auricle
j Left auricle

k Conus arteriosus
l Pulmonary trunk
m Left pulmonary a.
n Right pulmonary a.
o Lig. arteriosum

p Pulmonary vv.
q Caud. vena cava
r Cran. vena cava
s Costocervical v.
t Middle cardiac v.

u Great cardiac v.
v Right ventricular border
w Left ventricular border and intermediate groove
x Apex of heart
y Longus colli m.

Right atrium and Right ventricle

(Atrial surface)

Left auricle and Left ventricle

(Auricular surface)

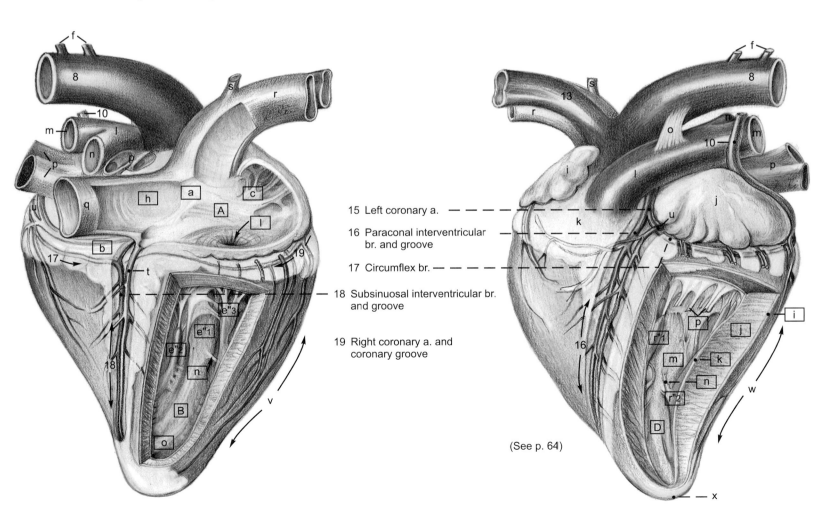

15 Left coronary a.
16 Paraconal interventricular br. and groove
17 Circumflex br.
18 Subsinuosal interventricular br. and groove
19 Right coronary a. and coronary groove

(See p. 64)

CHAPTER 7: ABDOMINAL WALL AND ABDOMINAL CAVITY

1. THE ABDOMINAL WALL

For demonstration of the five layers of the abdominal wall (a, b, d, e, f), the remaining skin is cut along the dorsomedian line and along the transverse plane of the tuber coxae, and reflected ventrally to the base of the udder or prepuce. Remnants of the cutaneus trunci, abdominal muscles, and internal fascia of the trunk are cut just ventral to the iliocostalis lumborum and reflected ventrally, one after the other, to the subcutaneus abdominal vein and the lateral border of the rectus abdominis.

a) The **SKIN (1)** of the lateral abdominal wall (flank) is easily moveable. Dorsally the *surgically important triangular* **paralumbar fossa (b)** is outlined by the ends of the transverse processes of the lumbar vertebrae, the last rib, and the prominent ridge formed by the part of the internal oblique that extends from the tuber coxae to the knee of the last rib. Ventrally, the subcutaneous **cranial superficial epigastric v.** ("milk vein"—3) *in the cow, is conspicuous, meandering, and 2–3 cm thick. It comes from the int. thoracic v. and emerges from the "milk well" (anulus venae subcutaneae abdominis) at the second tendinous intersection of the rectus, ventral to the 7th to 9th intercostal spaces. It joins the* **cranial mammary v.** *(caudal superficial epigastric v., p. 91, 12) at the udder.*

b) The **SYSTEM OF THE EXTERNAL FASCIA OF THE TRUNK** includes the superficial fascia and deep fascia.

I.   The **superficial fascia of the trunk** envelops the **cutaneus trunci** and the cranially related **cutaneus omobrachialis**, which are essentially the same as in the horse. The *strong* **cranial preputial muscles**, *present in the dog, but not in the horse, originate mainly from the region of the xiphoid cartilage and secondarily from the ventral border of the cutaneus trunci, and form a loop around the preputial orifice.* The **caudal preputial muscles** (see text figure p. 80) are inconspicuous in the dog and absent in the horse and polled breeds of cattle.* *They originate from the deep fascia, mainly lateral to the tunica vaginalis, but often also medial to it, and terminate at the loop formed by the cranial preputial muscles.*

The 8–12 cm long **subiliac lymph node (5)**, absent in the dog, differs from the multiple nodes of the horse. *It is a single large node above the patella on the abdominal wall near the cranial border of the tensor fasciae latae, easily palpable in the live ox. A small accessory node may be present.*

II.   The **deep fascia of the trunk** covers the external oblique, and on the ventrolateral abdomen is also known as the **yellow abdominal tunic (4)** due to the inclusion of yellow elastic fibers. With its collagenous laminae the deep fascia completely envelops the two abdominal obliques; whereas it covers only the external surface of the rectus and transversus. On both sides of the ventral median line the yellow tunic gives off the elastic **medial laminae** of the udder, or in the bull, radiates into the prepuce. The **linea alba** is the ventromedian fixation and interwoven seam of the fasciae and aponeuroses of the abdominal muscles. It extends from the sternum *through the prepubic tendon* to the pecten pubis and passes around both sides of the umbilicus.

c) The **NERVES OF THE ABDOMINAL WALL**

I.   The **dorsal branches** of spinal nerves T12–L3 divide into medial and lateral mixed motor and sensory branches. The lateral brr. (Tdl, Ldl) pass out between the longissimus and iliocostalis muscles and divide into **dorsomedial cutaneous brr.** and **dorsolateral cutaneous brr.** The latter innervate the skin of the abdomen down to the level of the patella. On p. 67 the small dorsomed. cut. brr. are mislabeled Ldl. The dorsolat. cut. brr. are cut off short. Those of T13 and L1 and L2 cross the paralumbar fossa to a line from the ventral end of the last rib to the patella, but cannot be traced that far by gross dissection. They must be blocked with the ventral brr. to provide anesthesia for flank incisions.

II.   The **ventral branches** of spinal nerves T12–L2 innervate the skin, abdominal mm., and peritoneum. The ventral br. of L1 is the **iliohypogastric n.** The ventral br. of L2, together with a communication from L3, forms the **ilioinguinal n.** The ventral brr. give off **lateral cutaneous branches (Tvl, Lvl)** which emerge through the external oblique on a line extending from the knees of the ribs to a point ventral to the tuber coxae at the level of the hip joint. Passing caudoventrally, they innervate the skin of the ventrolateral abdomen. The ventral brr. of T12–L2 communicate with each other at the origins of the lateral cutaneous brr. and continue ventrally on the external surface of the transversus. Near the milk vein they give off **ventral cutaneous branches (Tvc, Lvc)**** extending to the ventral midline and cranial portions of the prepuce or udder, and terminate in the rectus and parietal peritoneum. The relations of nerves T13–L2 to the transverse processes of the vertebrae are of great clinical importance for anesthesia of the abdominal wall. The **lateral cutaneous femoral n. (11)** comes from L3 and L4 through the lumbar plexus. It accompanies the caudal branches of the deep circumflex iliac a. and v., *at first medial then craniolateral to the tensor fasciae latae, down to the stifle.* (For the innervation of the udder see p. 90.)

d) The **SKELETAL MUSCLE LAYER** consists of four broad muscles.

I.   The **external oblique abdominal m. (2)**. The lumbar part originates on the last rib and thoracolumbar fascia and runs to the tuber coxae, and caudoventrally to the inguinal lig. and prepubic tendon (see p. 80). *The costal part begins with its digitations on the last 8–9 ribs, touching part of the ventral border of the latissimus dorsi.* It ends with the aponeurosis mainly on the linea alba, but also on the prepubic tendon by means of its abdominal and pelvic tendons (see pp. 79, 80). *The transition of the muscle to its aponeurosis follows the curve of the costal arch and continues to the tuber coxae. The aponeurosis is a component of the external lamina of the sheath of the rectus.*

II.   The **internal oblique abdominal m. (10)** originates mainly from the tuber coxae and the iliac fascia (see p. 81). It also takes origin from the thoracolumbar fascia and the lumbar transverse processes. The dorsal part ends on the last rib, and the portion running from the tuber coxae to the knee of the last rib forms the caudoventral border of the paralumbar fossa. The main termination is by its aponeurosis on the linea alba; the caudal border of the aponeurosis joins the abdominal and pelvic tendons of the ext. oblique and the tendon of the rectus in the prepubic tendon. The aponeurosis, unlike that of the dog, is involved only in the external lamina of the sheath of the rectus. (For its contribution to the deep inguinal ring see p. 80.)

III. The **transversus abdominis (7)** originates with a tendinous lumbar part from the lumbar transverse processes, and a fleshy costal part interdigitating with the diaphragm *on the last 7–8 costal cartilages.* It terminates on the linea alba, its aponeurosis forming the internal lamina of the sheath of the rectus. Its caudal extent is at the transverse plane of the tuber coxae.

IV. The **rectus abdominis (6)** takes origin from the 4th–9th costal cartilages *and has five tendinous intersections. The terminal tendons of the recti become abruptly narrower near the inguinal region and turn their inner surfaces toward each other, forming in the cow a narrow median trough. Near the prepubic tendon the rectus tendons twist into sagittal planes and fuse by decussation caudal to the intertendinous fossa (see p. 78 c). They form a common median tendon incorporated in the prepubic tendon and continuous with the symphyseal tendon.*

e) The **INTERNAL FASCIA OF THE TRUNK** (see p. 80) lines the transversus and rectus on the lateral and ventral abdominal wall as the **fascia transversalis**. Dorsally it covers the psoas and iliacus as iliac fascia. It joins the pelvic fascia on the pelvic wall.

f) The **PERITONEUM** (see also p. 80). The peritoneum extends into the pelvic cavity as the rectogenital, vesicogenital, and pubovesical pouches (excavations) and in the bull is evaginated *into the scrotum as the vaginal tunic.*

66

---

*   Long, and Hignett, 1970
** Schaller, 1956

Pectoral and abdominal regions

(lateral)

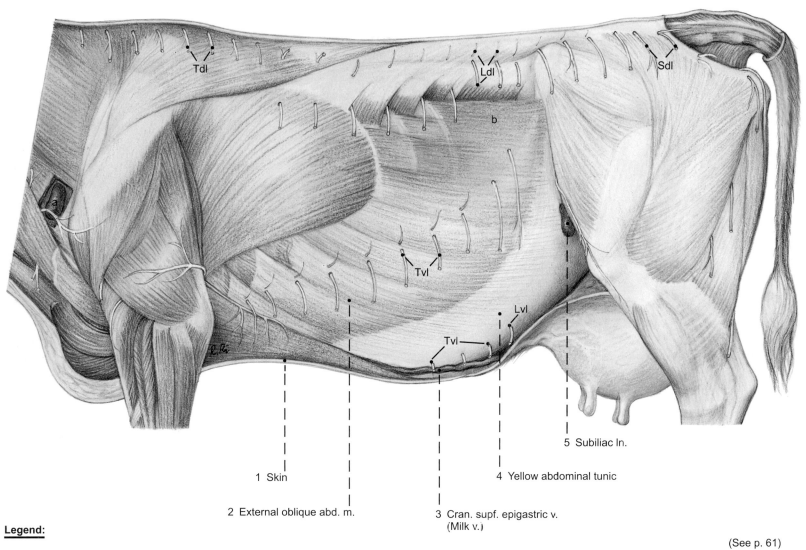

5 Subiliac ln.

1 Skin

4 Yellow abdominal tunic

2 External oblique abd. m.

3 Cran. supf. epigastric v.
(Milk v.)

Legend:

a Supf. cervical ln.
b Paralumbar fossa
c Rectus thoracis
d Int. intercostal mm.

(See p. 61)

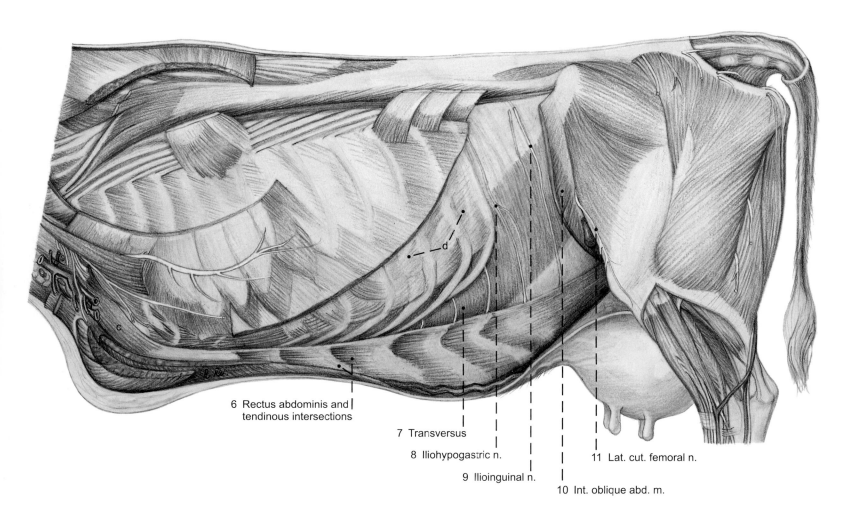

6 Rectus abdominis and
tendinous intersections

7 Transversus

8 Iliohypogastric n.

9 Ilioinguinal n.

10 Int. oblique abd. m.

11 Lat. cut. femoral n.

2. TOPOGRAPHY AND PROJECTION OF THE ABDOMINAL ORGANS ON THE BODY WALL

> The costal part of the diaphragm is detached from the ribs on both sides. A dorsoventral incision is made through the diaphragm on the right of the caudal vena cava and on the left of the adhesion with the spleen, and the severed parts of the diaphragm are removed. In the process, the falciform ligament and the round ligament of the liver, still intact in the young animal, can be seen on the right.

A knowledge of the topographic relations of the abdominal organs to the body wall is essential for their examination from the exterior as well as for laparotomy and rectal examination. The abdominal wall is divided into cranial, middle, and caudal regions, and these are subdivided on each side as follows: I. The large **cranial abdominal region** consists of a) left, and b) right caudoventral parts of the costal regions and the hypochondriac regions (covered by the costal cartilages), and c) the xiphoid region between the costal arches. II. The **middle abdominal region** consists of the a) left and b) right lateral abdominal regions (flanks) with the paralumbar fossae, and the c) umbilical region. III. The **caudal abdominal region** consists of right and left inguinal regions and the pubic region. In the costal and hypochondriac regions the intrathoracic abdominal organs are not in contact with the thoracic wall, but are separated from it by the lungs and diaphragm. The rumen extends from the diaphragm to the pelvic inlet. It takes up most the left half of the abdominal cavity. Its extension to the right and toward the pelvic inlet depends on the age of the animal, the kind of feed, and, if pregnant, the stage of gestation. These factors also affect the position and relations of all other abdominal organs.

I. a) In the **left costal** and **hypochondriac regions** the **atrium (3)** and **recess (6) of the rumen** are projected on the thoracic wall, as well as the **spleen (4)**, adherent to the dorsolateral surface of the atrium from the vertebral ends of the 12th and 13th ribs, over the middle of the 10th rib, to the level of the knees of the 7th and 8th ribs. The **reticulum (2)** is in contact with the left abdominal wall in the ventral third of the 6th and 7th intercostal spaces. Near the median plane it may extend caudally as far as the transverse plane of the 9th intercostal space, and ventrally to the level of the xiphoid cartilage. Of the **liver (1)**, only the left border is projected in the narrow space between the diaphragm and reticulum in the ventral 3rd of the 6th intercostal space. The **fundus of the abomasum (5)** lies on the left side between the reticulum and the atrium of the rumen.

I. b) In the **right costal and hypochondriac regions** the **liver (25)**, covered by the diaphragm, and mostly also by the lung, is projected on the thoracic wall, its border forming a caudally convex curve. It lies almost entirely on the right side, including the **left lobe (1)**, **right lobe (25)**, and **caudate process (24)**. It extends from the ventral end of the 6th intercostal space to the dorsal end of the 13th rib. The percussion field of the liver, however, is limited to a zone about a hand's breadth wide along the border of the lung in the last four intercostal spaces.

Ventral to the caudate process is the cranial part of the **descending duodenum (13)** with the **right lobe of the pancreas (15)** in the mesoduodenum. Ventral to the descending duodenum, covered by the **greater omentum**, are cranial loops of the **jejunum (19)** and cranial to them, the **gall bladder (27)** in the ventral part of the 10th intercostal space. Directly cranial to the gall bladder is the **cranial part of the duodenum (26)**, continuous ventrocaudally with the **pylorus**, which varies in position from the ventral end of the 9th to that of the 12th intercostal space.

Cranial to the **pyloric part of the abomasum (28)** is the **omasum (30)**, covered by the lesser omentum, between the transverse planes of the 7th and 11th ribs, but because of its spherical shape, it presses the lesser omentum against the thoracic wall in the 7th–9th intercostal spaces only.

II. a) In the **left lateral abdominal region** only rumen compartments adjoin the abdominal wall. The **dorsolateral abdominal wall** in the region of the **paralumbar fossa** is in contact with the **dorsal sac (7)** and the **caudodorsal blind sac (8)**. The **ventrolateral abdominal wall** is indirectly in contact, through the **superficial wall (21)** of the greater omentum, with the **ventral sac (9)** and the **caudoventral blind sac (10)** of the rumen.

II. b) In the **right lateral abdominal region**, projected from dorsal to ventral on the dorsolateral abdominal wall, are the **right kidney (14)** from the last rib to the 3rd lumbar vertebra, the **right lobe of the pancreas (15)** with the **descending duodenum (13)**, which passes into the **caudal flexure (12)** at the level of the tuber coxae, and immediately caudal to that, the **sigmoid part of the descending colon (11)**. Ventral to the duodenum, in the **supraomental recess (23)** of the greater omentum, are the **proximal loop of the ascending colon (16)** and the **cecum (17)**. The latter extends from the middle of the lumbar region to the pelvic inlet. The apex of the cecum projects caudally from the supraomental recess. (Relations between the descending duodenum and the parts of the large intestine may vary but are not necessarily abnormal.) The **ventrolateral abdominal wall** covers the **pyloric part of the abomasum (28)** ventrally along the right costal arch back to the knee of the 12th rib, and middle and caudal parts of the **jejunum (19)** from the last rib to the plane of the last lumbar vertebra. The jejunum overreaches the greater omentum caudally and passes into the straight **ileum (18)** just ventral to the cecum.

III. Ventrally in the xiphoid region, are the **reticulum (2)** cranially, more on the left than on the right; the **fundus of the abomasum (5)** caudal to the reticulum; the **omasum (30)** ventral to the right costal arch, covered by the lesser omentum, between the transverse planes of the 7th and 11th intercostal spaces; the **fundus of the abomasum** caudal to the reticulum; and the **atrium of the rumen** on the left. Ventrally in the middle abdominal region the **body of the abomasum (29)** lies on the median line with more of it on the left than on the right. At the **angle of the abomasum** the pyloric part (28) curves to the right around the omasum, with the greater curvature crossing the median line at the transverse plane of the last rib. The **jejunum (19)** is caudal to the abomasum on the right as far caudally as the last lumbar vertebra, partly within the supraomental recess. On the left of the median plane, caudally and also slightly to the right, the **ventral sac (9)** and **caudoventral blind sac (10)**, covered by the greater omentum, lie on the abdominal floor.

> Study of the abdominal organs is carried out by the students on both sides of the body at the same time. On the left side the stomach and spleen are studied and the adhesions of the organs with the abdominal wall and with other organs and structures are noted. The interior relations of the compartments of the stomach are exposed by fenestration of the dorsal sac of the rumen from the lumbar transverse processes to the left longitudinal groove of the rumen, and removal of the contents. Prepared demonstrations of the stomach are also studied. On the right side, before the study of the liver and intestines, the special relations of the greater omentum are examined and the omental foramen is explored. Then the superficial wall (21) of the greater omentum is cut ventral and parallel to the descending duodenum, opening the caudal recess of the omental bursa (22). The duodenum with the mesoduodenum and pancreas are carefully reflected dorsally to the ventral surface of the right kidney. After study of the liver and its vessels, nerves, and ducts, the common bile duct, hepatic a., portal v., portal lnn., and nerves are severed at the porta of the liver, and the hepatic ligaments and caudal vena cava, cranial and caudal to the liver, are cut and the liver is removed. After complete transection of the superficial wall down to the pylorus, the deep wall of the greater omentum is cut ventral to the distal loop of the ascending colon and the transverse colon, and the supraomental recess (23) is opened for study of the remaining intestines. The blood vessels, nerves, and lymph nodes are identified with attention to species-specific peculiarities. For final exenteration the duodenum between the cranial and descending parts, and the rectum caudal to the caudal mesenteric a. are double-ligated and cut. Also the cranial and caudal mesenteric aa. ventral to the aorta, and the splenic and gastroduodenal vv. at the portal v. are cut. While separating the mesentery and mesocolon from the dorsal abdominal wall, the intestinal mass is removed from the abdominal cavity and the parts of the intestines are identified on the isolated intestinal tract.

Abdominal cavity and Digestive system

(Left side)

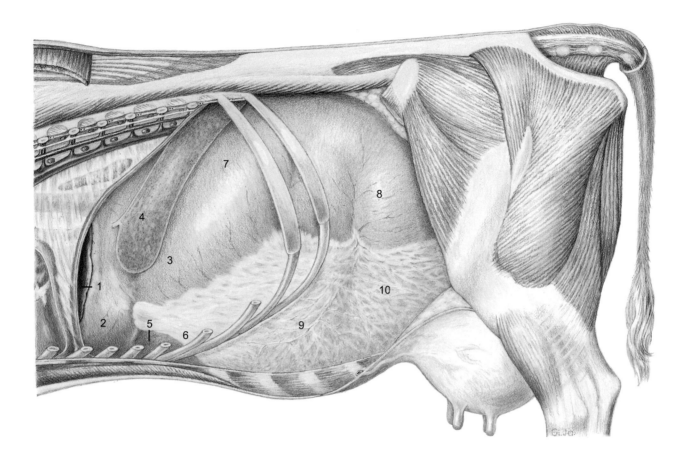

(Right side)

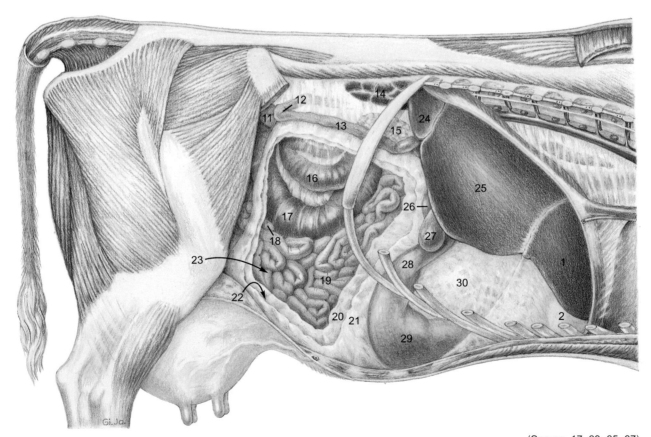

(See pp. 17, 63, 65, 67)

69

3. STOMACH WITH RUMEN, RETICULUM, OMASUM, AND ABOMASUM

The ruminant stomach is one compartmentalized complex stomach which consists of three nonglandular compartments lined with stratified squamous epithelium (rumen, reticulum, and omasum) and one compartment with glandular mucosa (abomasum). The individual compartments all develop from one spindle-shaped gastric primordium like that of the simple stomach. The total capacity of the stomach varies with body size from 100 to 200 l.

At about 18 months the compartments have reached the following approximate percentages of total stomach capacity: rumen 80 percent, reticulum 5 percent, omasum 7 percent, and abomasum 8 percent.* These postmortem measurements on isolated stomachs are not reliable indications of capacity in the live animal.

a) The capacity of the **RUMEN (A)** is 102–148 l. Most of the interior bears **papillae (21)**. Its **parietal surface** lies against the left and ventral abdominal wall and its **visceral surface** is in contact with the intestines, liver, omasum, and abomasum. The wide **ruminoreticular orifice (22)** and close functional relationship has given rise to the term ruminoreticulum. The **dorsal curvature (1)** is adherent to the internal lumbar muscles, right and left crura of the diaphragm, spleen, pancreas, and left adrenal gland. The left kidney with its fat capsule, almost completely surrounded by peritoneum, and pendulous, is pushed over to the right of the median plane by the rumen. The **ventral curvature (2)** lies on the ventral abdominal wall.

The surfaces of the rumen are divided by **right (16)** and **left (3) longitudinal grooves** connected by **cranial (5)** and **caudal (6) grooves** into a **dorsal sac (7)** and a **ventral sac (9)**. The dorsal sac contains a large gas bubble during life and its dorsal wall is free of papillae. The right longitudinal groove gives off dorsally a **right accessory groove (17)** that rejoins the main groove and with it surrounds an elongated bulge, the **insula ruminis (18)**. The left longitudinal groove gives off a dorsal branch, the **left accessory groove (4)**. Dorsal and ventral rumen sacs communicate through the wide **intraruminal orifice (19)**.

At the caudal end of the rumen on both sides the two rumen sacs are divided by **dorsal (11)** and **ventral (12) coronary grooves** from the **caudodorsal (13)** and **caudoventral (14) blind sacs**, both of which extend about the same distance toward the pelvis.

At its cranial end there are no coronary grooves; however the **atrium of the rumen (8)** can be recognized craniodorsal to the cranial groove, and the large **recess of the rumen (10)** is the cranial part of the ventral sac.

The external grooves of the rumen correspond to the internal muscular **pillars (20)** of the same names, covered by nonpapillated mucosa. The **ruminoreticular groove (15)** forms the internal **ruminoreticular fold (23)**.

b) The **RETICULUM (B)** has its cranial **diaphragmatic surface** in contact with the diaphragm and left lobe of the liver. Its caudal **visceral surface** is in contact with the rumen, omasum, and abomasum. Its **greater curvature** lies against the left abdominal wall, while its **lesser curvature** contains the reticular groove. The **fundus of the reticulum** is in the xiphoid region.

The mucosa forms a network of **crests (29)** in three orders of height. The crests contain muscle, are covered with **papillae**, and enclose four- to six-sided **cells (29)**, which become smaller and more irregular toward the reticular groove.

c) The **GASTRIC GROOVE** *is the shortest route between the esophagus and the pylorus. It consists of three segments: the reticular groove, the omasal groove, and the abomasal groove.*

It begins at the **cardia (24)**, which opens caudally, as determined by transruminal palpation in the live ox. Boluses expelled from the esophagus go directly over the ruminoreticular fold (23) into the atrium (8). From the cardia the 15–20 cm long **reticular groove (25)** runs ventrally along the lesser curvature (right wall) of the reticulum. Its muscular **right (26)** and **left (27) lips**, are named for their relation to the cardia, over which they are continuous. As the lips descend, the right lip becomes caudal and the left lip cranial, and they run parallel and straight to the **reticulo-omasal orifice (28)**, where the right lip overlaps the left. The **floor of the reticular groove** has longitudinal folds that increase in height toward the omasum and at the orifice bear long sharp **claw-like papillae** which continue into the omasum.

d) The **OMASUM (C)** is almost spherical with slightly flattened sides and lies on the right on the floor of the intrathoracic part of the abdominal cavity. The **parietal surface** is cranioventrolateral (see p. 69); the **visceral surface** is caudodorsomedial; and the **curvature (30)** is between them facing dorsally, caudally, and to the right. All of the omasum except the ventral part of the parietal surface is covered on the right by the lesser omentum (p. 69, 30). Cranioventrally the **base of the omasum (31)**, containing the omasal groove, contacts the reticulum, rumen, and abomasum. Cranially and dorsolaterally the omasum adjoins the liver, and medially, the rumen. From the externally visible **neck of the omasum** the internal **omasal groove (35)** leads to the **omasoabomasal orifice (36)**. This is bounded by two folds of mucosa, the **vela abomasica (45)**, which are covered on the omasal side by stratified squamous epithelium and on the abomasal side by glandular mucosa. The thick muscular **omasal pillar** runs across the floor of the groove.

About 100 **omasal laminae (32)** in four orders of size project from the curvature and the sides of the omasum toward the omasal groove. The groove and the free borders of the largest laminae form the **omasal canal**. Between the laminae are the **interlaminar recesses (33)**. The laminae are covered by conical **papillae (34)**.

e) The **ABOMASUM** is *thin-walled and capable of great distension and displacement. It has a capacity of up to 28 l. The drawing of the right surface of the stomach (p. 71) shows the organ after removal from the abdominal cavity and inflation, which distorts the relation of abomasum to omasum.* Its **parietal surface** and part of the **greater curvature (37)** lie on the ventral abdominal wall. The caudal part of the greater curvature is separated from the intestines by the greater omentum. The **visceral surface** is in contact with the rumen. The **lesser curvature (38)** bends around the omasum. The **fundus of the abomasum (39)** is a cranial recess in the left xiphoid region. It is continuous with the **body of the abomasum (40)** and both have internal permanent oblique, but not spiral, **abomasal folds (44)** of reddish-gray mucosa containing proper gastric glands. The folds begin at the omasoabomasal orifice and from the sides of the **abomasal groove (46)** and reach their greatest size in the body. The more lateral folds diverge toward the greater curvature, whereas the folds near the abomasal groove run more nearly parallel to it. The folds diminish toward the **pyloric part** which begins at the **angle of the abomasum** and consists of the **pyloric antrum, pyloric canal, and pylorus**. It is lined by wrinkled yellowish mucosa containing pyloric glands.

The **pyloric sphincter (43)** *and the* **torus pyloricus (42)** *that bulges from the lesser curvature into the pylorus can close off the flow from the abomasum to the duodenum.*

The abomasal groove runs along the lesser curvature, bordered by low mucosal folds, from the omasoabomasal orifice to the *pylorus.*

* Getty, 1975

Stomach [Ventriculus]

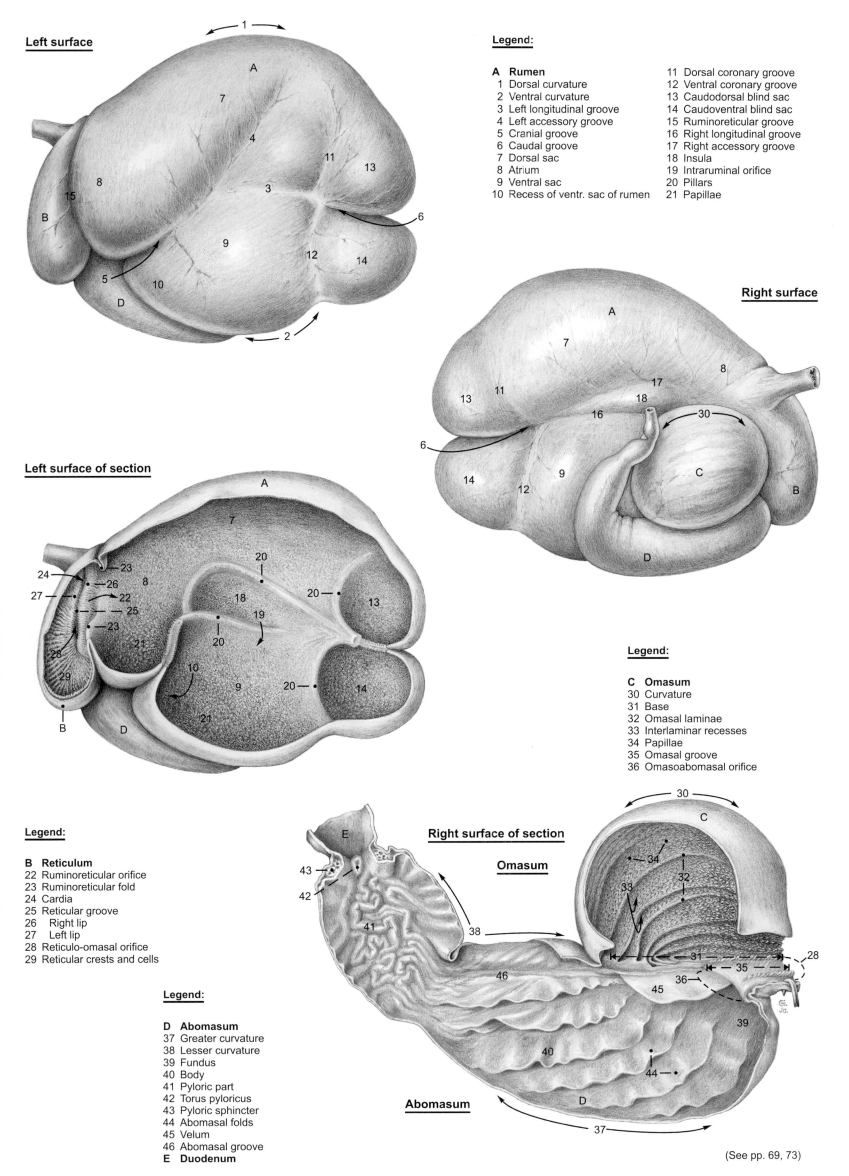

Left surface

1 Dorsal curvature
2 Ventral curvature

Legend:

A Rumen
1 Dorsal curvature
2 Ventral curvature
3 Left longitudinal groove
4 Left accessory groove
5 Cranial groove
6 Caudal groove
7 Dorsal sac
8 Atrium
9 Ventral sac
10 Recess of ventr. sac of rumen

11 Dorsal coronary groove
12 Ventral coronary groove
13 Caudodorsal blind sac
14 Caudoventral blind sac
15 Ruminoreticular groove
16 Right longitudinal groove
17 Right accessory groove
18 Insula
19 Intraruminal orifice
20 Pillars
21 Papillae

Left surface of section

Right surface

Legend:

C Omasum
30 Curvature
31 Base
32 Omasal laminae
33 Interlaminar recesses
34 Papillae
35 Omasal groove
36 Omasoabomasal orifice

Legend:

B Reticulum
22 Ruminoreticular orifice
23 Ruminoreticular fold
24 Cardia
25 Reticular groove
26   Right lip
27   Left lip
28 Reticulo-omasal orifice
29 Reticular crests and cells

Right surface of section

Omasum

Abomasum

Legend:

D Abomasum
37 Greater curvature
38 Lesser curvature
39 Fundus
40 Body
41 Pyloric part
42 Torus pyloricus
43 Pyloric sphincter
44 Abomasal folds
45 Velum
46 Abomasal groove
E Duodenum

(See pp. 69, 73)

71

4. BLOOD SUPPLY AND INNERVATION OF THE STOMACH; LYMPH NODES AND OMENTA

a) The **CELIAC A.** (1) originates from the aorta at the level of the first lumbar vertebra. *It has a relatively long course,* and after giving off phrenic arteries and adrenal branches, divides on the right dorsal surface of the rumen into hepatic, splenic, and left gastric aa. The arteries of the rumen and reticulum correspond to small branches of the splenic and left gastric aa. on the simple stomach.

The **splenic a.** (3) enters the dorsal part of the spleen. Near its origin it gives off the large **right ruminal a.** (4) to the right accessory groove as the main artery of the rumen. This gives off right dorsal and ventral coronary aa., goes through the caudal groove, and comes out on the left side of the rumen, where it gives off left dorsal and ventral coronary aa. and anastomoses with the **left ruminal a.** (5), which passes through the cranial groove of the rumen from right to left. Near its origin it gives off the **reticular a.** (6), which passes over the rumen, then ventrally in the ruminoreticular groove on the left side, and through the groove from left to right. The right and left ruminal aa. may originate either from the splenic or left gastric aa.

The **left gastric a.** (8) supplies the omasum and goes to the lesser curvature of the abomasum, where it anastomoses with the **right gastric a.** (11) from the **hepatic a.** (2). On the greater curvature of the abomasum, the **left** (9) and **right** (12) **gastroepiploic aa.** anastomose. They come from the left gastric a. and the gastroduodenal a. (a br. of the hepatic), respectively. The **accessory reticular a.** (10) arises from the left gastric or from the first part of the left gastroepiploic. It runs dorsally on the diaphragmatic surface of the lesser curvature of the reticulum. The veins, branches of the portal v., have a predominantly corresponding course.

b) The innervation by **AUTONOMIC NERVES** is accomplished in general as in the dog and horse.

The dorsal and ventral trunks of the vagus nn. are of special clinical interest in regulating the functions of each compartment of the stomach. The rumen is innervated mainly by the **dorsal vagal trunk (a)**, but the atrium of the rumen and the other three compartments are innervated by both vagal trunks. Individual brr. of these nerves may vary in location or extent. The dorsal vagal trunk supplies the right side of the atrium (h), the brr. to the celiac plexus (c), the dorsal ruminal brr. (d), and the right ruminal br. (b), which runs back in the right accessory groove, giving brr. to the dorsal and ventral sacs, and passing around in the caudal ruminal groove to the left side. A branch of the dorsal trunk is also given off to the cranial ruminal groove and left longitudinal groove (e) and to the greater curvature of the abomasum (g). Branches of the dorsal trunk (f) pass over the omasum and the visceral side of the lesser curvature of the abomasum, innervating the right lip of the reticular groove, the caudal (visceral) surface of the reticulum, both sides of the omasum, and the visceral surface of the abomasum to the pylorus.

The **ventral vagal trunk (j)** gives branches to the left side of the atrium (l), the diaphragmatic surface of the reticulum (k), and branches that run in the lesser omentum to the liver, cranial part of the duodenum, and pylorus (p). Branches of the ventral trunk (m) innervate the left lip of the reticular groove (see p. 70, c), and continue across the parietal side of the neck of the omasum and run in the lesser omentum along the parietal surface of the base of the omasum and the lesser curvature of the abomasum to the pylorus, innervating the parietal surface of the omasum and abomasum.

c) The **LYMPH NODES** of the stomach and spleen include the following: Celiac lnn. (p. 76, A) 2–5 are found with the cran. mesenteric lnn. (p. 77) at the origin of the aa. of the same names. **Splenic (or atrial) lnn.** (E) 1–7 are grouped dorsocranial to the spleen between the atrium of the rumen and the left crus of the diaphragm. Among the numerous gastric lymph nodes, the **reticuloabomasal (A), ruminoabomasal (B), left ruminal (C), right ruminal (D), cranial ruminal** (not illustrated), **reticular (F), omasal** (not illustrated), **dorsal abomasal (G),** and **ventral abomasal (H)** lie in the grooves and in the omental attachments of the stomach compartments. Their efferent lymphatic vessels go to the splenic nodes or nodes preceding them, gastric trunks, visceral trunks, or the cisterna chyli (p. 74).

d) **OMENTA.** The embryonic dorsal mesogastrium and ventral mesogastrium undergo important changes in form and position with the **development of the four compartments of the stomach.** *After the rotation of the spindle-shaped stomach primordium through about 90° to the left, with the axis of the stomach directed at first from craniodorsal to caudoventral, three protuberances appear on the greater curvature. In craniocaudal order they are the primordia of the rumen, reticulum, and greater curvature of the abomasum. The craniodorsal end of the rumen tube is divided by the future caudal groove into the future dorsal and ventral caudal blind sacs.*

The only protuberance on the lesser curvature is the primordium of the omasum. In the course of further development the reticulum moves cranially; the two blind sacs of the rumen turn dorsally and then caudally, so that cranial and caudal blind sacs become dorsal and ventral. The caudal groove is extended on both sides of the rumen as the right and left longitudinal grooves, and a flexure in the rumen tube becomes the cranial groove. The abomasum approaches the rumen and reticulum, and its greater curvature becomes ventral as it continues the rotation clockwise as viewed from the head. The omasum comes up on the right side.

In spite of these complicated translocations, the attachments of the dorsal and ventral mesogastria to the greater and lesser curvatures of the stomach primordium are maintained. The line of attachment of the **dorsal mesogastrium** on the stomach in the adult runs from the dorsal surface of the esophagus at the hiatus to the right longitudinal groove, through the caudal groove and the left longitudinal groove of the rumen, across a part of the left surface of the atrium and reticulum, and along the greater curvature of the abomasum to the cranial part of the duodenum.

The **greater omentum** (see the lower left figure) with its **deep wall (15)** and **superficial wall (14),** together with the **omental bursa,** is the main derivative of the dorsal mesogastrium. It extends caudally, ventrally, and to the right. **Caudally** near the pelvis, as in the dog, the deep wall is reflected as the supf. wall, forming a fold enclosing the **caudal recess of the omental bursa (16). Ventrally,** because the attachment of the dorsal mesogastrium to the rumen followed the right longitudinal, caudal, and left longitudinal grooves, the ventral sac is enclosed by the greater omentum and forms a part of the wall of the omental bursa. **On the right,** the greater omentum is adherent to the medial surface of the mesoduodenum from the cranial flexure, along the descending part, to the caudal flexure of the duodenum (p. 69, 12). In the sling formed by the deep and supf. walls of the greater omentum between the mesoduodenum and the right longitudinal groove of the rumen, is the **supraomental recess (13),** open caudally and containing the bulk of the intestines. The deep wall of the greater omentum passes from the mesoduodenum, ventral to the intestines, to its attachment in the right longitudinal groove of the rumen, whereas the supf. wall passes ventral to the intestines and the ventral sac of the rumen to the left longitudinal groove. Both walls of the omentum meet in the caudal groove. Cranial parts of the dorsal mesogastrium disappear or are shortened in the adult by expansion of the atrium and adhesion with its surroundings. The spleen on the left and the left lobe of the pancreas are held between the rumen and the diaphragm by adhesions. The line of origin of the dorsal mesogastrium is displaced to the right and runs obliquely craniocaudally from the level of the esophageal hiatus through the origin of the celiac a. to the level of the distal loop of the ascending colon.

The **ventral mesogastrium** is divided by the developing liver into the **lesser omentum** on the visceral surface of the liver and the **falciform lig.** (see p. 75, 13) on the diaphragmatic surface. The lesser omentum extends, as the **hepatogastric lig.,** from the porta of the liver ventrally to the esophageal hiatus, the lesser curvature of the reticulum, the base of the omasum, and the lesser curvature of the abomasum, covering the right surface of the omasum (p. 69, 30). The lesser omentum ends as a free border, the **hepatoduodenal lig.,** from the porta of the liver to the cranial flexure of the duodenum. It contains the portal vein and forms the ventral border of the **omental (epiploic) foramen,** which leads to the **vestibule of the omental bursa.** The vestibule opens into the caudal recess.

Gastric Vessels, Nerves, and Lymph nodes

(Left surface)

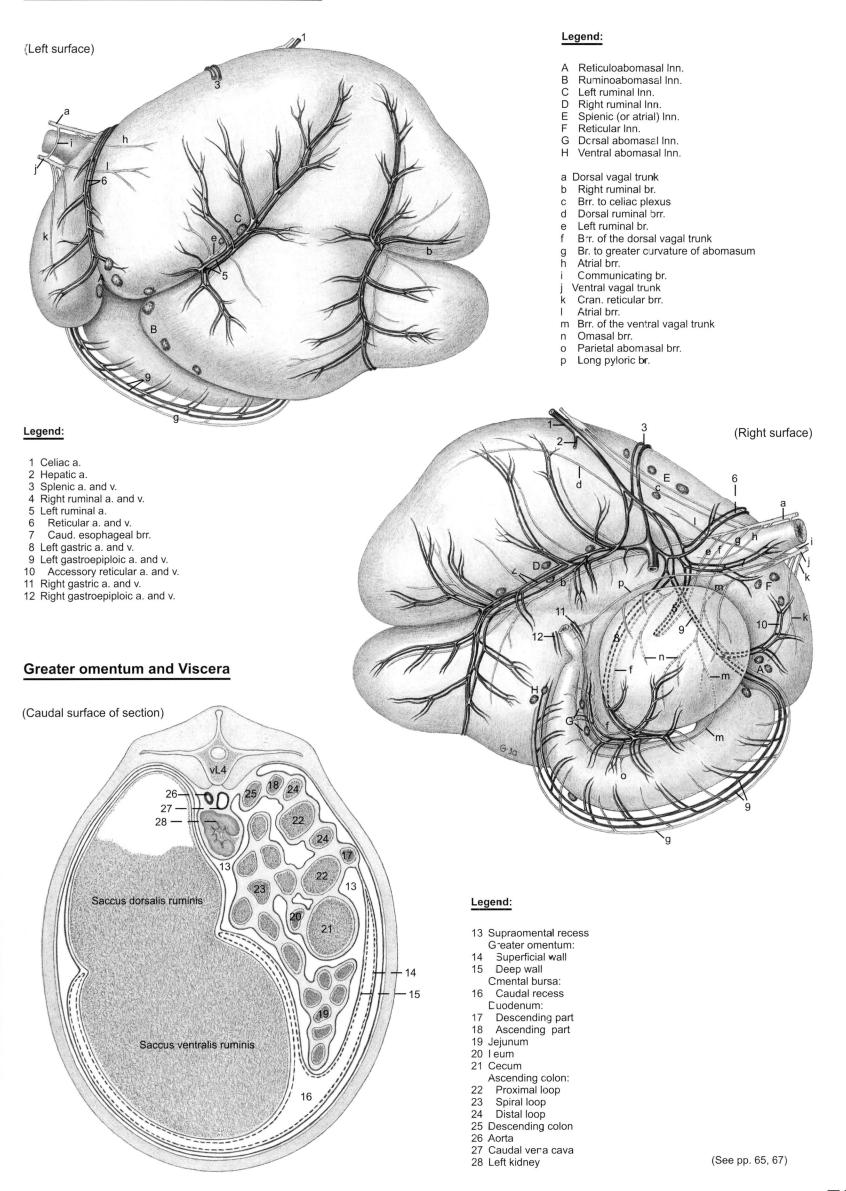

Legend:

A Reticuloabomasal lnn.
B Ruminoabomasal lnn.
C Left ruminal lnn.
D Right ruminal lnn.
E Splenic (or atrial) lnn.
F Reticular lnn.
G Dorsal abomasal lnn.
H Ventral abomasal lnn.

a Dorsal vagal trunk
b Right ruminal br.
c Brr. to celiac plexus
d Dorsal ruminal brr.
e Left ruminal br.
f Brr. of the dorsal vagal trunk
g Br. to greater curvature of abomasum
h Atrial brr.
i Communicating br.
j Ventral vagal trunk
k Cran. reticular brr.
l Atrial brr.
m Brr. of the ventral vagal trunk
n Omasal brr.
o Parietal abomasal brr.
p Long pyloric br.

(Right surface)

Legend:

1 Celiac a.
2 Hepatic a.
3 Splenic a. and v.
4 Right ruminal a. and v.
5 Left ruminal a.
6 Reticular a. and v.
7 Caud. esophageal brr.
8 Left gastric a. and v.
9 Left gastroepiploic a. and v.
10 Accessory reticular a. and v.
11 Right gastric a. and v.
12 Right gastroepiploic a. and v.

Greater omentum and Viscera

(Caudal surface of section)

Legend:

13 Supraomental recess
Greater omentum:
14 Superficial wall
15 Deep wall
Omental bursa:
16 Caudal recess
Duodenum:
17 Descending part
18 Ascending part
19 Jejunum
20 Ileum
21 Cecum
Ascending colon:
22 Proximal loop
23 Spiral loop
24 Distal loop
25 Descending colon
26 Aorta
27 Caudal vena cava
28 Left kidney

(See pp. 65, 67)

73

5. SPLEEN, LIVER, PANCREAS, AND LYMPH NODES

a) The **SPLEEN** is relatively small, red-brown in the bull and blue-gray in the cow. It is up to 50 cm long and its average weight varies with sex, age, and body size from 390 to 2000 g. It is an elongated oval, tongue-shaped organ of about equal width throughout. Its position is almost vertical (see p. 69, 4). The **dorsal end (2)** is near the vertebral column and the **ventral end (6)** is a hand's breadth dorsal to the 7th–8th costochondral junction. The **cranial (4) and caudal (5) borders** are rounded in the bull, acute in the cow. The spleen does not extend caudal to the line of pleural reflection. The **diaphragmatic surface** is applied to the diaphragm; the **visceral surface**, dorsomedially to the atrium of the rumen and cranioventrally to the reticulum. Both surfaces of the dorsal part are more or less extensively fused with the surroundings, so that a **phrenicosplenic lig. (1)** and a **gastrosplenic lig.** are only vestigial. The rather small **hilus (3)** is in the dorsal third of the cranial border in the area of adhesion to the rumen.

b) The **LIVER** reaches its adult size by the third year and after that its weight ranges from 4–10 kg depending on breed, age, and nutritional condition. The weight is relatively greater in the calf. Its color varies from yellowish in the calf to reddish-brown in the adult. *Because of the enlargement of the rumen it is almost entirely displaced to the right (see p. 69), except for a small portion ventral to the esophagus.*

The right lobe is caudodorsal and the left lobe is cranioventral. The thick **dorsal border (28)** *is almost in the median plane.* Here the caudal vena cava (h) runs in a groove inclined ventrally to the foramen venae cavae. Between the caudate lobe and the left lobe is the esophageal impression (w), distinct only in fixed livers. The acute **ventral border (27)** *is caudoventral on the right.* The fixed specimen shows a large omasal impression (q) and ventral to it, a reticular impression (r). In contrast to the dog and horse the liver is not distinctly lobated. Except for the **fissure for the round ligament (p)**, *interlobar notches are absent.* The **left lobe (26)** is not divided. The gallbladder fossa separates the **right lobe (17)**, undivided as in the horse, from the **quadrate lobe (22)**. The **caudate lobe** lies between the vena cava and the left (intrahepatic) branch of the portal vein. As in the dog it has a **papillary process (24)**, which overlaps the left branch of the portal vein. The short **caudate process (15)** overlaps the right lobe and is partially fused with it. Together they form the renal impression for the cranial end of the right kidney. On the visceral surface is the **porta hepatis** where the portal v., hepatic a., and autonomic nn. enter the liver, and the bile-carrying hepatic duct and lymph vessels leave the liver. Of the hepatic ligaments, the **right triangular lig. (7)** goes to the dorsal abdominal wall, and dorsomedial to it, the **hepato-renal lig. (8)** connects the caudate process to the right kidney. The **left triangular lig. (14)** is found on the diaphragm near the esophageal hiatus. The **coronary lig. (21)** attaches the liver to the diaphragm and connects the triangular ligg. and the falciform lig. Its line of attachment to the liver passes from the left triangular lig. around ventral to the caud. v. cava and along the right side of the caud. v. cava. On the right lobe it divides into two laminae that surround the **area nuda (16)**. The **falciform lig. (13)** with the **round lig.** in its free border is attached to the diaphragmatic surface of the liver on a line from the coronary lig. at the foramen venae cavae to the fissure for the round lig. It is attached to the diaphragm on a horizontal line from the foramen venae cavae to the costochondral junction. Unlike that of the horse, it does not go to the umbilicus. The diaphragmatic attachment is a secondary adhesion resulting from the displacement of the liver to the right, and in many adults the falciform and round ligg. have disappeared. The **gallbladder (25)** is pear-shaped with a total length of 10–15 cm. It extends beyond the ventral (right) border of the liver. The right and left hepatic ducts join to form the **common hepatic duct (18)**, which receives the **cystic duct (20)** and becomes the short, wide **common bile duct (19, ductus choledochus)**, which opens into the duodenum about 60 cm from the pylorus on the oblique **greater duodenal papilla**. Hepatocystic ducts open directly into the gall bladder.

c) *The main duct of the bovine* **PANCREAS** *is the* **accessory pancreatic duct (m)**, *which opens in the descending duodenum 30–40 cm from the greater duodenal papilla. The pancreatic duct is represented in the ox by small ducts that open into the common hepatic duct in its course across the pancreas.* The **left lobe (10)** extends to the spleen and is attached by connective tissue to the rumen and the left crus of the diaphragm. The **body of the pancreas**

(12) lies between the liver and the omasum ventral to the portal vein, which passes dorsally through the **pancreatic notch (11)** to the liver. The **right lobe (9)** is enclosed in the mesoduodenum descendens and extends to the plane of the right kidney.

d) The **LYMPH NODES** of the spleen, liver, and pancreas.

The **1–7 splenic lnn.** (p. 73) lie dorsocranial to the spleen between the atrium of the rumen and the left crus of the diaphragm, and *are regularly examined in meat inspection.*

The **6–15 hepatic (portal) lnn. (23)** are grouped around the porta of the liver and *are regularly examined in meat inspection.* The **accessory hepatic lnn. (29)** are found on the dorsal border of the liver near the caudal vena cava. The outflow of lymph occurs, together with that of the dorsal and ventral abomasal lnn., through the hepatic trunk. The **pancreaticoduodenal lnn.** (see p. 76, I) lie between the pancreas and descending duodenum and between the pancreas and transverse colon.

The lymph drainage is through the **intestinal trunk (A)** which joins the **hepatic trunk (B)**, and after receiving the **gastric trunk (C)** with lymph from the stomach and spleen, becomes the **visceral trunk (D)** and enters the **cisterna chyli (E)**. The valveless cisterna chyli receives the **lumbar trunk (F)**, which drains the lymph from the pelvic limbs, genital organs, and the pelvis.

The **thoracic duct (G)**, *emerging cranially from the cisterna chyli, passes in the ox through a slit in the muscle of the right crus of the diaphragm into the thorax. It does not pass through the aortic hiatus as in the horse and dog.* For lymph nodes of the pelvic cavity, see also pp. 82–83.

Lymph nodes and Lymphatic vessels*

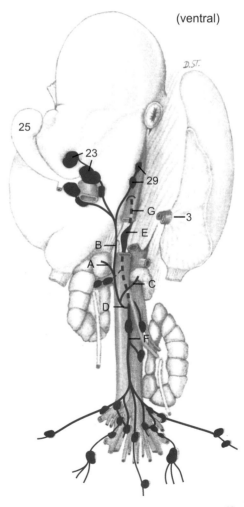

(ventral)

(See p. 82)

* see also Baum, 1912

Spleen, Liver, and Pancreas (Abdominal surface of diaphragm)

(dorsal)

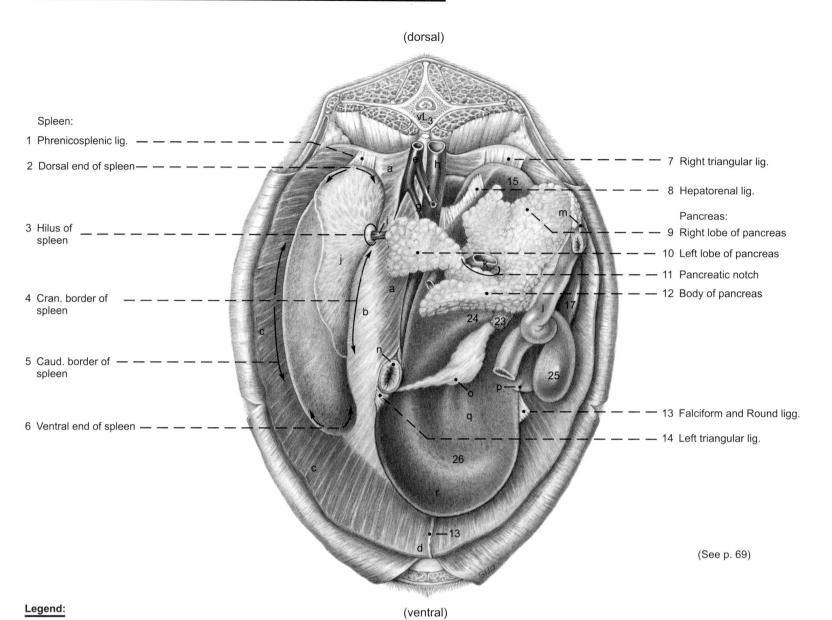

Spleen:
1 Phrenicosplenic lig.
2 Dorsal end of spleen
3 Hilus of spleen
4 Cran. border of spleen
5 Caud. border of spleen
6 Ventral end of spleen

7 Right triangular lig.
8 Hepatorenal lig.

Pancreas:
9 Right lobe of pancreas
10 Left lobe of pancreas
11 Pancreatic notch
12 Body of pancreas

13 Falciform and Round ligg.
14 Left triangular lig.

(See p. 69)

(ventral)

Legend:

Diaphragm:	e Aorta	j Splenico-ruminal adhesion
a Lumbar part	f Cran. mesenteric a.	k Portal v.
b Tendinous center	g Celiac a.	l Duodenum
c Costal part	h Caud. vena cava	m Accessory pancreatic duct
d Sternal part	i Splenic a. and v.	n Esophagus

o Lesser omentum	t Right gastric a.
p Fissure for round lig.	u Gastroduodenal a.
q Omasal impression	v Renal impression
r Reticular impression	w Esophageal impression
s Hepatic a.	(cut edge)

Liver

(Visceral surface)

(Diaphragmatic surface)

15 Caudate proc.
16 Bare area (Area nuda)
17 Right lobe
18 Common hepatic duct
19 Common bile duct (Ductus choledochus)
20 Cystic duct
21 Coronary lig.
22 Quadrate lobe
23 Hepatic lnn.
24 Papillary proc.
25 Gallbladder
26 Left lobe
27 Ventral border
28 Dorsal border

75

6. INTESTINES WITH BLOOD VESSELS AND LYMPH NODES

a) The **INTESTINAL TRACT** *is displaced to the right half of the abdominal cavity by the enormous expansion of the stomach, primarily the rumen, on the left. Most of the intestines, attached by the mesentery, lie in the supraomental recess. The intestinal tract has considerable length – 33–59 m, whereas the lumen, especially of the large intestine, is small compared to the horse.*

The **small intestine** has a total length of 27–49 m. The **duodenum** begins ventrally on the right at the pylorus with the **cranial part (1)**, which runs dorsally to the porta of the liver. Here it forms the **sigmoid flexure (1)**, turns caudally at the **cranial flexure**, and continues as the **descending part of the duodenum (2)** (see also p. 69). This runs caudodorsally, accompanied at first by the right lobe of the pancreas, to the plane of the tuber coxae. Here it turns sharply medially around the caudal border of the mesentery at the **caudal flexure (3)**, and continues cranially as the **ascending part of the duodenum (4)**. The **descending colon (17)** is dorsal to the ascending duodenum and adherent to it. The caudal free border of this adhesion is the **duodenocolic fold (5)**. Under the left lobe of the pancreas and on the left side of the cranial mesenteric a., the ascending duodenum passes through the duodenojejunal flexure into the **jejunum (6)**. This surrounds the disc of the coiled colon like a wreath. It begins cranially at the liver and pancreas and runs caudoventrally through many loops until it passes without a clear boundary into the ileum cranial to the pelvic inlet. The *caudal part, called the "flange" is of clinical significance because of its longer mesentery.* The **ileum (7)** is described as the part of the small intestine attached to the **ileocecal fold (8)**, *but in the ox the fold extends on the left side of the mesentery to the apex of the flange.* *There-fore by this definition the bovine ileum has a convoluted part as well as the 1 m long straight part near the cecum.* The ileum opens into the large intestine at the **ileal orifice**, on the **ileal papilla** (p. 77, lower figure) which marks the boundary between the cecum and colon at the transverse plane of the 4th lumbar vertebra.

The **large intestine** including the cecum, colon, and rectum has neither bands nor sacculations, unlike that of the horse. The **cecum** is cylindrical, 50–70 cm long, and slightly curved. It lies in the dorsal part of the right abdominal cavity and extends to the pelvic inlet with a free, rounded blind **apex (10)**. The **body of the cecum (9)** is attached by the common mesentery to the proximal and distal loops of the colon, and is *continuous with the colon, with no change in the lumen,* at the cecocolic orifice (p. 77, lower figure). The **colon** is about 7–9.5 m long, and consists of the ascending colon, transverse colon, and descending colon.* The **ascending colon**, the longest part of the large intestine, has three parts. The **proximal loop (11)** runs cranially for a short distance to the plane of the right kidney, where it doubles back dorsal to the first part and the cecum. It then turns mediodorsally around the caudal border of the mesentery and runs cranially on the left side of the mesentery. Near the left kidney it becomes narrower and turns ventrally into the elliptical coil formed by the **spiral loop**. This is variable, but usually consists of 1.5–2 **centripetal gyri (12)**, the **central flexure (13)**, and the same number of **centrifugal gyri (14)**. The last (outer)

centrifugal gyrus passes into the narrow **distal loop (15)** at the plane of the first lumbar vertebra. The distal loop runs first dorso-caudally on the left side of the mesentery, ventral to the ascending duodenum and dorsal to the proximal loop. At the plane of the 5th lumbar vertebra it turns sharply around the caudal border of the mesentery and runs forward on the right to the short **transverse colon (16)**. It turns around the cranial mesenteric a. from right to left and becomes the **descending colon (17)** that runs caudally ventral to the vertebral column. Its fat-filled mesocolon lengthens at the last lumbar vertebra, and the **sigmoid colon (18)** forms at the pelvic inlet. The **rectum (19)** begins at the pelvic inlet with a shortened mesorectum, but no structural transition.

b) The MESENTERY. The derivatives of the primitive dorsal mesentery that are attached to the parts of the small and large intestines are fused in the intestinal mass to form a **common mesentery**. Only the transverse and sigmoid colons have a free mesocolon. The proximal and distal loops and the cranial part of the descending colon are adherent to the cranial part of the cecum and ascending duodenum in a fat-filled mass around the root of the mesentery.

c) The BLOOD SUPPLY to the intestines comes from the cranial and caudal mesenteric aa. The long **cran. mesenteric a. (a)** gives off **pancreatic brr.** directly to the right lobe of the pancreas, and the **caud. pancreaticoduodenal a. (b)**. It also gives off the **middle colic a. (c)** directly. From the proximal part of the **ileocolic a. (d)** the **right colic aa. (e)** are given off to the distal loop of the colon and to the centrifugal gyri. From the distal part of the ileocolic a. the **colic branches (f)** go to the proximal loop of the colon and the centripetal gyri. All of the arteries of the spiral loop may originate from the ileocolic a. by a common trunk. They anastomose via collateral branches. The **cecal a. (g)** passes to the left of the ileocecal junction into the ileocecal fold and can give off an **antimesenteric ileal branch (h)**, which is constant in the dog. *In addition, the cranial mesenteric a. gives off a large* **collateral branch (i)**, *peculiar to the ox, that runs in the jejunal mesentery along the last centrifugal gyrus, to which it gives branches, and rejoins the cranial mesenteric a.* Both give off **jejunal aa. (f')** and finally anastomose with the **ileal aa. (k)**. The **mesenteric ileal branch (h')** from the ileocolic a. or cecal a. also supplies several branches to the neighboring parts of the spiral colon. The **caudal mesenteric a. (l)** gives off the **left colic a. (m)** to the descending colon, and the **cranial rectal a. (n)** and **sigmoidal aa. (o)**. The **portal v.** and its main branches are generally similar to those of the horse and dog. The veins predominantly follow the course of the corresponding arteries.

d) The LYMPH NODES. The **cranial mesenteric and celiac lnn. (A)** lie at the origin of the cranial mesenteric a. The *following are regularly examined in meat inspection:* the **jejunal lnn. (E)** are in the mesentery of the jejunum and ileum *near the intestinal border,* unlike the dog and horse. The **cecal lnn. (D)** are inconstant. Three groups of **colic lnn. (C)** are most numerous on the right surface of the spiral loop; others are present on the proximal and distal loops. The **caudal mesenteric lnn. (B)** are on the sides of the descending colon. The lymph drainage goes into the cisterna chyli.

Lymph nodes and Lymphatic vessels

Legend:

A   Celiac and cran. mesenteric lnn.
B   Caud. mesenteric lnn.
C   Colic lnn.
D   Cecal lnn.
E   Jejunal lnn.
F   Aortic lumbar lnn.
G   Proper lumbar lnn.
H   Renal lnn.
I   Pancreaticoduodenal lnn.
K   Anorectal lnn.
L   Gastric trunk
M   Hepatic trunk
N   Intestinal trunk
O   Cisterna chyli
P   Thoracic duct
Q   Lumbar trunk
R   Visceral trunk

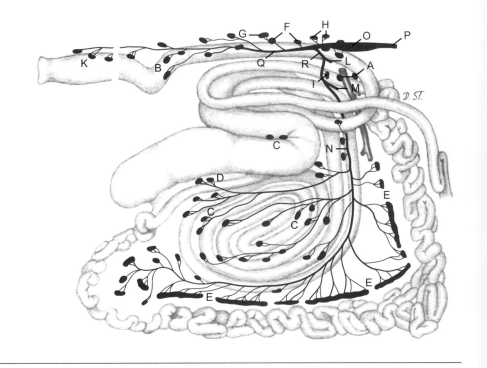

76

* Smith, 1984
** see also Baum, 1912

Intestines (Right surface)

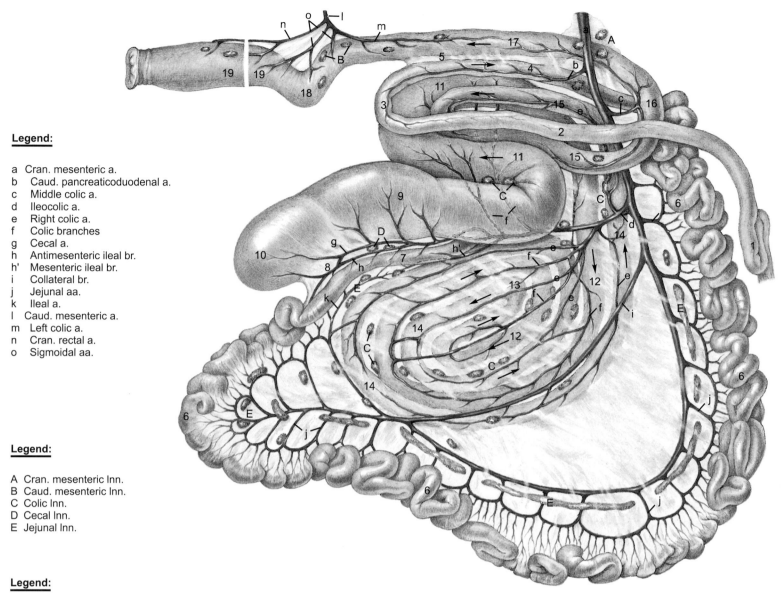

Legend:

a   Cran. mesenteric a.
b   Caud. pancreaticoduodenal a.
c   Middle colic a.
d   Ileocolic a.
e   Right colic a.
f   Colic branches
g   Cecal a.
h   Antimesenteric ileal br.
h' Mesenteric ileal br.
i   Collateral br.
j   Jejunal aa.
k   Ileal a.
l   Caud. mesenteric a.
m   Left colic a.
n   Cran. rectal a.
o   Sigmoidal aa.

Legend:

A   Cran. mesenteric lnn.
B   Caud. mesenteric lnn.
C   Colic lnn.
D   Cecal lnn.
E   Jejunal lnn.

Legend:

Duodenum:
1   Cran. part and
    Sigmoid loop
2   Descending part
3   Caud. flexure
4   Ascending part
5   Duodenocolic fold

6   **Jejunum**
7   **Ileum**
8   Ileocecal fold
    Cecum:
9   Body of cecum
10 Apex of cecum

Colon:
   Ascending colon:
11   Prox. loop of colon
     Spiral loop of colon
12   Centripetal gyri
13   Central flexure
14   Centrifugal gyri

15   Distal loop of colon
16   **Transverse colon**
17   **Descending colon**
18   Sigmoid colon
19   **Rectum**

Cecum, Ileum, and Prox. loop of colon (cut open)

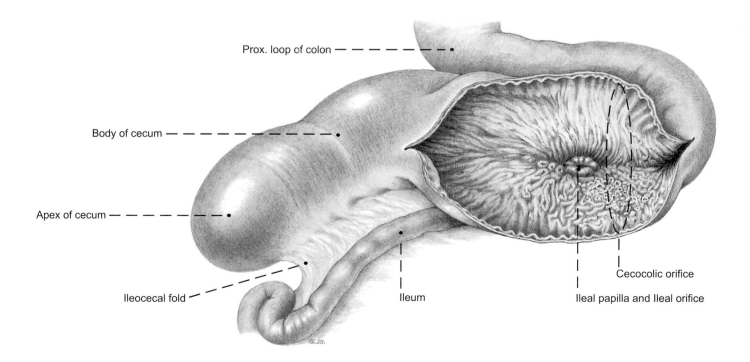

Prox. loop of colon

Body of cecum

Apex of cecum

Ileocecal fold

Ileum

Cecocolic orifice

Ileal papilla and Ileal orifice

77

CHAPTER 8: PELVIC CAVITY AND INGUINAL REGION, INCLUDING URINARY AND GENITAL ORGANS

1. PELVIC GIRDLE WITH THE SACROSCIATIC LIG. AND SUPERFICIAL STRUCTURES IN THE PUBIC AND INGUINAL REGIONS

a) The **PELVIC GIRDLE** consists of the two hip bones (ossa coxarum), each composed of the fused ilium, pubis, and ischium. The two hip bones are joined in the pelvic symphysis, which ossifies progressively with age.

I. On the **ilium** the **tuber coxae (13)** *is thick in the middle and undivided*, and the **gluteal surface (17)** *faces dorsolaterally*. The **wing of the ilium (10)** is broad, but smaller than in the horse. On the **sacropelvic surface (18)** the **auricular surface (19)** and the **iliac surface (20)** *are separated by a sharp crest*.

II. On the **ischium** the **ischial tuber (28)** has three processes, and the **ischial arch (29)** is deep.

III. The right and left **pubic bones** join in the pubic symphysis to form a **ventral pubic tubercle (35)** and an *elongated* **dorsal pubic tubercle (35')**. The **iliopubic eminence (34)** *is an imposing large rough tubercle*. The **pelvic symphysis (1)** is composed of the pubic symphysis and the ischial symphysis. *The latter is marked by a ventral* **symphyseal crest (1')** *with a prominent caudal tubercle*. The **sciatic spine (7)** *is high, with a sharp edge, and inclined slightly medially*. In the **acetabulum (3)** the **lunar surface (6)** *is divided by an additional cranioventral notch into a lateral* **greater part (6')** *and a medial* **lesser part (6")**. The **oval obturator foramen (2)** *is especially large, with a sharp margin*. The pelvic floor slopes medioventrally, is excavated by a deep transverse trough, and rises caudodorsally. Sexual dimorphism is not as striking as in the horse. The transverse trough is broader in the cow.

Hip bone

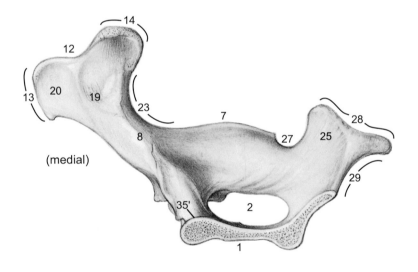

(medial)

The bony pelvis is the solid framework of the birth canal which is evaluated by measurements (pelvimetry). The **transverse diameter** between the right and left **psoas tubercles (22)** is significant because constriction occuring there is a hindrance to the birth process. The **vertical diameter** extends from the cranial end of the pelvic symphysis to the dorsal wall of the pelvis. The farther caudally the vertical diameter meets the dorsal wall, the more this tight passage in the birth canal can be enlarged by drawing the pelvic floor cranially. (The pelvic ligg. are relaxed in parturition.) On the whole, the pelvis of the cow is not as well adapted to parturition as that of the mare.

b) The **SACROSCIATIC LIGAMENT (LIG. SACROTUBERALE LATUM)** *extends from the lateral part of the sacrum to the ilium and ischium*. The cranial part is attached to the **sciatic spine (7)** as far as the **greater sciatic notch (23)**. Ventral to the sacral tuber it leaves the **greater sciatic foramen (A)** free for passage of the sciatic nerve and the cranial gluteal a., v., and n. The caudal (sacrotuberous) part of the ligament extends to the dorsal process of the tripartite **ischial tuber (28)**. Cranial to that, in the **lesser sciatic notch (27)**, is the **lesser sciatic foramen (B)** for the passage of the caudal gluteal a. and v. Because of *the absence of vertebral heads of the caudal thigh muscles*, the caudal part of the sacrosciatic lig. is the dorsolateral boundary of the ischiorectal fossa between the root of the tail and the ischial tuber. The fossa is also present in the dog, but not in the horse.

c) **SUPERFICIAL STRUCTURES IN THE PUBIC AND INGUINAL REGIONS**

The **intertendinous fossa (2)**, *open ventrally, is cranial to the ventral pubic tubercle and contains the terminal part of the linea alba (b). The fossa lies between bilateral semiconical pillars converging toward the symphyseal tendon at the apex of the prepubic tendon. These pillars are covered by the yellow abdominal tunic (a) and are formed by the abdominal tendons of the external oblique muscles sheathing the ventral borders of the rectus tendons. The latter fuse and terminate in the symphyseal tendon and on the symphyseal* **crest (1')**.

Sacrosciatic ligament

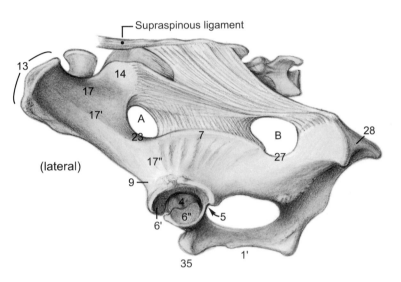

Supraspinous ligament

(lateral)

The **gracilis muscles (5)** originate mainly from the symphyseal tendon. The **external pudendal a. and v. (1)** pass through the **superficial inguinal ring (8)** as in the dog and horse. The caudomedial angle of the ring is close to the median plane.

The **lacuna vasorum (9)** is a space between the caud. border of the pelvic tendon of the ext. oblique and the ilium. It conducts the **femoral a. and v. (4)** through its lateral part *and the caudal (larger) head of the* **sartorius (14)** *through its medial part. Cranial and caudal heads of the muscle embrace the femoral vessels and then unite below them to form a single muscle belly. The femoral a. and v. and saphenous n. pass laterally through the sartorius into the* **femoral triangle** (p. 18, a) *and are therefore covered medially by the muscle and not by fascia alone as in the dog and horse*. (The lacuna vasorum was formerly called the femoral ring, and the femoral triangle was called the femoral canal by many veterinary anatomists, but the terms femoral ring and femoral canal are preempted for their meaning in human anatomy: the ring is in the medial angle of the lacuna vasorum, covered by transversalis fascia and peritoneum, and leads to the canal, which is only 1.25 cm long in man and contains nothing but fat and a lymph node. In adult domestic mammals the femoral ring is usually obscured by the **deep femoral (h)** and **pudendoepigastric (g) vessels**.) The large deep femoral vessels (h) usually originate from the external iliac vessels, give off the pudendoepigastric trunk and vein (g) in the abdominal cavity (p. 81, s, t), and pass out through the medial part of the lacuna vasorum, but the origin of the deep femoral vessels is variable. They may come from the femoral vessels in the femoral triangle, so that the pudendoepigastric a. and v. must pass back into the abdominal cavity through the femoral ring to reach the inguinal canal. They divide into the **caudal epigastric a. and v.** (p. 81, u) and the external pudendal a. and v. (1). The latter vessels always exit through the inguinal canal.

Through the **lacuna musculorum (10)** between the inguinal lig. and the ilium pass the iliopsoas, *the smaller cranial head of the* **sartorius (14)**, the **femoral n. (13)**, divided into its branches, and the **saphenous n. (6)**. Ventrally the lacuna musculorum is covered by the yellow abdominal tunic and by the tendinous **femoral lamina (12)** from the **external oblique (7)**, as in the horse.

Bones of the pelvic girdle

Hip bone (Os coxae)
Pelvic symphysis (1)
  Symphysial crest (1')
Obturator foramen (2)
Acetabulum (3)
  Acetabular fossa (4)
  Acetabular notch (5)
  Lunar surface (6)
    Greater part (6')
    Lesser part (6")
Sciatic spine (7)

Ilium
Body of the ilium (8)
  Ventr. caud. iliac spine (9)
Wing of the ilium (10)
  Iliac crest (12)
    Tuber coxae (13)
  Sacral tuber (14)
  Gluteal surface (17)
    Ventr. gluteal line (17')
    Caud. gluteal line (17")
  Sacropelvic surface (18)
    Auricular surface (19)
    Iliac surface (20)
Arcuate line (21)
  Tubercle of psoas minor (22)
Greater sciatic notch (23)

Ischium
Body of the ischium (24)
Tabula of the ischium (25)
Ramus of the ischium (26)
  Symphysial surface
Lesser sciatic notch (27)
Ischial tuber (28)
Ischial arch (29)

Pubis
Body of the pubis (30)
Caud. ramus of the pubis (31)
  Symphysial surface
Cran. ramus of the pubis (32)
Pecten pubis (33)
Iliopubic eminence (34)
Ventr. pubic tubercle (35)
Dors. pubic tubercle (35')

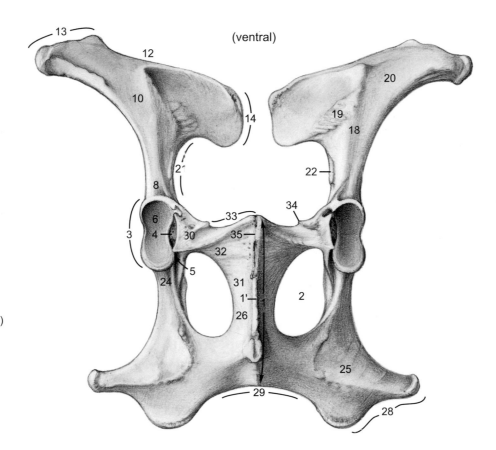

(ventral)

Pubic and inguinal regions

Legend:

a Yellow abdominal tunic
b Linea alba
c Cremaster m. and cranial br. of genitofemoral n.
d Tunica vaginalis

e Transversalis fascia
f Transverse acetabular lig.
g Pudendoepigastric a. and v.
h Deep femoral a. and v.

i Pectineus (and long adductor)
j Cran. femoral a. and v.
k Vastus medialis
l Rectus femoris

m Tensor fasciae latae
n Deep circumflex iliac a.
    and v. and lat. cut. femoral n.
o Internal oblique m.

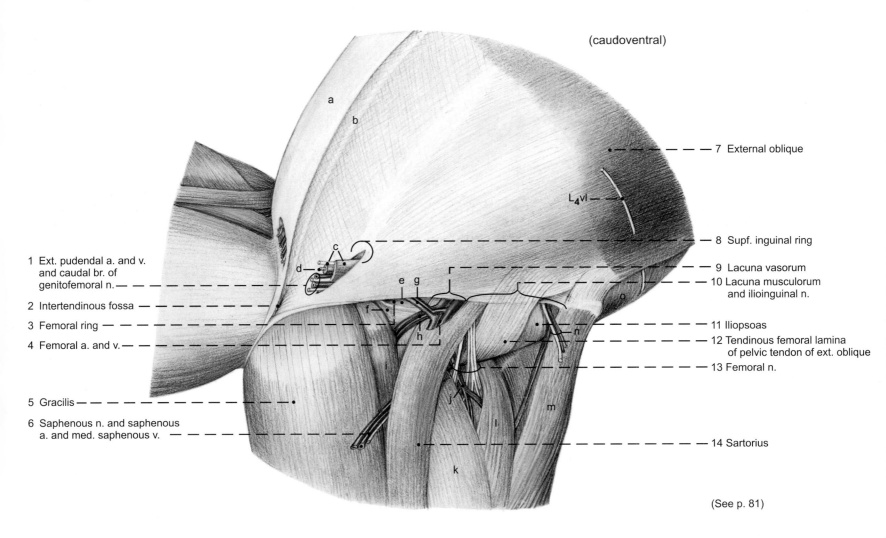

(caudoventral)

1 Ext. pudendal a. and v. and caudal br. of genitofemoral n.
2 Intertendinous fossa
3 Femoral ring
4 Femoral a. and v.
5 Gracilis
6 Saphenous n. and saphenous a. and med. saphenous v.

7 External oblique
8 Supf. inguinal ring
9 Lacuna vasorum
10 Lacuna musculorum and ilioinguinal n.
11 Iliopsoas
12 Tendinous femoral lamina of pelvic tendon of ext. oblique
13 Femoral n.
14 Sartorius

(See p. 81)

2. INGUINAL REGION WITH INGUINAL CANAL, INGUINAL LIG., AND PREPUBIC TENDON

a) The **INGUINAL CANAL** extends from the **deep inguinal ring** (13) to the **superficial inguinal ring** (8). In the bull the **vaginal tunic** (18) with its contents and the **cremaster muscle** (19) pass through the canal. *In the cow the vaginal tunic and the cremaster are absent. The round lig. of the uterus, unlike that of the bitch and mare, ends on the internal surface of the abdominal wall near the inguinal canal without passing through it.* In both sexes, the inguinal canal, as in the dog and horse, conducts the external pudendal a. and v., the lymphatics, and the **genital branch of the genitofemoral n.** from L2, L3, L4. The latter is divided into **cranial** (19) and **caudal** (11) **branches.** *In the ox the angles of the deep inguinal ring are medial and dorsolateral; whereas those of the superficial ring are caudal and cranial.* The distance between the inguinal rings is much shorter medially than craniolaterally.

The length of the inguinal canal, as in the horse, is about 15 cm from the dorsolateral angle of the deep ring to the caudal angle of the superficial ring.

I. The **skin** is not involved in the formation of the inguinal canal. It is continuous with the skin of the scrotum or vulva.

II. The **yellow abdominal tunic** (7) is the deep elastic lamina of the external fascia of the trunk. At the level of the superficial inguinal ring it gives off the *elastic* **external spermatic fascia** (7'), *reinforces both angles of the ring*, and ensheathes the structures that pass through the ring. In the bull the **caudal preputial muscle** (see p. 66) *originates on the deep (spermatic) fascia mainly lateral to the vaginal tunic.* In the cow the yellow abdominal tunic forms the medial laminae and part of the lateral laminae of the **suspensory apparatus of the udder** (see p. 88). In the bull it gives off the **fundiform lig.** (from Latin: *funda* = sling): bilateral elastic bands that pass around the penis and blend with the scrotal septum. From the fascia on the lateral crus of the superficial inguinal ring, the **fascial femoral lamina** (10)* is given off toward the thigh as in the horse. *In the bull it is thick and elastic; in the cow it is thin and collagenous.* In the inguinal groove the fascia passes to the medial surface of the thigh as the femoral fascia. The **linea alba** (6) enters the prepubic tendon and splits into a dorsal (internal) part to the pecten pubis and a ventral (external) part to the symphyseal tendon and crest.

III. The aponeurosis of the **external oblique abdominal m.** (3) is divided by the **superficial inguinal ring** (8) into an abdominal tendon whose border is the **medial crus** of the ring, and a pelvic tendon whose border is the **lateral crus** of the ring. The two tendons overlap and join the prepubic tendon.

The aponeurosis of the **internal oblique abdominal m.** (12) and the abdominal tendon of the **external oblique** (5) form the cranial border of the **deep inguinal ring** (13). The caudal border is the pelvic tendon of the **external oblique** (4). The vaginal tunic with its contents and the cremaster pass through the **dorsolateral angle** (14) which is fixed by the origin of the internal oblique from the iliac fascia near the external iliac vessels. The ext. pudendal vessels and the genital branches of the genitofemoral n. go through the ring more medially. The **medial angle** (15) *lies close to the median line against the prepubic tendon. The label, 2, marks only the caudal part of the prepubic tendon, which extends to the junction of the aponeurosis of the int. oblique (12) and the fused tendons of the* **rectus abdominis mm.** (17). (See c) Prepubic tendon.) The caudal border of the **transversus** (16) is in the plane of the tuber coxae and has no relation to the inguinal canal.

The **cremaster** (19) originates from the inguinal ligament and runs parallel to the caudal border of the internal oblique.

IV. The **fascia transversalis** (B) evaginates at first as the covering of the vaginal process of the peritoneum—the **internal spermatic fascia** (B') and after a short course becomes loose connective tissue. The bull lacks the annular thickening peculiar to the horse at the beginning of the evagination.

V. The **peritoneum** (A) evaginates at the **vaginal ring** (A') as the **vaginal process of the peritoneum** (A"), becoming the vaginal tunic after descent of the testis, passing through the inguinal canal into the scrotum, and covering the testis and epididymis.

b) The **INGUINAL LIG.** (20)** *consists of a twisted cord of fibers of the tendon of origin of the internal oblique that begins at the tuber coxae, is interwoven with the iliac fascia in its course, and, giving origin to the cremaster, ends lateral to the passage of the ext. iliac a. and v. through the lacuna vasorum. Unlike the condition in the dog and horse, the inguinal lig. does not join the caudal border of the pelvic tendon of the ext. oblique at this point to form a continuous inguinal arch from the tuber coxae to the prepubic tendon.*

Inguinal canal (transverse section)

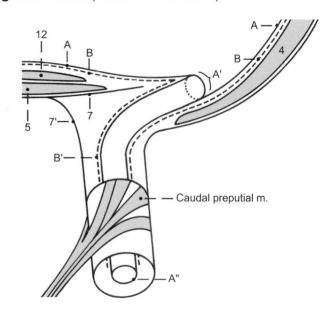

Ligamentous fibers that radiate into the pelvic tendon as in the dog and horse *do not exist in the ox. In this region only the thickened caudal border of the pelvic tendon is functionally important.*

c) The **PREPUBIC TENDON** (2) is attached to the pubic bones, primarily on the iliopubic eminences and the ventral pubic tubercle. It is also attached to the symphyseal tendon. It extends to junction of the aponeurosis of the **int. oblique** (12) and the fused tendons of the **recti** (17), but is not visible interiorly, except for its attachment on the pelvis. It consists of the crossed and uncrossed tendons of origin of the pectineus muscles and of the cranial parts of the gracilis muscles, and the pubic and symphyseal tendons of the recti and oblique abdominal muscles. The linea alba and the yellow abdominal tunic are also incorporated in it. Contrary to some authors, transverse ligamentous fibers connecting *right and left iliopubic eminences do not exist.* ***

* No tendinous lamina radiates from the lateral crus (it is composed of fascia).
** Traeder, 1968   *** Habel and Budras, 1992

(cranial)

♀

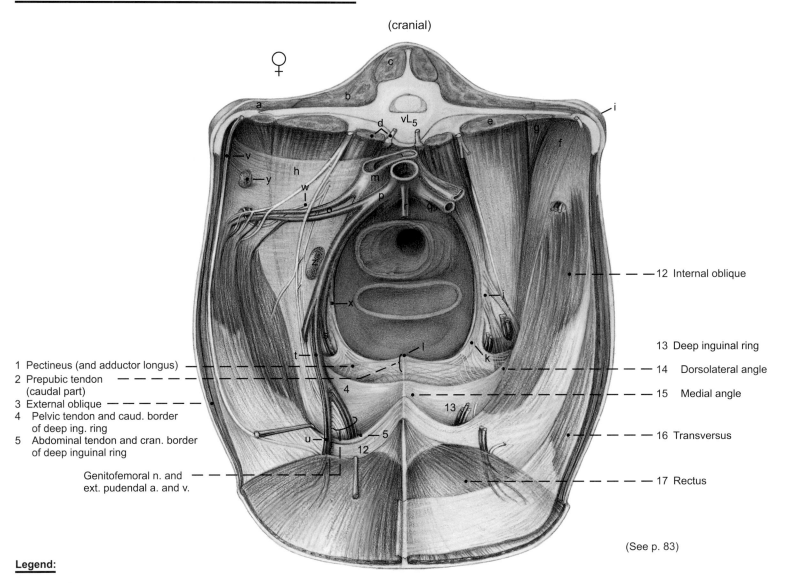

vL₅

12 Internal oblique

13 Deep inguinal ring

1 Pectineus (and adductor longus)

14 Dorsolateral angle

2 Prepubic tendon
(caudal part)

15 Medial angle

3 External oblique

4 Pelvic tendon and caud. border
of deep ing. ring

16 Transversus

5 Abdominal tendon and cran. border
of deep inguinal ring

17 Rectus

Genitofemoral n. and
ext. pudendal a. and v.

(See p. 83)

Legend:

a Iliocostalis	g Quadratus lumborum	n Aorta	u Caudal epigastric a. and v.
b Longissimus dorsi	h Internal iliac fascia	o Deep circumflex iliac vessels	v Iliohypogastric n.
c Multifidus	i Tuber coxae	p External iliac a.	w Lat. cut. femoral n.
d Psoas minor and	j Psoas minor tubercle	q Internal iliac a.	x Obturator n.
sympathetic trunk	k Iliopubic eminence	r Caudal mesenteric a.	y Lat. iliac ln.
Iliopsoas	l Dorsal pubic tubercle	s Deep femoral a. and v.	z Iliofemoral ln.
e Psoas major	m Caudal vena cava	t Pudendoepigastric vessels	
f Iliacus			

♂

(caudoventral)

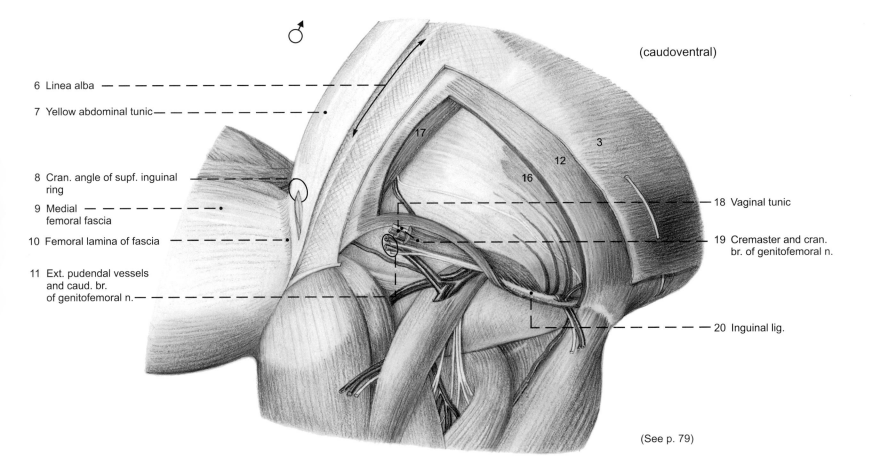

6 Linea alba

7 Yellow abdominal tunic

8 Cran. angle of supf. inguinal
ring

9 Medial
femoral fascia

10 Femoral lamina of fascia

11 Ext. pudendal vessels
and caud. br.
of genitofemoral n.

18 Vaginal tunic

19 Cremaster and cran.
br. of genitofemoral n.

20 Inguinal lig.

(See p. 79)

81

3. LYMPHATIC SYSTEM, ADRENAL GLANDS, AND URINARY ORGANS

> After the study of the topography of the lymph nodes, adrenals, and urinary organs, the kidneys are removed with attention to their coverings, and their peculiarities in the ox are studied.

a) The **LYMPHATIC SYSTEM** in the dorsal abdominal and pelvic cavities includes the following lymph nodes.

The 12–15 small **lumbar aortic lnn.** (8) lie dorsal and ventral to the aorta and caudal vena cava and are *examined in meat inspection in special cases.* There are also *up to 5 inconstant unilateral or bilateral proper lumbar lnn. between the lumbar transverse processes.* The 1–4 **renal lnn.** (9) are found on both sides between the **renal a. and v.** (2). *They are routinely examined in meat inspection.* The lymph drainage is through the lumbar trunk or directly into the cisterna chyli. The **medial iliac lnn.** (4), 1–5 in number, lie at the origin of the **external iliac aa.** (f). The **lateral iliac ln.** (12) at the bifurcation of the **deep circumflex iliac a.** (11) may be double. *Both groups are routinely examined in meat inspection.* The **sacral lnn.** (5), 2–8 in number, lie in the angle between the **internal iliac aa.** (h). The **sciatic ln.** (p. 17, B) is in the lesser sciatic foramen or dorsal to it on the outside of the sacrosciatic ligament. The **anorectal lnn.** (p. 77) are dorsal and lateral to the rectum and anus. The **iliofemoral ln.** (6) is up to 9 cm long and located in the angle between the deep circumflex iliac and external iliac vessels. It is clinically important because it receives lymph from the superficial inguinal (mammary) lnn. and can be palpated per rectum cranial to the shaft of the ilium. *It is examined in meat inspection in cases of mastitis.* The lymph drainage from the iliac, sacral, sciatic, anorectal, and iliofemoral lnn. passes through the medial iliac lnn., the iliofemoral ln., or the lumbar trunk into the **cisterna chyli,** which is 1.5–2 cm long and extends from the last thoracic vertebra to the 1st or 2nd lumbar vertebra, dorsal to the vena cava and aorta.

b) The **ADRENAL GLANDS** (7) are 5–8 cm long, flattened, relatively smooth, and reddish brown to dark gray, sometimes also with black spots. Each weighs 15–23 g. They are retroperitoneal and covered ventrally by fat. The **right adrenal** is more or less heart-shaped and located at the 12th intercostal space craniomedial to the right kidney. It is partly covered ventrally by the caudal vena cava and attached to it by connective tissue. The **left adrenal** is comma-shaped and larger and heavier than the right. It lies in the plane of the 1st lumbar vertebra on the left side of the vena cava, to which it also is attached by connective tissue. It is usually several cm cranial to the left kidney.

c) The **URINARY ORGANS**

I. The **kidneys** differ remarkably in position as a result of the developmental expansion of the rumen.

The flat elongated oval **right kidney** (1) is retroperitoneal and extends from the 12th intercostal space to the 2nd or 3rd lumbar vertebra. The pit-like **hilus** is medial. The cranial end is in contact with the liver (see p. 75, v). The **dorsal surface** is applied to the right crus of the diaphragm and the lumbar muscles. The **ventral surface** lies on the pancreas, cecum, and ascending colon.

The **left kidney** (10) is not illustrated in its normal position. In the live ox *it is pushed to the right side by the rumen. It is almost completely surrounded by peritoneum and therefore pendulous, and lies ventral to lumbar vertebrae 2–5, and caudal to the right kidney,* from which it is separated by the descending mesocolon. *Because the left kidney undergoes a 90-degree rotation on its long axis, its hilus (24) is dorsal.* Medially it adjoins the rumen and laterally, the intestinal mass.

The kidneys are red-brown; their combined weight is 1200–1500 g. *They are marked on the surface by the* **renal lobes** (26), *unlike any other domestic mammal. In the ox, two or more fetal lobes remain distinct; others are partially or completely fused in the cortex, resulting in 12–15 simple or compound lobes of various sizes.* The actual boundaries of the lobes can be seen only by the course of the **interlobar aa. and vv.** (19). On the cut surface the reddish light brown **renal cortex** (23) with its distinct **renal columns** (21) *contrasts with the dark red* **external zone** (17) *and the light* **internal zone** (18) of the **renal medulla** (15). The **renal pyramids** (16) *project with their prominent* **renal papillae** (20) *into the urine collecting* **renal calices** (25). *These open into* cranial and caudal **collecting ducts** *which join within the irregular fat-lined* **renal sinus** *to form the ureter. The ox lacks a renal pelvis.*

II. In the standing live ox the **right ureter** (3) takes a course on the ventral surface of its kidney and *dorsal to the left kidney* toward the pelvic cavity. The **left ureter** *runs along the dorsal surface of the caudal half of its kidney, inclines to the left of the median plane and enters the urinary bladder.* *

III. The **urinary bladder** (n) (see also text figure) is relatively large. When moderately filled it extends into the ventral abdominal cavity farther than in the horse. The **apex** (27) and **body** (28) are covered with peritoneum. The **neck** (31) is extraperitoneal and attached to the vagina by connective tissue. On the apex there is a distinct conical vestige of the urachus, which in the three-month-old calf can still be as long as 4 cm. The ureters open close together in the middle of the neck of the bladder. The **ureteric folds** (30) run caudally from there inside the bladder and converge to form the *narrow* **vesical triangle** (29). The **lateral ligaments of the bladder** (13) contain in their free border the *small, in old age almost obliterated, umbilical artery* (**round lig. of the bladder;** p. 87, t). The **middle lig. of the bladder** (14) runs from the ventral wall of the bladder to the pelvic symphysis and to the ventromedian abdominal wall.

IV. The **male urethra** (see p. 92, K) consists of a **pelvic part** surrounded by a stratum spongiosum, and a **penile part** surrounded by the **corpus spongiosum penis.** The pelvic part is also surrounded by the disseminate prostate (see p. 92), and *ventrally and laterally* by the thick striated urethral muscle (93, g). Just inside the ischial arch is the **urethral recess,** *present in ruminants and swine; it opens caudally and practically prevents catheterization. The recess is dorsal to the urethra and separated from it by a fold of mucosa that bifurcates caudally into lateral folds on which the ducts of the bulbourethral glands open. The lumen of the urethra passes through the narrow slit between the folds.*

V. The **female urethra** (see text figure) *is about 12 cm long and attached to the vagina by connective tissue and the urethral muscle.* The **urethral crest** (32), 0.5 cm high, passes through the urethra on its dorsal wall *to the slit-like urethral orifice, which is on the cranial side of the neck of the clinically important, blind,* **suburethral diverticulum** (33). The latter extends cranially for 2 cm from its common opening with the urethra on the floor of the vestibule, and must be avoided in catheterization. (See p. 87, x.)

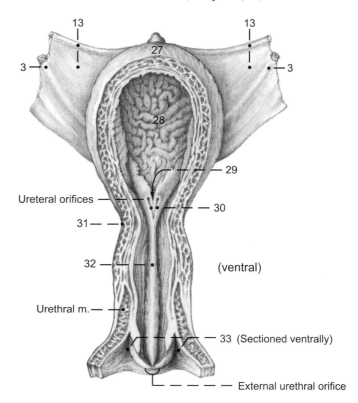

13   13
27
3
28
29
Ureteral orifices
31 —   — 30
32 —   (ventral)
Urethral m. —
33 (Sectioned ventrally)
External urethral orifice

* Fabisch, 1968

Abdominal cavity and Urinary organs as seen at autopsy, in dorsal recumbency with stomach and intestines removed

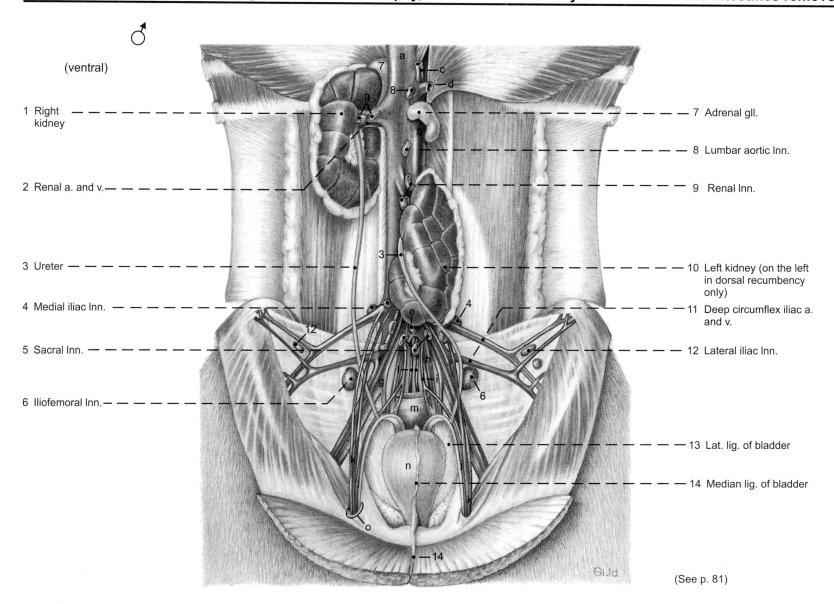

♂

(ventral)

1 Right
   kidney

2 Renal a. and v.

3 Ureter

4 Medial iliac lnn.

5 Sacral lnn.

6 Iliofemoral lnn.

7 Adrenal gll.

8 Lumbar aortic lnn.

9 Renal lnn.

10 Left kidney (on the left
   in dorsal recumbency
   only)

11 Deep circumflex iliac a.
   and v.

12 Lateral iliac lnn.

13 Lat. lig. of bladder

14 Median lig. of bladder

(See p. 81)

Legend:

a Caud. vena cava	d Cran. mesenteric a.	g Common iliac v.	j Ductus deferens and A. ductus deferentis	m Rectum
b Aorta	e Caud. mesenteric a.	h Int. iliac a.	k Testicular a. and v.	n Urinary bladder
c Celiac a.	f Ext. iliac a.	i Umbilical a.	l Median sacral a. and v.	o Vaginal ring

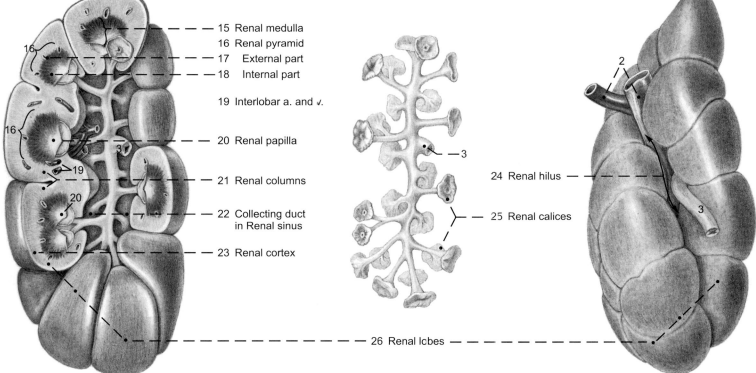

Right kidney (Sectioned)   ### Ureter and Calices (Right kidney)   ### Left kidney

15 Renal medulla
16 Renal pyramid
17   External part
18   Internal part

19 Interlobar a. and v.

20 Renal papilla

21 Renal columns

22 Collecting duct
   in Renal sinus

23 Renal cortex

24 Renal hilus

25 Renal calices

26 Renal lobes

83

5. ARTERIES, VEINS, AND NERVES OF THE PELVIC CAVITY

a) The **ABDOMINAL AORTA** (1) gives off the paired external iliac aa. at the level of the 6th lumbar vertebra, and the paired internal iliac aa. and the dorsally directed unpaired **median sacral a.** (13) at the level of the sacral promontory.

The **external iliac a.** (5), while still in the abdominal cavity, gives off the **deep circumflex iliac a.** (6) and shortly before entering the femoral triangle, it gives origin to the **deep femoral a.** with the attached **pudendoepigastric trunk** (7), which divides into the **caudal epigastric a.** (8) and the **external pudendal a.** (9). The latter passes through the inguinal canal and gives off branches to the scrotum or udder (see also p. 91). The **internal iliac a.** (15) is, in contrast to that artery in the dog and horse, *a long vessel that extends to the lesser sciatic notch and ends there by dividing into the caudal gluteal and internal pudendal aa.* Its first branch is the **umbilical a.** (17), which gives off the **a. of the ductus deferens** in the bull and the **uterine a.** (18) in the cow, and in both sexes the **cranial vesical a.** (19) with the obliterated termination of the umbilical a. as the **round lig. of the bladder.**

Also originating from the internal iliac a. are the iliolumbar a. (16) and the cranial gluteal a. (i). The **vaginal a.** (23) or **prostatic a.** originates at the level of the hip joint. Together with the internal pudendal a. their branches supply most of the pelvic viscera. The vaginal or prostatic a. supplies the **uterine br.** (24) or the **br. to the ductus deferens**, the **caudal vesical a.** (25) (which can also come indirectly from the int. pudendal a.), the **urethral br.** (27), the **middle rectal a.** (28), and, in the cow, the **dorsal perineal a.** (28), which ends as the **caudal rectal a.** (30). The dorsal perineal a. may give off the mammary br. (37).

The **int. pudendal a.** (32) gives off the **urethral a.** (33), the **vestibular a.** (34), the dorsal perineal a. in most bulls, and the **ventral perineal a.** (36) with its **mammary br.** (37), and ends as the **a. of the clitoris** or **a. of the penis** (35). *The obturator a. is absent.*

The **caudal gluteal a.** (31) *emerges from the pelvis through the lesser sciatic foramen. It supplies the deep gluteal m., cran. part of the gluteobiceps, the gemelli, and the quadratus femoris.*

b) The **VEINS** run generally parallel to the corresponding arteries; therefore only the important exceptions will be mentioned here.

The terminal division of the **caudal vena cava** (1) into paired common iliac vv. *occurs at the level of the first sacral vertebra.* The **median sacral v.** (13) comes from the caudal vena cava, and the **deep circumflex iliac v.** (6) comes from the **common iliac v.** The *left common iliac v. gives off the left **ovarian** or **testicular v.** (2). Medial to the ilium the common iliac v. divides into the external and internal iliac vv.*

Shortly before its entry into the femoral triangle the **external iliac v.** (5) gives off the pudendoepigastric v. (7) which may arise from the **deep femoral v.** The **internal iliac v.** (15) gives off the **obturator v.** (20), which runs to the obturator foramen, and the **accessory vaginal vein** (22) *neither has an accompanying artery.* (See e) veins of udder.)

The **v. of the ductus deferens** (24) comes from the prostatic v.; the **uterine br.** (24), from the vaginal v., from which the **caudal vesical v.** (25) also arises.

The blood supply of the penis, uterus, and udder follows.

c) The **BLOOD SUPPLY OF THE PENIS** is provided by the internal pudendal a. It ends as the **a. of the penis** (35) and this gives off the **a. of the bulb of the penis** (38) for the corpus spongiosum and bulb; the **deep a. of the penis** (39), which enters the corpus cavernosum at the root of the penis; and the **dorsal a. of the penis** (40), which runs to the apex of the penis. The veins ramify in the same way as the arteries of the same name.

d) The **BLOOD SUPPLY OF THE UTERUS** is provided mainly by the **uterine a.** (18), *which originates from the first part of the umbilical a., near the internal iliac a.* It runs on the mesometrial border of the uterine horn in the parametrium. Its branches form anastomotic arches with each other and cranially with the **uterine br.** (2') of the **ovarian a.** and caudally with the **uterine br.** (24) of the **vaginal a.** In the cow the uterine a. is palpable per rectum after the third month of pregnancy as an enlarged vessel with a characteristic thrill (fremitus) in addition to the pulse. The **uterine v.** is an insignificant vessel that comes from the internal iliac v. and accompanies the uterine a. The main veins are the **uterine br. of the ovarian v.** (2), the **uterine br. of the vaginal v.** (24), and the **accessory vaginal v.** (22), *which comes from the internal iliac v. and has no accompanying a.*

e) The **BLOOD SUPPLY OF THE UDDER** comes mainly from the external pudendal a. (9), and additionally from the internal pudendal a. (32) via the ventral perineal a. (36). The external pudendal a., with a sigmoid flexure, enters the base of the udder dorsally and divides into the cranial and caudal mammary aa. The **cran. mammary a.** (caud. supf. epigastric a., 10) supplies the cranial and caudal quarters, including the teats. The **caud. mammary a.** (11) goes mainly to the caudal quarter. A third (middle) mammary artery may be present, arising from the other two or from the external pudendal a. at its bifurcation. There are many variations in all three arteries.

The cranial and caudal mammary vv. are branches of the external pudendal. The **cranial mammary v.** (10) *is also continous with the caud. supf. epigastric v., which joins the cran. supf. epigastric v. to form the large, sinous milk vein (***subcutaneous abdominal v.***). The **caudal mammary v.** (11) joins the large **ventral labial v.** (37), which is indirectly connected to the internal pudendal v.* Further details of the mammary vessels will be discussed with the udder (p. 90).

f) The **SACRAL PLEXUS** is joined to the lumbar plexus in the lumbosacral plexus. The **cranial gluteal n.** (i) issues cranially from the **lumbosacral trunk** at the greater sciatic foramen and runs with the branches of the cran. gluteal vessels to the middle, accessory, and deep gluteal muscles, as well as the tensor fasciae latae, fused with the supf. gluteal muscle.

The **caudal gluteal n.** (j) arises caudodorsally from the lumbosacral trunk near the greater sciatic foramen, but emerges through the lesser sciatic foramen and innervates the parts of the gluteobiceps that originate from the sacrosciatic ligament.

The **caudal cutaneous femoral n.** (k) *is small in the ox.* It arises from the lumbosacral trunk just caudal to the caudal gluteal n. and runs outside the sacrosciatic lig. to the lesser sciatic foramen, where it divides into medial and lateral brr. The medial br. (communicating br.) passes into the foramen and joins the pudendal n. or its deep perineal br. *In the ox the lateral br. of the caud. cut. femoral n. may be absent; it may join the proximal cutaneous br. of the pudendal n.; or it may contribute to the cutaneous innervation of the caudolateral thigh, which is supplied mainly by the proximal and distal cutaneous brr. of the pudendal n.*

The **sciatic n.** (f) is the direct continuation of the lumbosacral trunk. It runs caudally over the deep gluteal m. and turns ventrally behind the hip joint to supply the pelvic limb. It is the largest nerve in the body.

The **pudendal n.** (h) originates from sacral nn. 2–4. It runs caudoventrally on the inside of the sacrosciatic lig., and near the lesser sciatic foramen gives off two cutaneous brr. (p. 95): the **proximal cutaneous br.** emerges through, or caudal to, the gluteobiceps, and runs distally on the semitendinosus; the **distal cutaneous br.** emerges from the ischiorectal fossa and runs distally on the semimembranosus. It also supplies the **supf. perineal n.** to the skin of the perineum. In the bull, this provides the dorsal scrotal nn., and in the cow, the labial nn., and branches that extend on the ventral labial v. to the caudal surface of the udder.

The pudendal n. gives off the **deep perineal n.** (p. 95) to the striated and smooth perineal muscles, and continues with the internal pudendal vessels around the ischial arch, and ends by dividing into the **dorsal n. of the clitoris** and the **mammary br.** The latter is closely associated with the loops of the ventral labial v. In the bull the pudendal n. divides into the **dorsal n. of the penis** and the **preputial and scrotal br.**

The **caudal rectal nn.** (30) are the last branches of the sacral plexus. They have connections with the pudendal n. and supply the rectum, skin of the anus, and parts of the perineal musculature.

g) **AUTONOMIC NERVOUS SYSTEM.** The sympathetic division includes the **caudal mesenteric ganglion** on the caudal mesenteric a. cranial to the pelvic inlet. The paired **hypogastric nn.** leave the ganglion and run on the dorsolateral pelvic wall to the level of the vaginal or prostatic a. to join the pelvic plexus. The **sympathetic trunk** in the sacral region has five vertebral ganglia and in the coccygeal region, four or five ganglia.

The **parasympathetic nn.** from sacral segments 2–4 leave the vertebral canal with the ventral roots of the pudendal n. and form the **pelvic nn.**, which, from a dorsal approach, join the **pelvic plexus** with its contained ganglion cells. (See also p. 56.)

Pelvic arteries, veins, and nerves (left side)

Legend:

Arteries, veins:

 1 Abd. aorta and caud. vena cava
 2 Ovarian or testicular a. and v.
 2' Uterine br.
 3 Caud. mesenteric a. and v.
 4 Cran. rectal a. and v.
 5 Ext. iliac a. and v.
 6 Deep circumflex iliac a. and v.
 7 Pudendoepigastric trunk and v.
 8 Caud. epigastric a. and v.
 9 Ext. pudendal a. and v.
10 Caud. supf. epigastric a. and v.
   (Cran. mammary a. and v.)
11 Caud. mammary a. and v. or
   Ventr. scrotal br. and v.
12 Lumbar aa. and vv.
13 Median sacral a. and v.
14 Median caud. a. and v.
14' Ventrolat. caudal a. and v.
14" Dorsolat. caudal a. and v.
15 Int. iliac a. and v.
16 Iliolumbar a. and v.
17 Umbilical a.
18 Uterine a. or a. of ductus deferens
19 Cran. vesical a.
20 Obturator v.
21 Cran. gluteal a. and v.
22 Accessory vaginal v.
23 Vaginal or prostatic a. and v.
24 Uterine br. and v. or v. of ductus deferens
25 Caud. vesical a. and v.
26 Ureteric br.
27 Urethral br.
28 Middle rectal a. and v.
29 Dors. perineal a. and v.
30 Caud. rectal a. and v.
31 Caud. gluteal a. and v.
32 Int. pudendal a. and v.
33 Urethral a. and v.
34 Vestibular a. and v.
35 A. and v. of clitoris or penis
36 Ventr. perineal a. and v.
37 Ventr. labial v. and mammary br.
   of ventr. or dors. perineal a.
   In bull, br. and v. from ventr. perineal vessels
38 A. and v. of bulb of penis
39 Deep a. and v. of penis
40 Dors. a. and v. of penis

Nerves:

a Iliohypogastric n.
b Ilioinguinal n.
c Genitofemoral n.
d Lat. cut. femoral n.
e Femoral n.
f Sciatic n.
g Obturator n.
h Pudendal n.
i Cran. gluteal n.
j Caud. gluteal n.
k Caud. cut. femoral n.
l Caud. rectal nn.
m Caudal mesenteric plexus
n Hypogastric n.
o Pelvic plexus
p Pelvic n.

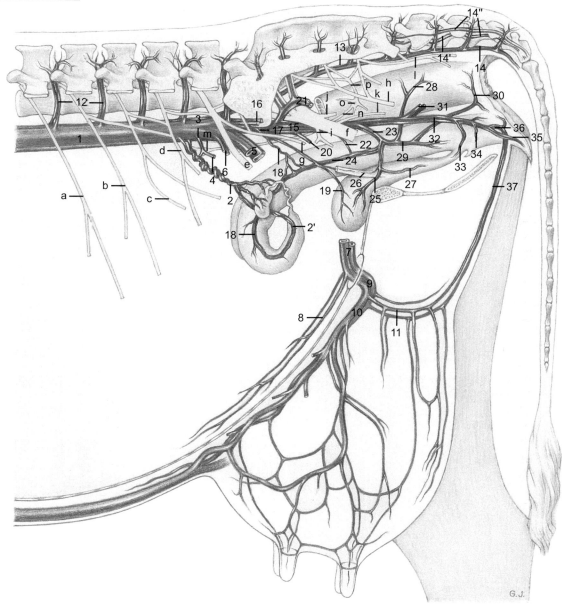

(See pp. 17, 19, 21, 91)

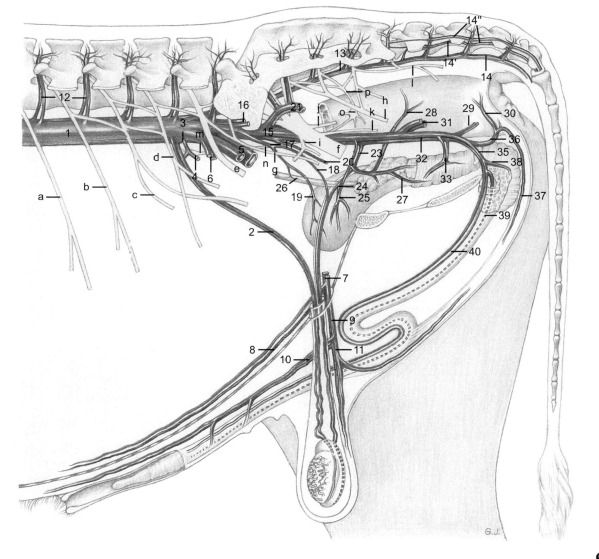

85

5. FEMALE GENITAL ORGANS

a) The **OVARY** (6) has a different position from that of the bitch and mare because of the *longer developmental "descent" of the ovary and parietal attachment of the* **mesovarium** (2) *toward the pelvis. This results in the spiral of the uterine horn and gives the long axis of the ovary an obliquely transverse direction. The tubal end of the ovary is dorsolateral and the uterine end is ventromedial. The ovary lies near the lateroventral part of the pelvic inlet, cranial to the external iliac a. In the pregnant cow it is drawn cranioventrally.* The mesovarium contains the ovarian a., coming from the aorta, and gives off laterally the thin **mesosalpinx** (3) for the uterine tube. The cranial border of the mesovarium is the **suspensory lig. of the ovary** (1). Caudally the mesovarium is continuous with the **mesometrium** (4). The mesovarium, mesosalpinx, and mesometrium together form the **broad ligament (lig. latum uteri)** which contains smooth muscle.

The **ovary** *measures 3.5 x 2.5 x 1.5 cm, about the size of the distal segment of the human thumb. Compared to that of the mare it is relatively small. It is covered by peritoneum on the mesovarian margin only, and by the superficial epithelium elsewhere. There is no ovarian fossa, which is a peculiarity of the mare. The* **cortex** *and* **medulla** *are arranged as in the bitch. On the irregularly tuberculated surface there are always follicles and* **corpora lutea** *of various stages of the estrous cycle which can be palpated per rectum. A follicle matures to about 2 cm; a corpus luteum can reach the size of a walnut. The single corpus luteum changes color during the cycle from yellow or ocher-yellow to dark red, red-brown, gray-white, and black. This can be seen on a section through the ovary.*

Ovary

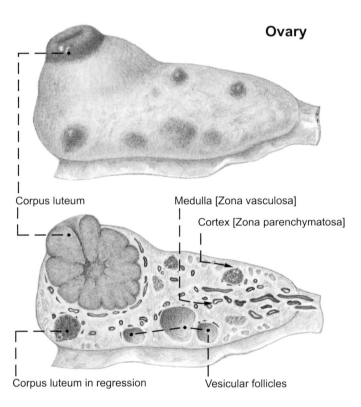

Corpus luteum

Medulla [Zona vasculosa]

Cortex [Zona parenchymatosa]

Corpus luteum in regression

Vesicular follicles

b) The **UTERINE TUBE** (14) *is somewhat tortuous and at 28 cm, relatively long.* The **mesosalpinx** (3) with the uterine tube surrounds the ovary cranially and laterally like a mantle and forms with the mesovarium the flat voluminous **ovarian bursa** (13) *with a wide cranioventromedial opening.* The **infundibulum of the tube** (16) with its fimbriae surrounds the ovary. It funnels into the **abdominal orifice of the tube** (15). The ampulla and isthmus of the tube *do not show any great difference in the size of the lumen.* The uterine tube ends, unlike that of the bitch and mare, *without a uterine papilla* at the **uterine orifice of the tube** (7) in the apex of the uterine horn. Here the **proper ligament of the ovary** (8) ends and the **round lig. of the uterus** begins. The latter is attached by a serosal fold to the lateral surface of the mesometrium and extends to the region of the inguinal canal. Both ligaments develop from the **gubernaculum of the ovary**. (The mammalian uterine tube differs in form and function from the oviduct of lower animals.)

c) The **UTERUS**, as in all carnivores and ungulates, is a uterus bicornis. The horns of the uterus (**cornua uteri**, 9) *are 30–40 cm long, rolled through cranioventral to caudodorsal, and fused caudally into a 10–15 cm long double cylinder.* Cranial to the union the horns are connected by the dorsal and ventral intercornual ligg. (11). Internally the true, undivided **body of the uterus** (12) is only 2–4 cm long. The **neck of the uterus (cervix uteri,** 26) with the **cervical canal** (26) begins at the **internal uterine orifice** (27) and ends at the **external uterine orifice** (25) on the **vaginal part of the cervix (portio vaginalis,** 25). The cervix is 8–10 cm long and can be distinguished from the body of the uterus and the vagina by its firm consistency.

The three layers of the wall of the uterus are formed by the peritoneum (perimetrium), the muscular coat (myometrium), and the mucosa (endometrium). The mucosa of the uterus forms longitudinal and transverse folds and *in each uterine horn four rows of 10–15 round or oval* **caruncles** (10)* *of various sizes. These project dome-like on the internal surface, and in the pregnant uterus can reach the size of a fist. The total number of caruncles in the uterus, including the body, is about 100.*

Placentome

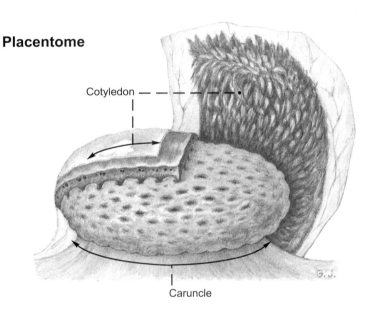

Cotyledon

Caruncle

During pregnancy they form, together with the **cotyledons,**** the **placentomes**. *Cotyledons are bunches of villi on the fetal amniochorion and allantochorion that invade the caruncles.* (See text figure.) The cervical mucosa presents **longitudinal folds** and, with the support of the musculature, bulges into the lumen, usually in *four characteristic* circular folds, and closes the cervical canal. This is clinically important. The last **circular fold** projects into the vagina as the **portio vaginalis cervicis** (25).

d) *The* **Vagina** (18), *30 cm long, is longer than in the mare, hollow* and its **fornix** (17) *arches over the portio vaginalis cervicis dorsally.* The cranial part of the vagina is covered by peritoneum in the area of the **rectogenital excavation** (5) which extends caudally to the middle of the pelvic cavity or to the first caudal vertebra. Caudally the vagina joins the **vestibule** (23), sometimes *without a distinct boundary,* sometimes with only *a faint transverse fold, the* **hymen** (19). The **external urethral orifice** (20) opens into the cranial end of the vestibule 7–11 cm from the ventral commissure of the labia. The **suburethral diverticulum** (x) *lies ventral to the urethral orifice.*

The openings of the vestigial deferent ducts (remnants of the caudal parts of the mesonephric ducts) are found on each side of the urethral orifice. The ducts run between the mucosa and the musculature and can reach a considerable length. They end blindly and can become cystic. The **major vestibular gland** (w) is cranial to the **constrictor vestibuli** (m). It is 3 cm long and 1.5 cm wide, and has 2–3 ducts that open in a small pouch (24) lateral to the urethral orifice. The microscopic minor vestibular glands open on the floor of the vestibule cranial to the clitoris.

e) The **VULVA** surrounds with its thick **labia** (22) the **labial fissure (rima pudendi).** The **dorsal commissure** of the labia is, in contrast to the mare, more rounded, and the **ventral commissure** is pointed, with a tuft of long coarse hairs.

The **clitoris** (21) *is smaller than in the mare, although 12 cm long and tortuous. The end is tapered to a cone.* The **glans** is indistinct. The **prepuce** is *partially adherent to the apex of the clitoris so that an (open)* fossa clitoridis is almost absent.

* Caruncula -ae, L. = papilla
** Cotyledo(n) -onis L., Gr. = cup

Female genital organs

(Left side)

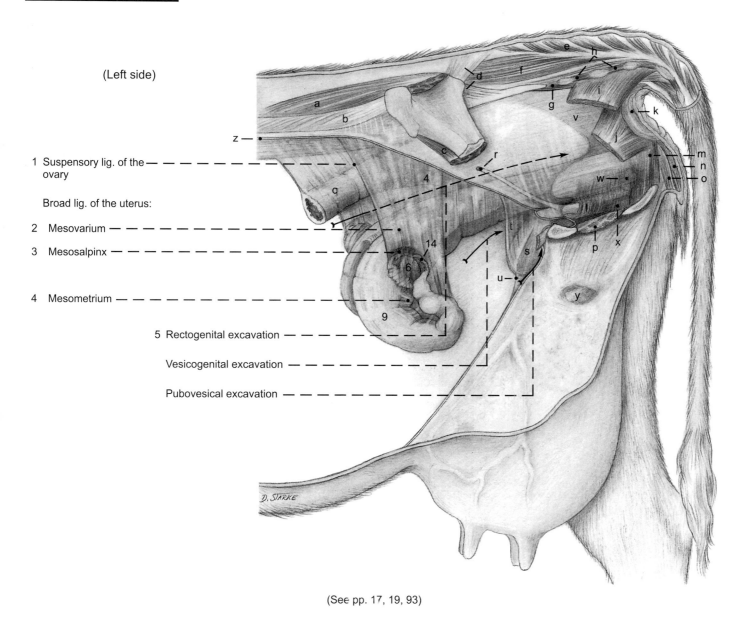

1 Suspensory lig. of the ovary

Broad lig. of the uterus:

2 Mesovarium
3 Mesosalpinx

4 Mesometrium

5 Rectogenital excavation

Vesicogenital excavation

Pubovesical excavation

(See pp. 17, 19, 93)

Legend:

a Middle gluteal m.	f Sacrocaudalis dorsalis lateralis	l Urethralis	q Descending colon	v Rectum
b Longissimus lumborum	g Sacrocaudalis ventralis lateralis	Bulbospongiosus:	r Ureter	w Major vestibular gl.
c Iliacus	h Intertransversarii	m Constrictor vestibuli	s Urinary bladder	x Suburethral diverticulum
d Sacroiliac ligg.	i Coccygeus	n Constrictor vulvae	t Lat. lig. and round	y Supf. inguinal lnn.
e Sacrocaudalis dorsalis medialis	j Levator ani	o Retractor clitoridis	lig. of bladder	z Peritonum (Sectio)
	k Ext. anal sphincter	p Intrapelvic part of ext. obturator	u Median lig. of bladder	

(dorsal)

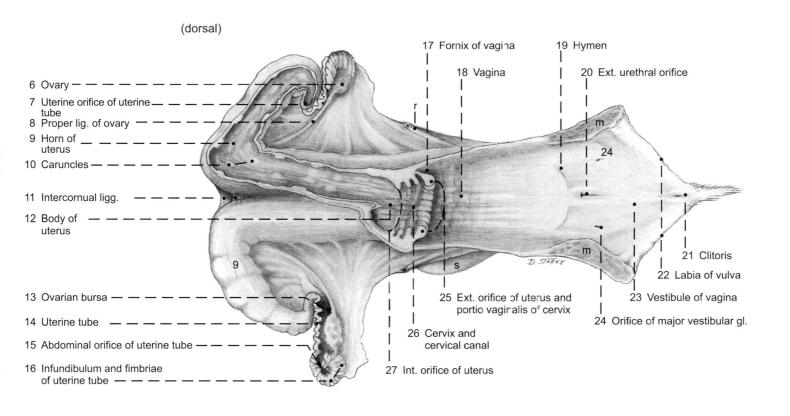

6 Ovary
7 Uterine orifice of uterine tube
8 Proper lig. of ovary
9 Horn of uterus
10 Caruncles

11 Intercornual ligg.

12 Body of uterus

13 Ovarian bursa
14 Uterine tube
15 Abdominal orifice of uterine tube
16 Infundibulum and fimbriae of uterine tube

17 Fornix of vagina
18 Vagina

19 Hymen
20 Ext. urethral orifice

21 Clitoris
22 Labia of vulva
23 Vestibule of vagina
24 Orifice of major vestibular gl.

25 Ext. orifice of uterus and portio vaginalis of cervix
26 Cervix and cervical canal
27 Int. orifice of uterus

6. THE UDDER

The **udder** is composed of four **mammary glands**—modified skin glands that occur in this form only in true mammals (Eutheria). The mammary secretion is **milk (lac).** The first milk secreted after parturition is **colostrum,** containing a high concentration of antibodies, which give the newborn passive immunity. Cow's milk and also milk from sheep and goats, is a valuable human foodstuff. It contains proteins, fats, sugar, and minerals (for example, calcium and phosphorus). Therefore milk production is of great economic significance in agriculture. Diseases of the udder lead directly to reduced milk production that persists throughout the lactation period. For that reason early treatment of udder diseases is especially important in veterinary practice. The diagnosis of udder diseases and the possible need for surgery, such as removal of half of the udder (mastectomy) or the amputation of a teat, require anatomical knowledge of the structure of the udder, its suspensory apparatus, blood vessels, lymph drainiage, and innervation.

The four **mammary glands** of the bovine udder are attached to the body in the inguinal region and are commonly called quarters. At the height of lactation each quarter may reach enormous size.

Each mammary gland consists of a **teat (papilla mammae, 5)** and a **body (corpus mammae, 4).** The size of the body and the length of the teat vary with the individual cow, functional status, and form. The teats are about as thick as the thumb and as long as the index finger. The teat canal, with its orifice on the end of the teat, may be incompletely closed, permitting ascending bacterial inflammation of the udder (mastitis). A narrow, partly blocked teat canal will restrict the flow of milk. Rudimentary accessory glands and teats occur and are not rare. They are usually caudal to the normal teats, but may be between them or cranial to them. Rudimentary teats occur in the bull cranial to the scrotum. The right and left halves of the udder are divided by a **median intermammary groove.** The udder is covered by modified skin that is hairless and without skin glands on the teat, and sparsely haired elsewhere. The skin of the healthy udder is easily slipped on the subcutis, but this mobility is lost in inflammation, and together with pain, edema, and heat serves to diagnose mastitis. **Suspensory apparatus: lateral laminae (1)** of fascia pass over the surface of the udder from the symphyseal tendon and the lateral crus of the superficial inguinal ring in a mainly cranioventral direction. The **medial laminae (2)** separate the right and left halves of the udder. (This median separation can be demonstrated by blunt dissection between the medial laminae from their caudal borders.) Composed mostly of elastic tissue, they originate as a paired paramedian **suspensory lig. (2).** This comes from the yellow abdominal tunic on the exterior surface of the prepubic tendon (p. 66) at its junction with the symphysial tendon.[*] From both the lateral and the medial laminae, thin **suspensory lamellae (3)** penetrate the mammary gland, separating the parenchyma into curved, overlapping **lobes (7).**[**] When filled with milk the udder has considerable weight, which stretches the suspensory apparatus, especially the medial laminae. Therefore the teats of the tightly filled udder project laterally and cranially because the elastic medial laminae are stretched more than the lateral laminae, which consist mainly of regular dense collagenous tissue.

In contrast to the bitch and mare, each mammary gland of the cow contains only one duct system and the associated glandular tissue. In addition the gland contains interstitial connective tissue with nerves, blood vessels, and lymphatics. The duct system ends on the apex of the teat with the **orifice (5")** of the narrow **teat canal (papillary duct, 5')**, surrounded by the **teat sphincter (b).**

The teat canal drains the lactiferous sinus with its **papillary part (teat sinus, 9")** and **glandular part (gland sinus, 9).** The boundary between the parts is marked by the **annular fold (9')** of mucosa, containing a venous circle (of Fuerstenberg). A **venous plexus (a)** in the wall of the teat forms an erectile tissue that makes hemostasis difficult in injuries or surgery. The mucosa of the teat canal bears **longitudinal folds (11),** and the proximal ends of the folds form a radial structure called Fuerstenberg's rosette at the boundary between the teat sinus and the teat canal.

In the gland sinus are the openings of several large **collecting ducts (ductus lactiferi colligentes, 8).** Each of these receives milk from one of the numerous lobes through **small lactiferous ducts (14)** and **alveolar lactiferous ducts (13),** which drain the **lobules (10).** A lobule resembles a bunch of grapes, measures 1.5 x 1.0 x 0.5 mm, and consists of about 200 alveoli.[***] Many alveoli are connected directly, and this construction has led to the term, "storage gland". The alveoli are surrounded by septa containing nerves and vessels. The duct systems are separate for each quarter, as demonstrated by injections of different colored dyes, even though quarters on the same side have no septum between them. Therefore ascending infections may be limited to one quarter. The separate medial laminae make it possible to amputate one lateral half of the udder. The teat canal has a defensive mechanism in its lining of stratified squamous epithelium that produces a plug of fatty desquamated cells in the canal between milkings. This is *an important factor in resistance to infection.*[****]

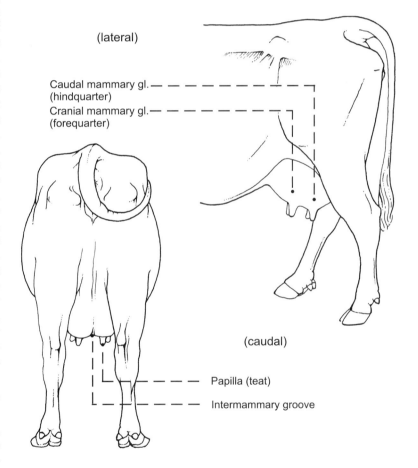

(lateral)

Caudal mammary gl. —
(hindquarter)
Cranial mammary gl.—
(forequarter)

(caudal)

Papilla (teat)

Intermammary groove

*   Habel and Budras, 1992   *** Weber et al., 1955
** Ziegler and Mosimann, 1960   **** Adams and Rickard, 1963

Udder

Transverse section through forequarters, cranial surface

(cranial)

Suspensory apparatus:

1 Lateral lamina

2 Medial laminae
(Suspensory lig.)

3 Suspensory lamellae

4 Body (Corpus)
of right forequarter

5 Teat (Papilla)

5' Teat canal
(Ductus papillaris)

5" Teat orifice

6 Yellow abdominal tunic

1

Cran. mammary a. and
v. and cran. br. of
genitofemoral n.

7 Lobe of
mammary gl.

8 Collecting duct

Lactiferous sinus:

9 Glandular part (Gland sinus)

9' Annular fold and
Venous circle

9" Papillary part (Teat sinus)

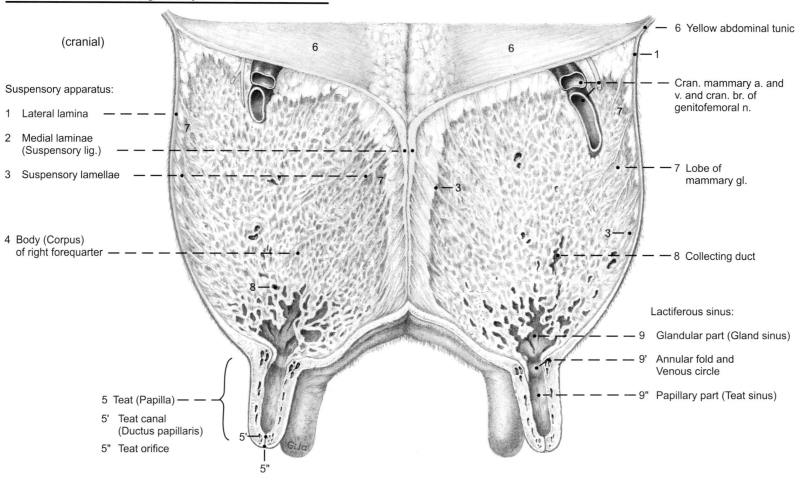

Mammary gland and Teat

Legend:

10 Lobule
11 Longitudinal folds

12 Alveoli
13 Alveolar lactiferous ducts
14 Lactiferous duct

a Venous plexus of the teat
b Teat sphincter muscle
c Lactocyte

d Fat droplet
e Myoepithelial cell
f Basement membrane

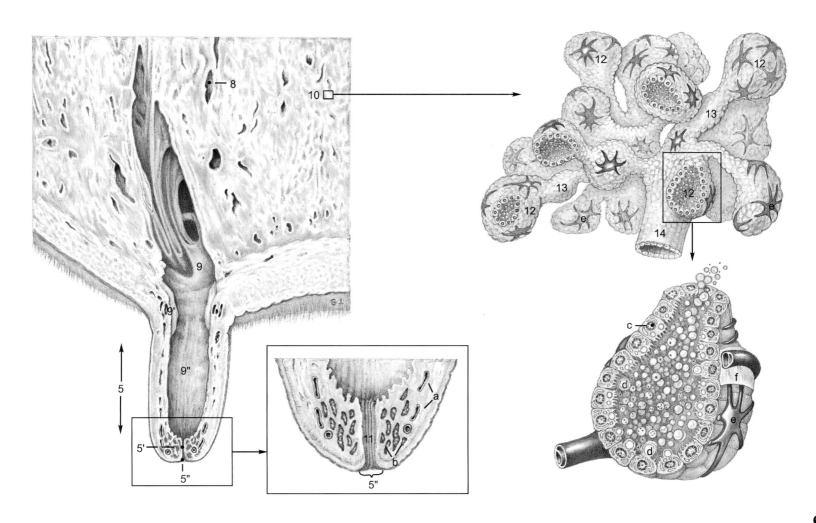

7. THE UDDER WITH BLOOD VESSELS, LYMPHATIC SYSTEM, NERVES, AND DEVELOPMENT

I. The **blood vascular system** is adapted to the high milk production of the udder. Up to 600 liters of blood must flow through the udder to produce one liter of milk. Therefore the blood vessels are remarkable for their large calibre, and they have received additional names. The ext. pudendal a. and v. bifurcate into the **cran.** (12) and **caud.** (11) **mammary a. and v.** The cran. mammary vessels are also known as the caud. supf. epigastric vessels. The caud. mammary a. and v. are continuous with the **mammary br. and ventral labial v.** (5), which usually come from the ventral perineal vessels, but in some cows they come from the dorsal perineal vessels (see p. 95, 16).

The **cran. supf. epigastric vein** in milk cows can be seen bulging under the skin of the ventral abdominal wall. It is therefore called the **subcutaneous abdominal v.** (18). The place where it perforates the abdominal wall in the xiphoid region from the int. thoracic v. is the "milk well" [anulus venae subcutaneae abdominis]. The **caud. supf. epigastric v.** is also called the **cran. mammary v.** (12). The caudal and cranial supf. epigastric vv. anastomose end-to-end and form the "milk vein". This is enlarged during the first lactation and its valves become incompetent, making blood flow possible in either direction. The right and left cran. mammary vv. anastomose on the cran. border of the udder. This connection, with that of the caudal mammary vv., completes the venous ring around the base of the udder. Many veins of the udder join this ring. The **vent. labial v.** is large and tortuous in the dairy cow (see p. 95, 16). In most of its extent the valves indicate that blood flows toward the **caud. mammary v.**

II. The **lymph** from the udder is conducted to 1–3 **supf. inguinal lnn.** (mammary lnn., B). They lie caudally on the base of the udder (the surface applied to the body wall) and can be palpated between the thighs about 6 cm from the skin at the caudal attachment of the udder. Small intramammary lnn. may be present. The lymph flows to the **iliofemoral ln. (deep inguinal ln., A).** *These lnn. are routinely incised in meat inspection.*

III. The **innervation** of the udder is sensory and also autonomic (sympathetic). The skin and teats of the forequarters and the cranial part of the base of the udder are supplied by the **iliohypogastric n.** (a), **ilioinguinal n.** (b), and the **cran. br. of the genitofemoral n.** (c'). The skin and teats of the hindquarters are innervated by the **caud. br. of the genitofemoral n.** (c") and the **mammary br.** of the **pudendal n.** (f). The cran. and caud. brr. of the genitofemoral n. pass through the inguinal canal into the body of the udder. The sensory innervation of the teats and skin of the udder is the afferent pathway of the **neurohormonal reflex arc,** which is essential for the initiation and maintenance of milk expulsion from the mammary glands. The stimulus produced by sucking the teats and massaging the mammary gll. is conducted by the afferent nerves to the CNS, where, in the nuclei of the hypothalamus, the hormone oxytocin is produced. The afferent nervous stimulus causes the hormone to be released through the neurohypophysis into the blood, which carries it into the mammary gll. Here oxytocin causes contraction of the myoepithelial cells on the alveoli, by which milk is pressed into the lactiferous ducts and sinus. This expulsion of milk is disturbed under stress by secretion of the hormone adrenalin, which suppresses the action of oxytocin on the myoepithelial cells. (For details, see textbooks of histology and physiology.)

IV. The **prenatal development of the udder** begins in the embryo in both sexes on the ventrolateral body wall between the primordia of the thoracic and pelvic limbs. This linear epidermal thickening is the **mammary ridge.** It is shifted ventrally by faster growth of the dorsal part of the body wall. Local epithelial sprouts grow down into the underlying mesenchyme from the ridge, forming the **mammary buds** in the location and number of mammary glands of each species. The mesenchyme surrounding the epithelial sprout is called the areolar tissue. Each mammary bud is bordered by a slightly raised ridge of skin. The teat develops in ruminants, as in the horse, by the growth of this areolar tissue, as a proliferation teat. The surrounding skin ridge is completely included in the formation of the teat. (For details see the textbooks of embryology.)

Postnatally the mammary glands are inconspicuous in calves of both sexes because the teats are short and the mammary glands are hardly developed. The duct system consists only of the teat canal, the sinus, and the primordia of the collecting ducts, which are short solid epithelial cords. Normally, the male udder remains in this stage throughout life. During puberty some bull calves can undergo a further temporary growth of the mammary glands under the influence of an elevated level of estrogen, as is natural in females. In young heifers during pubertal development ovarian follicles ripen and cause the level of estrogen in the blood to rise. In the udder this results in an increase of connective and adipose tisssue, and also further proliferation of the epithelial buds as primordia of the lactiferous ducts, which divide repeatedly, producing the small collecting ducts. The mammary gland primordia rest in this stage of proliferation until the first pregnancy.

During the first pregnancy further generations of lactiferous ducts develop by growth and division of the epithelial cords. In the second half of pregnancy the still partially solid glandular end-pieces are formed, while space-occupying adipose tissue is displaced. Toward the end of gestation (about 280 days) under the influence of progesterone and estrogen, a lumen develops in these glandular end-pieces, and under the influence of prolactin the lactocytes begin the secretion of milk (lactogenesis). In the first five days after parturition the milk secreted is colostrum. This is rich in proteins; it contains immunoglobulins, and it may be reddish due to an admixture of erythrocytes. In addition to the passive immunization of the newborn, colostrum has another function: it has laxative properties that aid in the elimination of meconium (fetal feces). Lactation can begin a few days or a few hours before parturition, and the first drops of milk on the end of a teat are taken as an indication of impending birth.

After birth milk secretion is maintained only in the quarters that the suckling uses. The unused quarters rapidly undergo involution. This occurs naturally when the calf is weaned by the dam, but in U.S. dairy practice the calf is removed from the dam and fed artificially, beginning with colostrum from the dam. Milk secretion is maintained by milking twice a day. After about ten months, lactation is stopped by decreasing the ration and reducing the milking to provide a dry period of about 60 days before calving.* During involution the secretory cells in the alveoli and in the alveolar lactiferous ducts degenerate. The glandular tissue is replaced by fat and connective tissue. This is important for the clinical evaluation of the consistency of individual quarters. The size of the udder decreases, but never returns to the small size of an udder that has not yet produced milk.

Accessory (supernumerary) mammary gll. may be present on the udder, a condition called hypermastia. The presence of supernumerary teats is called hyperthelia (Gk. thele, nipple). They may be located before, between, or behind the main teats. If they occur on a main teat *they interfere with* milking and must be removed.

* Ensminger, 1977

Arteries, Veins, and Nerves of the Udder

Left side

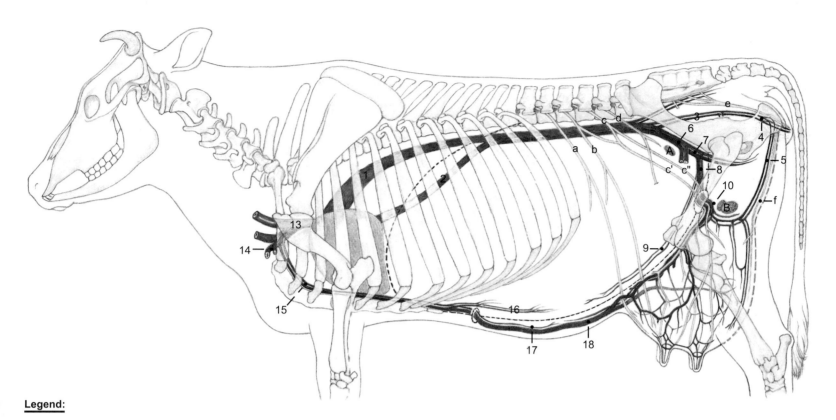

Legend:

1 Aorta
2 Caud. vena cava
3 Int. iliac a. and v.
4 Int. pudendal a. and v.
5 Vent. labial v. and mammary br.
  of vent. perineal a.
6 Ext. iliac a. and v.
7 Deep femoral a. and v.
8 Pudendoepigastric vessels
9 Caud. epigastric a. and v.
10 Ext. pudendal a. and v.
11 Caud. mammary a. and v.
12 Cran. mammary a. and v.
   [Caud. supf. epigastric a. and v.]
13 Brachiocephalic trunk and
   cran. vena cava
14 Left subclavian a. and v.
15 Int. thoracic a. and v.
16 Cran. epigastric a. and v.
17 Cran. supf. epigastric a.
18 Subcutaneous abdominal v.
   [Cran. supf. epigastric v.]

A Iliofemoral ln.
   [Deep inguinal ln.]
B Mammary lnn.
   [Supf. inguinal lnn.]
C Afferent lymphatic vessels
C' Efferent lymphatic vessels

a Iliohypogastric n.
b Ilioinguinal n.
c Genitofemoral n.
c' Cran. branch
c" Caud. branch
d Lat. cut. femoral n.
e Pudendal n.
f Mammary br. of pudendal n.

Left cran. and caud. mammary gll.

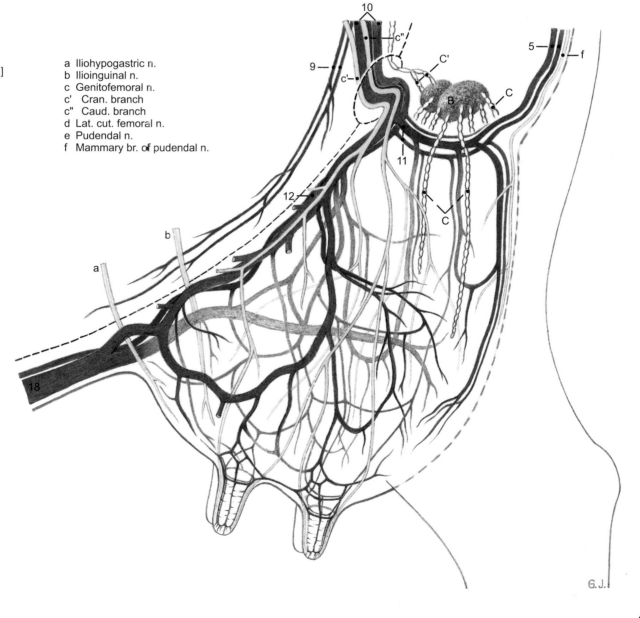

91

8. MALE GENITAL ORGANS AND SCROTUM

a) The **SCROTUM** (5) *is attached in the cranial pubic region. It is elongated dorsoventrally and bottle-shaped. It is generally flesh-colored and fine-haired, and bears two rudimentary teats on each side of the cranial surface of the neck.*

b) The elongated oval **TESTES** (4 and 16) *hang vertically in the scrotum and weigh about 300 g each.* The **capital end** is *proximal* and the **caudate end** is *distal.* (Names derived from the head and tail of the epididymis.) *In ruminants the* **epididymal border** *of the testis is medial or caudomedial and the* **free border** *is lateral.* The part of the **mesorchium (p)** between the vaginal ring and the testis contains the testicular vessels and nerves. It is covered by the visceral lamina of the vaginal tunic, which is attached to the parietal lamina along the caudomedial surface. The ductus deferens runs in the **mesoductus deferens (q)**, a narrow fold attached to the cranial surface of the mesorchium. This location is important for vasectomy. The **spermatic cord** (10) extends from the **vaginal ring** (d) to the testis and consists of the mesorchium and its contents, the ductus deferens, and the mesoductus deferens. The mesorchium continues distally along the epididymal border of the testis. At the tail of the epididymis the mesorchium ends in a short free fold, **the lig. of the tail of the epididymis (o)**, the vestige of the distal part of the gubernaculum testis. Between the testis and the tail of the epididymis is the very short **proper lig. of the testis (n)**, the vestige of the proximal part of the gubernaculum.

c) The **EPIDIDYMIS** begins with a *long* head (caput, 12) on the capital end *and adjacent free boder of the testis. The head consists of a descending limb, and an ascending limb that crosses the mesorchium to the slender* **body of the epididymis** (14). This descends medial to the testis along the caudal side of the mesorchium to the *prominent* **tail of the epididymis** (19). Between the body of the epididymis and the testis is the **testicular bursa** (17), often obliterated by adhesion.

d) The **DUCTUS DEFERENS** (e) ascends in its mesoductus *on the medial side of the testis,* cranial to the mesorchium, to the **spermatic cord** (10), which is *longer and narrower than in the horse.* After it enters the abdominal cavity the duct crosses the lateral lig. of the bladder and the **ureter** (f) and enters the genital fold. It ends in the urethra on the colliculus seminalis in a common orifice with the duct of the vesicular gland.

e) The **ACCESSORY GENITAL GLANDS** are all present as in the horse, *but fully developed only in the bull—not in the steer.* The bilateral **vesicular gland** (11) *is the largest accessory genital gland in the bull. It is a lobated gland of firm consistency—not vesicular.* It is 10–20 cm long and lies dorsal to the bladder and lateral to the ureter and the **ampulla of the ductus deferens** (13). The ductus deferens narrows again caudal to the ampulla and, with the duct of the vesicular gland, passes under the body of the prostate. The two ducts open on the colliculus seminalis (see above). The **body of the prostate** (15) projects on the dorsal surface of the urethra between the vesicular glands and the urethral muscle. The **disseminate part of the prostate**, 12–14 cm long, is concealed in the wall of the urethra and covered ventrally and laterally by the urethral muscle. The bilateral **bulbourethral gland** (18) is the size of a walnut. It lies on each side of the median plane dorsal to the urethra in the transverse plane

of the ischial arch. *It is mostly covered by the bulbospongiosus muscle. Its duct opens on the lateral fold that extends caudally from the septum between the urethra and the urethral recess (see p. 82).*

f) The **PENIS** *of the bull belongs to the fibroelastic type. It extends from its* **root** (h) *at the ischial arch to the* **glans penis** (A) *in the umbilical region. It is covered by skin, is about one meter long, and in the* **body** [corpus penis (i)], *has a* **sigmoid flexure** (j) *that is caudal to the scrotum. The proximal bend is open caudally and the distal bend, open cranially, can be grasped through the skin caudal to the thighs.* The penis is sheathed by telescoping fascia. The short collagenous **suspensory ligg. of the penis** (l) are attached close together on the ischial arch, and the dorsal nn. and vessels of the penis pass out between them. They should not be confused with the fundiform lig. of the penis (p. 80). The penis consists of the dense **corpus cavernosum penis**, which begins at the junction of the **crura penis** (7), attached to the ischial arch. *It is surrounded by a thick* **tunica albuginea** (F) *containing cartilage cells. The cavernae are mainly peripheral, and axially there is a dense* **connective tissue strand** (J). The **free part of the penis** (k), 8 cm long, is distal to the attachment of the internal lamina of the **prepuce** (2). *It is twisted to the left as indicated by the oblique course of the* **raphe of the penis** (D) *from the midventral* **raphe of the prepuce** (D") *to the* **external urethral orifice** (B) *on the right side. Just before ejaculation an added left-hand spiral of the free part of the penis is caused by the internal pressure acting against the right-hand spiral of the collagenous fibers of the subcutaneous tissue and tunica albuginea, and against the* **apical lig.** *The latter originates dorsally from the tunica albuginea, beginning distal to the sigmoid flexure.* Midventral on the penis is the **penile urethra**, surrounded by the **corpus spongiosum penis** (K). The **urethral process** (C) lies in a shallow groove between the raphe and the cap-like **glans penis** (A), which is connected to the corpus spongiosum, but *contains little erectile tissue.* The **prepuce** consists, as in the dog, of an **external lamina** (1) and an **internal lamina** (2), and has bristle-like hairs at the **preputial orifice** (3). The **frenulum of the prepuce** (D') connects the raphe of the prepuce to the raphe of the penis. The **muscles of the penis:** The **ischiocavernosus** (7) extends from the medial surface of the ischial tuber to the body of the penis, covering the crus penis. The **bulbospongiosus** (6) covers the bulb of the penis and a large part of the bulbourethral gland and extends to the beginning of the body of the penis. During erection *both muscles regulate the inflow and outflow of blood.* The paired smooth muscle **retractor penis** (8) originates from the caudal vertebrae, *receives reinforcing fibers from the internal anal sphincter, extends across the first bend of the sigmoid flexure and is attached to the second bend. The two muscles then approach each other on the ventral surface and terminate on the tunica albuginea 15–20 cm proximal to the glans. In erection these muscles relax, permitting the extension of the sigmoid flexure and elongation of the penis.*

The **lymphatic vessels** of the scrotum, penis, and prepuce drain to the **superficial inguinal lnn.** (9) which lie dorsolaterally on the penis at the transverse plane of the pecten pubis, just caudal to the spermatic cord. The lymph vessels of the testes go to the medial iliac lnn. (p. 82).

Penis

(Cross section cranial to sigmoid flexure)

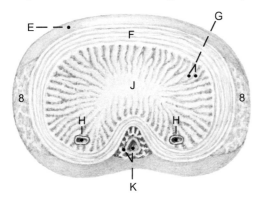

(Right surface)

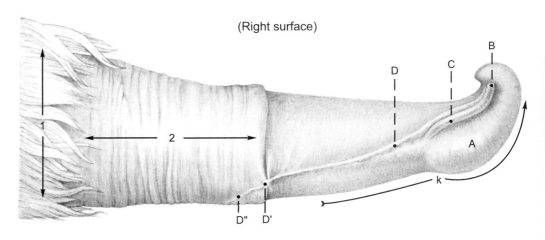

Legend:

A Glans penis	D Raphe of penis	F Tunica albuginea	J Corpus cavernosum
B Ext. urethral orifice	D' Frenulum of prepuce	G Trabeculae of J	K Corpus spongiosum and urethra
C Urethral process	D" Raphe of prepuce	H Deep veins of penis	k Free part of penis
	E Fascia of penis		

* Ashdown, 1958; Ashdown 1969; Seidel and Foote, 1967

Male genital organs

(Left side)

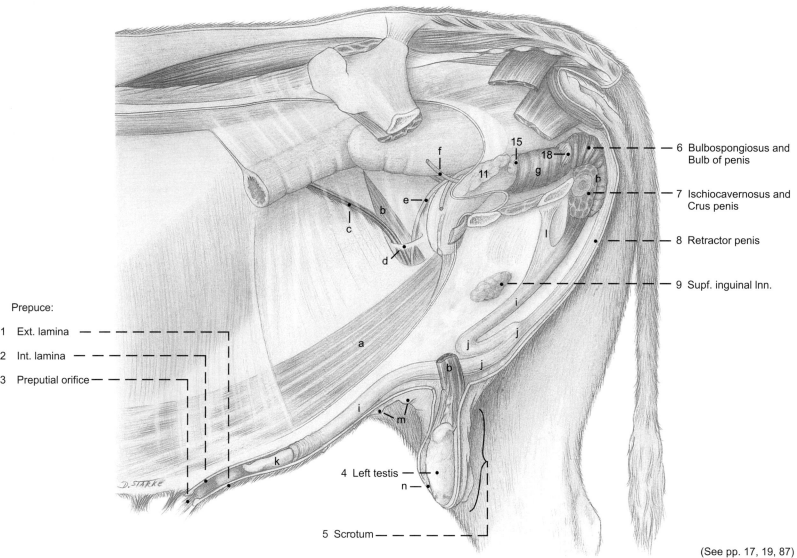

6	Bulbospongiosus and Bulb of penis
7	Ischiocavernosus and Crus penis
8	Retractor penis
9	Supf. inguinal lnn.

Prepuce:

1 Ext. lamina

2 Int. lamina

3 Preputial orifice

4 Left testis

5 Scrotum

(See pp. 17, 19, 87)

Legend:

a Rectus abdominis
b Cremaster
c Testicular a. and v.
d Vaginal ring
e Ductus deferens

f Ureter
g Urethralis
Penis:
h Root of the penis
i Body of the penis

j Sigmoid flexure
k Free part of penis
l Suspensory ligg. of penis
m Male mammary gl.
n Proper lig. of testis

o Lig. of the tail of the epididymis
p Mesorchium
q Mesoductus deferens
r Mesofuniculus
s Pampiniform plexus

Testis and Epididymis

(caudal)

Accessory genital gll.

(dorsal)

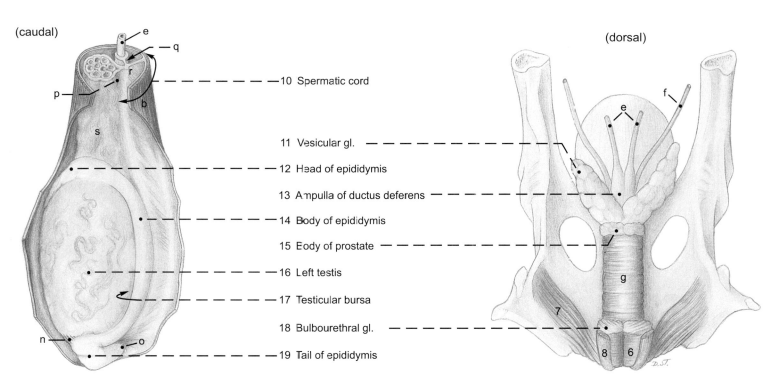

10 Spermatic cord

11 Vesicular gl.

12 Head of epididymis

13 Ampulla of ductus deferens

14 Body of epididymis

15 Body of prostate

16 Left testis

17 Testicular bursa

18 Bulbourethral gl.

19 Tail of epididymis

9. PERINEUM, PELVIC DIAPHRAGM, ISCHIORECTAL FOSSA, AND TAIL

The clinically important perineum is studied by first removing the skin from the perineal region to see the superficial muscles, nerves, and vessels. The fat is removed from the ischiorectal fossa, exposing the **distal cutaneous br. of the pudendal n.** (19) where it emerges on the medial surface of the tuber ischiadicum and supplies the **superficial perineal nn.** (4). The **caudal rectal a.** (21) is exposed in its course along the lateral border of the ext. anal sphincter, and branches of the **dorsal and ventral perineal aa.** are seen. The superficial fascia is incised from the labia to the udder to expose the large, convoluted, and often double **ventral labial v.** (16), draining blood from the perineum to the **caudal mammary v.** The **mammary brr. of the pudendal nn.** are traced on the lateral borders of the vein. The corresponding nerve in the bull is the preputial and scrotal br., and the vein is the ventral scrotal. In deeper dissections the fascia is removed from the terminations of the **coccygeus** (2) and **levator ani** (3) and from the **constrictor vestibuli** (13) and **constrictor vulvae** (14). The smooth muscle **retractor clitoridis** (15) is seen between the constrictor vestibuli and constrictor vulvae in the cow, and the **retractor penis** between the bulbospongiosus and ischiocavernosus in the bull.

a) The **PERINEUM and PERINEAL REGION.** The **perineum** is the part of the body wall that closes the pelvic outlet, bounded by the first caudal vertebra, the **sacrosciatic ligg.** (1), the **tubera ischiadica** (b), and the ischial arch. The part of the perineum dorsal to a line connecting the tubera ischiadica is the anal triangle, surrounding the anal canal and closed by the pelvic diaphragm. The part of the perineum ventral to the line is the urogenital triangle, surrounding the urogenital tract and closed by the perineal membrane. A more restricted definition includes only the perineal body between the anus and the urogenital tract. The **perineal region** is the surface area over the perineum and adjacent parts. In the ox it is bounded dorsally by the root of the tail and ventrally by the attachment of the scrotum or udder. The lateral border is formed by the sacrosciatic ligament, tuber ischiadicum, and a line from the tuber to the scrotum or udder. The perineal region is divided into anal and urogenital regions by a line connecting the medial processes of the tubers. *The urogenital region is greatly elongated in ruminants by the ventral position of the scrotum and udder.*

b) The **ANAL TRIANGLE.** The **pelvic diaphragm** is composed of right and left **coccygeus** (2) and **levator ani** (3) muscles and the **external anal sphincter** (12), together with the deep fascia on their external and internal surfaces. Each half of the diaphragm is oblique, extending caudomedially from the origin of the muscles on the medial surface of the sciatic spine, to the termination of the coccygeus on the caudal vertebrae and of the levator ani on the external anal sphincter. The **perineal body** [centrum tendineum perinei], is the fibromuscular mass between the anus and the urogenital tract.

c) The **UROGENITAL TRIANGLE.** The **perineal membrane** in the cow is a strong sheet of deep perineal fascia extending from the ischial arch to the ventral and lateral walls of the vestibule, cranial to the **constrictor vestibuli** (13) and caudal to the **major vestibular gland** (10). Together with the urogenital muscles it closes the urogenital triangle, joining the pelvic diaphragm at the the level of the perineal body and anchoring the genital tract to the ischial arch.

d) The **ISCHIORECTAL FOSSA** is a fat-filled, wedge-shaped space lateral to the anus. The laterodorsal wall is the **sacrosciatic lig.**, the caudal border of which, the **sacrotuberous lig** (1), is easily palpable. The lateroventral wall is the tuber ischiadicum and the obturator fascia. The medial wall is the deep fascia covering the coccygeus, levator ani, and constrictor vestibuli. In the ox, unlike the horse, the sacrotuberous lig. and tuber ischiadicum are subcutaneous (see p. 16).

e) **NERVES AND VESSELS.** For the intrapelvic origins of the perineal nerves and vessels, see pp. 84–85. The **pudendal n.** (9) gives off the **proximal** and **distal cutaneous branches** and the **deep perineal n.** (20), and continues caudally on the pelvic floor with the **internal pudendal a. and v.** (9), supplying the vestibule and the **mammary br.** (25) and terminating in the clitoris. In the bull, the pudendal n. gives off the **preputial** and **scrotal brr.** and continues as the **dorsal n. of the penis.** The deep perineal n. supplies the vagina, major vestibular gland, and perineal muscles, and ends in the labium and the skin lateral to the perineal body. The **caudal rectal n.** (17), which may be double, supplies branches to the rectum, coccygeus, levator ani, ext. anal sphincter, retractor clitoridis (penis), perineal body, constrictor vestibuli, roof of the vestibule, and labium. Anesthesia of the penis and paralysis of the retractor penis, or anesthesia of the vestibule and vulva can be produced by blocking bilaterally the pudendal and caudal rectal nn. and the communicating br. of the caud. cutaneous femoral n. (p. 84) inside the sacrosciatic lig.* The **internal iliac a.** (6), at the level of the sciatic spine, gives off the vaginal or prostatic a. (These arteries may originate from the internal pudendal a.) The internal iliac ends by dividing at the lesser sciatic foramen into the caud. gluteal a. and **internal pudendal a.** (9). The latter supplies the coccygeus, levator ani, ischiorectal fossa, vagina, urethra, vestibule, and major vestibular gl. The internal pudendal a. ends by dividing into the **ventral perineal a.** (23) and the **a. of the clitoris** (24). The ventral perineal a. usually gives off the **mammary branch** (25). In some cows the ventral perineal a. and mammary br. are supplied by the dorsal labial br. of the dorsal perineal a. The **vaginal a.** (7), after giving off the uterine br., divides into the middle rectal a. and the **dorsal perineal a.** (8). The latter divides into the **caud. rectal a.** (21) and the **dorsal labial br.** (22), which gives off the perineal br. seen on the tuber ischiadicum, and runs ventrally in the labium. It may also supply the mammary br. and the ventral part of the perineum. The dorsal labial br. may be cut in episiotomy. In the male, the **prostatic a.** gives branches to the urethra, prostate, and bulbourethral gl., and may terminate as the dorsal perineal a., but the latter usually comes from the internal pudendal a.**

f) The **TAIL** contains 16–21 caudal vertebrae. The **rectocaudalis** is longitudinal smooth muscle from the wall of the rectum, attached to caud. vertebrae 2 and 3. The smooth muscle retractor clitoridis (penis) originates from caud. vertebrae 2 and 3 or 3 and 4. The **caudal nerves** in the cauda equina run in the vertebral canal. The **median caudal a. and v.** on the ventral surface are convenient for the veterinarian working behind stanchioned cows. The pulse is best palpated between the vertebrae or about 18 cm from the root of the tail to avoid the hemal processes. Tail bleeding is done by raising the tail and puncturing the median caudal v. between hemal processes.

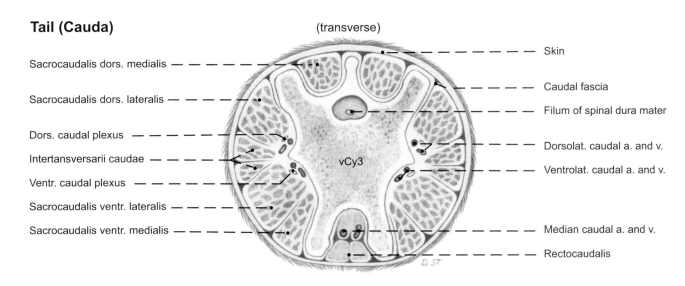

Tail (Cauda)   (transverse)

Sacrocaudalis dors. medialis — — — — — — — — — — — Skin

Sacrocaudalis dors. lateralis — — — — — — — — — — — Caudal fascia

Dors. caudal plexus — — — — — — — — — — — — Filum of spinal dura mater

Intertransversarii caudae — — — — — — — — — — Dorsolat. caudal a. and v.

Ventr. caudal plexus — — — — — — — — vCy3 — — — Ventrolat. caudal a. and v.

Sacrocaudalis ventr. lateralis — — — — — — — —

Sacrocaudalis ventr. medialis — — — — — — — — — — Median caudal a. and v.

                                                    — — — — — Rectocaudalis

* Larson, 1953
** Erasha, 1987

Perineal region

♀

(Caudal aspect)

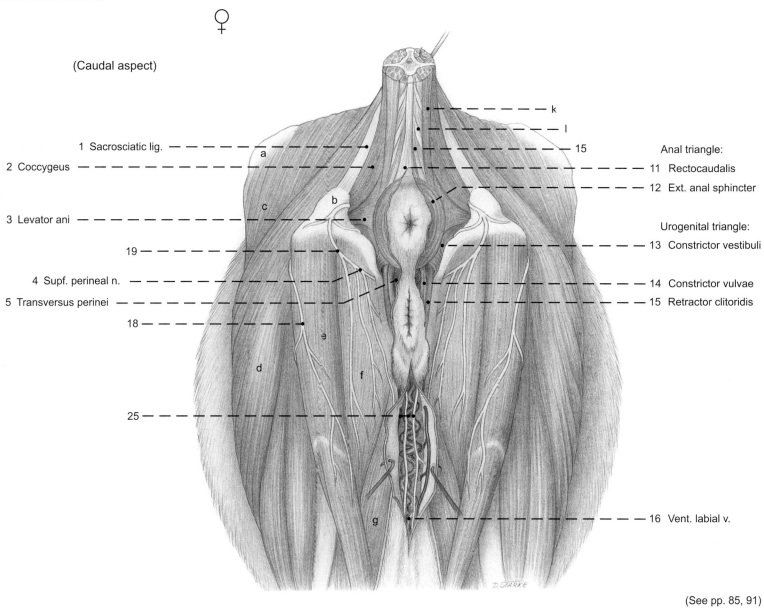

1 Sacrosciatic lig.
2 Coccygeus
3 Levator ani
19
4 Supf. perineal n.
5 Transversus perinei
18
25

k
l
15

Anal triangle:
11 Rectocaudalis
12 Ext. anal sphincter

Urogenital triangle:
13 Constrictor vestibuli
14 Constrictor vulvae
15 Retractor clitoridis

16 Vent. labial v.

(See pp. 85, 91)

Legend:

a Tuber coxae
b Tuber ischiadicum
c Gluteus medius
c Retractor clitoridis

d Biceps femoris
e Semitendinosus
f Semimembranosus

g Gracilis
h Intertransversarii
i Sacrocaudalis dors. med.

j Sacrocaudalis dors. lat.
k Sacrocaudalis vent. lat.
l Sacrocaudalis vent. med.

(Lateral aspect)

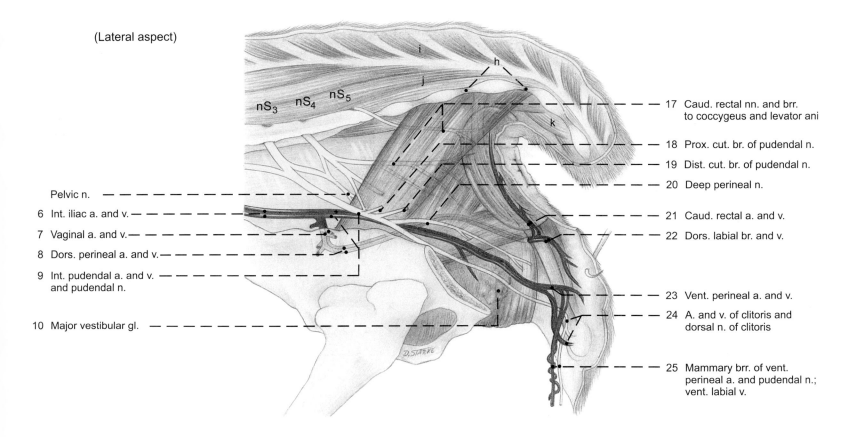

nS_3 nS_4 nS_5

17 Caud. rectal nn. and brr.
   to coccygeus and levator ani
18 Prox. cut. br. of pudendal n.
19 Dist. cut. br. of pudendal n.
20 Deep perineal n.

Pelvic n.
6 Int. iliac a. and v.
7 Vaginal a. and v.
8 Dors. perineal a. and v.
9 Int. pudendal a. and v.
   and pudendal n.

10 Major vestibular gl.

21 Caud. rectal a. and v.
22 Dors. labial br. and v.

23 Vent. perineal a. and v.
24 A. and v. of clitoris and
   dorsal n. of clitoris

25 Mammary brr. of vent.
   perineal a. and pudendal n.;
   vent. labial v.

ANATOMICAL ASPECTS OF BOVINE SPONGIFORM ENCEPHALOPATHY (BSE)

NATURE OF THE DISEASE

The term spongiform encephalopathy refers to spongy changes in the brain. BSE is one of a group of diseases called transmissible spongiform encephalopathies (TSE), of which scrapie of sheep has been know for a long time, is widely distributed, and has been intensively investigated. The TSE are caused by **prion proteins (PrP)** – minute proteinaceous infectious particles 4–6 nm in diameter. They occur in normal and pathogenic forms on the surface of nerve cells and various cells of lymphatic tissue. In normal PrP the amino acid chains are predominantly wound up in **alpha-helices.** By unknow processes, often by mutation in the controlling gene, pathogenic PrP develop, whose amino acids in some regions of the molecule are refolded from alpha helices into **beta-sheets** layered antiparallel on each other.* The misfolded, pathogenic PrP cause BSE by imposing their structure on normal PrP, thereby multiplying the pathogen. They enter the lysosomes of nerve cells, where they are not decomposed, but accumulate in amyloid plaques and cause the death of the nerve cells.**

Models of prion proteins (purple = alpha-helix structure, blue = beta sheet structure

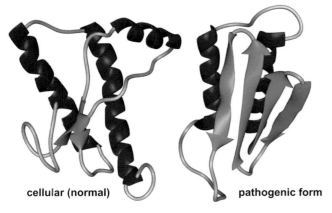

cellular (normal)   pathogenic form

SPECIES DISTRIBUTION OF PRION DISEASES

Prion diseases have been found in sheep, goats, cattle, zoo and wild ruminants, mink, great cats, and rhesus monkeys. Human prion diseases are Creutzfeldt-Jakob disease, Gerstmann-Straeussler syndrome, fatal familial insomnia, and kuru. BSE is of great importance because:

1. Its causative agent can overcome the species barrier and become very dangerous to man.

2. Cattle are significant sources of human food, and an undiagnosed BSE infection is a danger to man.

THE SIGNS OF BSE DISEASE

The average age of cattle affected with BSE is about 3 years, but the first signs may appear at 20 months. As a result of the brain disorder, the following signs appear: hypersensitivity to stimuli (e. g. noise), anxiety, aggression, and locomotor disturbance progressing to collapse. The terminal stage is prostration until death. There is no cure.

DIAGNOSIS OF BSE

A suspected clinical diagnosis is possible in the terminal stage, but a certain diagnosis can be made only after death. For the rapid test, parts of the brainstem are removed, homogenized, and digested by proteinases. After digestion, only the pathogenic PrP remain intact, and can be identified by a specific antibody. If the results are doubtful, further tests by immunohistological or cytological (E/M) methods are required.

POSSIBLE CAUSES FOR THE APPEARANCE OF NEW PRION DISEASES

The PrP of scrapie in sheep could have mutated in cattle to the PrP of BSE. Scrapie was widely distributed in Great Britain, and carcasses of affected sheep were reduced in rendering plants to fat and tankage in large autoclaves (tanks). The tankage (meat and bone meal) was a common source of protein in animal feed, including cattle feed. Transmission by feed was later made highly probable by the success of a ban on tankage in animal feed.**

In Germany BSE was probably spread by feeding calves a milk substitute made by replacing milk fat with tallow from adult bovine mesenteric and abdominal fat.

Failure to observe proper procedures in the operation of the tank (addition of lye and detergents and maintenance of heat at 130 °C for 20 min.) could have led to survival of pathogenic PrP.

PATHWAYS OF INFECTION

The probable mode of infection in sheep and cattle is intestinal. Precise information on infection of cattle is not available, but inferences can be drawn from experiments on rodents, which have a much shorter incubation period. Also, possible parallels can be drawn to scrapie in sheep.

TRANSPORT THROUGH THE AUTONOMIC SYSTEM

At least three routes to the CNS have been proposed on the basis of experiments on rodents: ***

1. The vagus conducts **parasympathetic fibers** that bypass the spinal cord. The vagal efferents have their nerve cell bodies in the dorsal motor nucleus in the obex region of the medulla. Vagal afferents have their nerve cell bodies in the proximal and distal vagal ganglia. They send their short axons to the obex region.

2. An alternative route goes from the enteric plexuses through prevertebral ganglia and the **splanchnic nerves** to the **sympathetic trunk**, thence through the communicating branches and spinal nerve roots to the tracts of the spinal cord leading to and from the brain.

3. A third possibility is passage from the sympathetic trunk through the cervicothoracic ganglion, ansa subclavia, and **vago-sympathetic trunk** to the head.

Sympathetic system

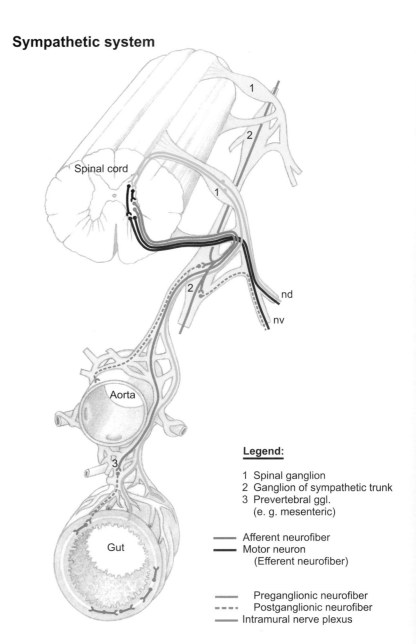

Legend:

1 Spinal ganglion
2 Ganglion of sympathetic trunk
3 Prevertebral ggl.
   (e. g. mesenteric)

――― Afferent neurofiber
――― Motor neuron
      (Efferent neurofiber)

――― Preganglionic neurofiber
- - - Postganglionic neurofiber
――― Intramural nerve plexus

*   Borchers, 2002   *** McBride et al., 2001
**   Hoernlimann et al., 2001

AREAS OF HIGHEST CONCENTRATION IN THE BRAIN

The primary site of pathogenic prions is the region of the obex between the medulla oblongata and the spinal cord. The dorsal vagal nucleus and other important nuclei here show typical spongiform changes. Other regions of the brainstem display lesions. Spongiform encephalopathy of the cerebellar cortex explains the locomotor disturbances and ataxia. Insoluble amyloid forms in the nerve cells, with high concentration of pathogenic prions and spongiform changes. Neighboring glia cells are also affected.

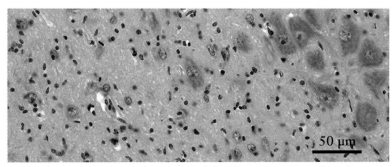

Normal nervous tissue in the region of the obex (dorsal vagal nucleus).
Preparation: Prof. G. Boehme, Inst. of Vet. Anatomy, FU-Berlin

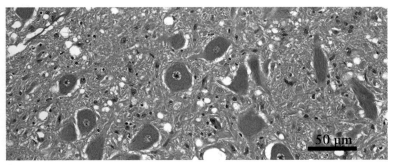

Nervous tissue of the region of the obex in BSE.
Preparation: Prof. F. Ehrensperger, Inst. of Vet. Pathology, Zürich

Another TSE, chronic wasting disease (CWD) of North American deer and elk, discovered in Colorado in 1967, has been found in wild or farmed deer and elk in Wyoming, Nebraska, South Dakota, Oklahoma, Montana, Wisconin, and one case in Illinois. (The North American elk, a misnomer, is *Cervus canadensis*, not *Alces alces*—the European Elch and the North American moose.) There is no evidence that other species, including man, are infected through contact with CWD.[****] In experimental deer inoculated orally with infective deer brain, pathogenic PrP were first found in lymphoid tissues of the alimentary system and then in autonomic nerves leading from the gut to the brainstem, where they appeared first in the dorsal motor nucleus of the vagus. Other peripheral nerves, such as the brachial plexus and sciatic nerve, were tested and found negative.[*****]

REMOVAL OF THE BRAINSTEM FOR LABORATORY TESTS

After slaughter and decapitation, brainstem tissue can be removed with a curette through the foramen magnum. If the head is bisected, the myelencephalon and metencephalon are separated from the more rostral parts of the brain (see p. 51, below by a transverse cut through 13 and 14, and by cutting the roots of cranial nn. V-XII and the cerebellar peduncles to release the sample of the brainstem. The material of the obex region is used for the BSE rapid test. If the results are positive, histopathologic, immunohistochemical, and E/M investigations follow, for which more rostral parts of the brainstem are used.

TRANSMISSION OF BSE TO MAN

Human infection with the agent of BSE and consequent illnes with the variant of Creutzfeld-Jacob disease (vCJD) is highly probable. In vCJD the multiplication of the agent also occurs outside the brain and spinal cord in the lymphatic organs (e.g. tonsils); whereas in the sporadic (classical) CJD the pathological changes remain restricted to the CNS. The likelihood of transmission from BSE-infected cattle to man is supported by the fact that the agents of BSE and vCJD are biologically and biochemically identical. The connection of time and place between occurences of BSE and vCJD in Great Britain supports this probability. Apparently a genetically determined susceptibility plays a role in transmission because, so far, only a few people have contracted vCJD, and only a few of the cattle in a herd contract BSE.

DANGERS OF EATING MEAT AND MEAT PRODUCTS FROM BSE-INFECTED CATTLE OR CATTLE SUSPECTED OF EXPOSURE TO BSE

The risks increase with the amount of infective material consumed and its concentration of pathogenic misfolded prions. Of the components of nervous tissue, the perikarya and therefore the ganglia and nuclei may present a greater danger than axons, and thus more than nerves and fiber tracts. The perikarya occupy a much larger volume and have a concentration of prions in the lysosomes, which are not present in the processes. The danger is increased, the nearer the ganglia lie to valuable cuts of meat; for example, the sympathetic trunk and ganglia are closely associated with the tenderloin (iliopsoas and psoas minor; see p. 81, upper fig.) The spinal ganglia lie in the intervertebral foramina and are included with the bone in steaks cut from the rib and loin regions (see text fig.). Regarding the concentration of pathogenic misfolded prions the following list presents the opinion of the European Union on the possible risk of infectivity in various tissues (including experiments with scrapie).

1. **Highly infectious tissues:** brain and spinal cord together with surrounding membranes, eyes, spinal ganglia.
2. **Tissues of intermediate infectivity:** intestine, tonsils, spleen, placenta, uterus, fetal tissue, cerebrospinal fluid, hypophysis, and adrenal gl.
3. **Tissues of lower infectivity:** liver, thymus, bone marrow, tubular bones, nasal mucosa, peripheral nerves.
4. **Infectivity was not demonstrated in the following tissues and organs:** skeletal muscle, heart, kidneys, milk, fat (exept mesenteric fat), cartilage, blood, salivary gll., testis, and ovary.

Spinal cord and sympathetic trunk after removal of the left side of the vertebral arches and the musculature

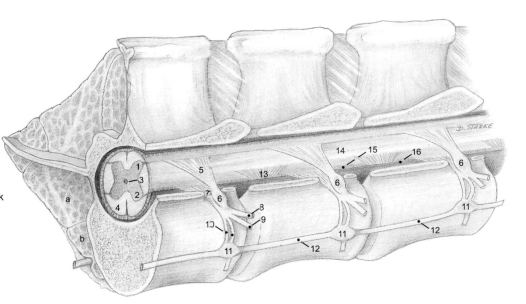

Legend:

	Gray matter		
	Gray matter		
1	Dorsal horn	10	Communicating brr.
2	Ventral horn		white and gray
3	Central canal	11	Ganglia of sympathetic trunk
4	White matter	12	Sympathetic trunk
5	Dorsal root	13	Denticulate lig.
6	Spinal ganglion	14	Pia mater
7	Ventral root	15	Arachnoidea
8	Dorsal br.	16	Dura mater
9	Ventral br.	a	Psoas major
		b	Psoas minor

[****]   JAVMA, 2002
[*****] Sigurdson et al., 2001

SPECIAL ANATOMY, TABULAR PART

1. MYOLOGY

MUSCLE / FIG.	ORIGIN	TERMINATION	INNERVATION	FUNCTION	REMARKS
MEDIAL MUSCLES OF THE SHOULDER AND ARM (p. 4)					
Teres major (5.2)	Caudal border of scapula and subscapualis	Teres major tuberosity of humerus	Axillary n.	Flexor of shoulder joint	Joined by terminal tendon of latissimus dorsi
Subscapularis (5.4)	Subscapular fossa of scapula	Minor tubercle of humerus	Subscapular and axillary nn.	Mainly an extensor of shoulder jt.	3–4 distinct parts; tendon acts as med. collat. lig. of shoulder joint
Coracobrachialis (5.16)	Coracoid process of scapula	Small part prox. and large part dist. to teres major tuberosity of humerus	Musculocutaneous n.	Extensor of shoulder joint and adductor and supinator of brachium	Two bellies; synovial bursa under tendon of origin
Articularis humeri	Inconstant in the ox.				
Biceps brachii (5.26)	Supraglenoid tubercle of scapula	Radial tuberosity, cranial surface of radius, fleshy on med. collat. lig. of elbow joint	Musculocutaneous n.	Extensor of shoulder joint, flexor of elbow joint	Intertubercular bursa under tendon of origin; thin lacertus fibrosis to antebrachial fascia
Brachialis (5.21)	Caud. surface of humerus, close to neck	*Radial tuberosity and med. collat. lig. of elbow joint*	Musculocutaneous n.; for distal parts, radial n.	Flexor of elbow joint	Spiral course in brachialis groove of humerus, added innervation from radial n. in 50 %
Tensor fasciae antebrachii (5.22)	Caud. border of scapula, latissimus dorsi	Medially on olecranon and antebrachial fascia	Radial n.	Tensor of fascia of forearm and extensor of elbow joint	
LATERAL MUSCLES OF SHOULDER AND ARM (p. 4)					
Deltoideus			Axillary n.		
Clavicular part (Cleidobrachialis) (5.23)	Clavicular intersection	Crest of humerus		Advances limb	Part of brachiocephalicus; see p. 60
Scapular part (5.6)	Caud. border of scapula, aponeurosis from scapular spine	Deltoid tuberosity of humerus, *fascia of triceps*		Flexor of shoulder joint	Small flat muscle
Acromial part (5.7)	Acromion	Deltoid tuberosity of humerus		Flexor of shoulder joint	Interspersed with tendinous strands
Teres minor (5.12)	Distal half of cd. border of scapula	Prox. to deltoid tuberosity of humerus on *teres minor tuberosity*	Axillary n.	Flexor of shoulder joint	
Supraspinatus (5.1)	Supraspinous fossa, *cran. border of scapula*	Major and minor tubercles of humerus	Suprascapular n.	Extensor and stabilizer of shoulder jt.; also flexor dependent on state of joint	Tendon of origin of biceps passes between the terminal tendons
Infraspinatus (5.11)	Infraspinous fossa and spine of scapula	Deep part on prox. border and med. surface of major tubercle; supf. part distal to tubercle	Suprascapular n.	Abductor and lateral rotator of arm; acts as lat. collateral lig.	Largely tendinous, flat; supf. tendon passes over infraspinatus bursa
Triceps brachii		All heads together on olecranon	Radial n.	Extensor of elbow joint; long head also flexes shoulder joint; stabilizer of elbow	Relatively flat
Long head (5.18)	Caud. border of scapula				
Lat. head (5.17)	Lateral on humerus				
Med. head (5.19)	Medial on humerus				
Accessory head	Caudal on humerus				Partially separable from med. head
Anconeus (5.25)	Borders of olecranon fossa	Lateral on olecranon	Radial n.	Extensor of elbow joint	Separable with difficulty from lat. head of triceps

MUSCLE / FIG.	ORIGIN	TERMINATION	INNERVATION	FUNCTION	REMARKS
CRANIOLATERAL MUSCLES OF THE FOREARM					
Generally extensors, which originate predominantly on the lateral epicondyle of the humerus (p. 4)					
Common digital extensor (5.40)			Radial n.		Extensor of the digits and carpus
Medial head (Proper extensor of digit III, Med. digital extensor)	*Lateral epicondyle of humerus*	*Middle and distal phalanges of digit III*		*Extensor of fetlock and pastern joints of digit III*	*Receives extensor branches of interosseus III*
Lateral head (Common extensor of digits III and IV)	*Lateral epicondyle of humerus, head of ulna*	*Branches to extensor processes of dist. phalanges of digits III & IV*		*Extensor of coffin joints*	*Narrow muscle; humeral and ulnar heads unite in a common tendon*
Lateral digital extensor *(Proper extensor of digit IV)* **(5.41)**	*Proximal on radius and ulna*	*Middle and distal phalanges of digit IV*	Radial n.	*Extensor of fetlock and pastern joints of digit IV*	Unified; corresponds to medial dig. extensor, with extensor branches from interosseus IV
Extensor carpi radialis (5.35)	Lat. supracondylar crest and radial fossa of humerus	Tuberosity of Mc III	Radial n.	Extensor and stabilizer of carpus	Has synovial bursae on carpus and at termination; may have rudimentary extensor digiti I
Ulnaris lateralis (Extensor carpi ulnaris) (5.38)	Lateral epicondyle of humerus	Accessory carpal bone and Mc V	Radial n.	Flexor (!) of the carpus	
Ext. carpi obliquus (Abductor pollicis longus) (5.39)	Craniolat. in middle third of radius	Mc III	Radial n.	Extensor of the carpus	Terminal tendon has synovial bursa
CAUDOMEDIAL MUSCLES OF THE FOREARM					
Generally FLEXORS, which originate predominantly on the medial epicondyle of the humerus (p. 4)					
Superficial digital flexor (5.36 and 5.37)	Med. epicondyle of humerus	Flexor tuberosities of middle phalanges	Ulnar n.	Flexor of the carpus and digits	Larger supf. belly supf. to flexor retinaculum; deep belly within carpal canal

MUSCLE / FIG.	ORIGIN	TERMINATION	INNERVATION	FUNCTION	REMARKS
Deep digital flexor (5.34)		Flexor tubercles of distal phalanges		Flexor of coffin jts.; support of fetlock jts.	The single deep flexor tendon is surrounded by a synovial bursa in the carpal canal
Humeral head	Med. epicondyle of humerus		Ulnar and median nn.		The humeral head is tripartite and interspersed with many tendinous strands
Ulnar head	Olecranon		Ulnar n.		Ulnar head is small
Radial head	Caudomedial on prox. third of radius		Median n.		
Flexor carpi ulnaris (5.29)		Accessory carpal bone	Ulnar n.	Flexor of carpus	
Humeral head	Medial epicondyle of humerus				
Ulnar head	Medially on olecranon				Ulnar head is small
Flexor carpi radialis (5.28)	Medial epicondyle of humerus	*Proximopalmar on Mc III*	Median n.	Flexor of carpus	Surrounded by a tendon sheath in carpal canal
Pronator teres (5.27)	Medial epicondyle of humerus	Craniomedial on radius	Median n.	Pronator of forearm and manus	Weakly muscular

METACARPUS (p. 4 and 18)

MUSCLE / FIG.	ORIGIN	TERMINATION	INNERVATION	FUNCTION	REMARKS
Interflexorii	Muscle fibers connecting the supf. and deep digital flexors as well as their tendons, in and near the carpal canal		Median n.	Auxiliary flexors of the digits	
Interosseus III and Interosseus IV (p. 18)	Prox. end of mtc. bone; deep palmar carpal lig.	Prox. sesamoid bones; branches to proper extensor tendons; accessory lig. to supf. flexor	Palmar branch of ulnar n.	Support fetlock joints; oppose tension of deep flexor on distal phalanx	Predominantly tendinous in older cattle

MUSCLES OF THE HIP JOINT (p. 16)

MUSCLE / FIG.	ORIGIN	TERMINATION	INNERVATION	FUNCTION	REMARKS
Tensor fasciae latae (17.5)	Tuber coxae	By the fascia lata on the patella, lat. patellar lig., and cran. border of tibia	Cran. gluteal n.	Flexor of hip joint, advances limb; extensor of stifle; tensor of fascia lata	Includes cran. parts of gluteus supf.; especially robust in cattle
Gluteus superficialis	Tuber coxae (gluteal fascia)	Cran. part of biceps femoris and fascia lata	Cran. and caud. gluteal nn.	*Extensor of hip joint; retractor of limb*	Not separable from the total mass of the gluteobiceps
Gluteus medius (17.1)	*Gluteal surface of ilium*	Major trochanter of femur	Cran. gluteal n.	Extensor of hip joint; abductor of limb	Has a lumbar process on the longissimus lumborum
Gluteus accessorius (17.3)	Gluteal surface of ilium	*Craniolat. on femur just distal to maj. trochanter*	Cran. gluteal n.	Same as gluteus medius	Clearly separable from gluteus medius; trochanteric bursa under terminal tendon
Gluteus profundus (17.4)	Sciatic spine, *lat. on body of ischium, sacrosciatic lig.*	*Craniolat. on femur, distal to gluteus accessorius*	Cran. gluteal n.	Abductor of limb	Synovial bursa under terminal tendon

MUSCLE / FIG.	ORIGIN	TERMINATION	INNERVATION	FUNCTION	REMARKS
CAUDAL THIGH MUSCLES (p. 16)					
Gluteobiceps (Biceps femoris) (17.7)	Vertebral head: caud. part of *median sacral crest* and last transverse processes; sacrosciatic lig.; and *tuber ischiadicum*. Pelvic head: tuber ischiadicum	Patella; *lat. patellar lig.*; cran. border of tibia (by fascia cruris and fascia lata); common calcanean tendon	Vert. head: caud. gluteal n. Pelvic head: tibial n.	Extensor of hip and stifle; with caud. part, flexor of stifle; abductor of limb; extensor of hock	Not clearly separable into cran. and caud. parts; almost complete fusion with gluteus supf.
Semitendinosus (17.20)	*Tuber ischiadicum*	Cran. border of tibia, *terminal aponeurosis of gracilis,* common calcanean tendon	*Tibial n.*	In supporting limb: extensor of hip, stifle and hock; in swinging limb: flexor of stifle; also adductor and retractor of limb	No vertebral head; transverse intersection between prox. and middle thirds.
Semimembranosus (17.18)	*Tuber ischiadicum*	Med. condyles of femur and tibia	*Tibial n.*	In supporting limb: extensor of hip and stifle; in swinging limb: retractor, adductor, and pronator of limb	No vertebral head. Belly divides into two branches
DEEP MUSCLES OF THE HIP JOINT (p. 16, 18)					
Gemelli (17.25)	Lesser sciatic notch	Trochanteric fossa of femur	Muscular brr. of sciatic n.	Rotate thigh laterally	Thick, unified muscle plate
Internal obturator is absent in the ox.					
Quadratus femoris (17.26)	Ventral surface of ischium	Lat. surface of body of femur	Muscular brr. of sciatic n.	Supinator of thigh, auxiliary extensor of hip joint	
External obturator (19.7)	Outer and inner surface of ischium around obturator for.	Trochanteric fossa of femur	Obturator n.	Supinator of thigh; adductor of limb	The intrapelvic part is small and not homologous to internal obturator
MEDIAL THIGH MUSCLES: Adductors (p. 18)					
Gracilis (19.10)	*Prepubic tendon; by symphysial tendon from pelvic symphysis*	*Fascia cruris*	Obturator and saphenous nn.	Adductor (and extensor of stifle jt.)	Right and left tendons of origin fused to form symphyseal tendon; terminal tendon fused with that of sartorius
Adductor magnus (et brevis) (19.9)	Symphyseal tendon; ventrally on pelvis	Facies aspera of femur	Obturator n.	Adductor and retractor of the limb	Joined by connective tissue with semimembranosus; on split carcass cut surface of adductor in bull is triangular; in cow it is bean-shaped
Pectineus (et adductor longus) (19.8)	Contralateral pubis: iliopubic eminence; ilium up to tubercle of psoas minor	Caudomedial on femur	Adductor part: obturator n.; pectineus part: saphenous n.	Adductor of limb, flexor of hip	More robust than in horse; crossed tendons of origin form the bulk of the prepubic tendon
EXTENSORS OF THE STIFLE (p. 18)					
Sartorius (19.3)	*Cranial: iliac fascia and tendon of psoas minor; caudal: iliopubic eminence and adjacent ilium*	Fascia cruris	Saphenous n.	Flexor of hip joint; protractor and adductor of limb; extensor of stifle	Lacuna vasorum for femoral vessels lies between the two tendinous heads
Quadriceps femoris		By middle patellar lig. on the tibial tuberosity	Femoral n.	Flexor of the hip joint (rectus); extensor and stabilizer of the stifle	Very large and clearly four heads
Rectus femoris (19.1)	Ilium: *main tendon from med. fossa cran. to acetabulum; small tendon from lat. area near acetab.*				
Vastus lateralis (17.29)	Proximolateral on femur				
Vastus medialis (19.2)	Proximomedial on femur				
Vastus intermedius	Proximocranial on femur				

MUSCLE / FIG.	ORIGIN	TERMINATION	INNERVATION	FUNCTION	REMARKS
SPECIAL FLEXOR OF THE STIFLE: Caudal to the stifle (p. 18)					
Popliteus (29.4)	Lateral femoral condyle	Proximomedial on caud. surface of tibia	Tibial n.	Flexor of stifle	
EXTENSORS OF THE HOCK AND FLEXORS OF THE DIGITS: Caudal on the crus (p. 18)					
Gastrocnemius (19.11) Lateral head Medial head	On both sides of supracondylar fossa of the femur	By the common calcanean tendon on calcanean tuber	Tibial n.	Extensor of the hock, flexor of the stifle	Very tendinous; intermediate fleshy tract connects origin of lat. head to tendon of med. head
Soleus (17.31)	Prox. rudiment of the fibula	Joins common calcanean tendon	Tibial n.	Auxiliary extensor of the hock	Fused with the lat. head of gastrocnemius
Supf. digital flexor (19.22)	Supracondylar fossa of femur	Flexor tuberosities of middle phalanges	Tibial n.	Extensor of hock; digital flexor; and flexor of the stifle	Very tendinous, fused proximally with lat. head of gastroc.; tendon caps calcaneus
Deep digital flexors		Distal phalanges	Tibial n.	Flexors of coffin joints; support of hock and fetlock joints	Tendons join to form the common deep flexor tendon in the metatarsus
Lat. digital flexor (17.32)	Lat. condyle and caud. surface of tibia				Passes over sustentaculum tali
Caudal tibial m. (17.33)	Lat. condyle of tibia				Passes over sustentaculum tali
Med. digital flexor (19.5)	Lat. condyle of tibia				Crosses hock separately
FLEXORS OF THE HOCK AND EXTENSORS OF THE DIGITS: Craniolateral on the crus (p. 16)					
Tibialis cranialis (17.8)	*Cran. border and proximolat. surface of tibia; prox. rudiment of fibula and replacement ligament*	*T I; proximomedial on Mt III and Mt IV*	Deep peroneal n.	Flexor of hock	Smaller than in horse; perforates terminal tendon of peroneus tertius; smaller head corresponds to extensor digiti I
Peroneus tertius (17.10)	*Extensor fossa of femur*	*Prox. on Mt III and Mt IV; T II and T III*	Deep peroneal n.	Flexor of hock	*Large and fleshy; completely fused at origin with long digital extensor*
Long digital extensor (17.13)	*Extensor fossa of femur*		Deep peroneal n.	Extensor of digits and flexor of hock	Mostly covered by peroneus tertius
Medial head (Proper extensor of digit III, Med. digital extensor)		*Middle and distal phalanges of digit III*			*Receives extensor branches of interosseus III*
Lateral head (Extensor of digits III and IV)		*Branches to extensor processes of distal phalanges of digits III and IV*			

MUSCLE / FIG.	ORIGIN	TERMINATION	INNERVATION	FUNCTION	REMARKS
Lateral digital extensor (Proper extensor of digit IV) (17.12)	Lat. collateral lig. of stifle; lat. condyle of tibia	*Middle and distal phalanges of digit IV*	Deep peroneal n.	Extensor of digit IV and flexor of hock	Relatively large and pennate; receives extensor branches from interosseus IV
Extensor digitalis brevis (17.15)	*Ligamentous mass on dorsal surface of tarsus*	Joins tendon of long digital extensor	Deep peroneal n.	Digital extensor	Small
Peroneus longus (17.11)	Lat. condyle of tibia, rudiment of fibula	Tendon crosses lat. surface of hock and tendon of lat. dig. ext. and plantar surface of hock to T I	Deep peroneal n.	Flexor of hock	Small, with long thin tendon

METATARSUS:
Interossei III and IV: (see Muscle tables, p. 100 and p. 18)

MUSCLES INNERVATED BY THE FACIAL NERVE (p. 36 and 37)

MUSCLE / FIG.	ORIGIN	TERMINATION	INNERVATION	FUNCTION	REMARKS
Cervicoauricularis superficialis	Nuchal lig.	Dorsolat. surface of auricle	Caud. auricular n. from facial nerve	Raises auricle	
Cervicoauricularis profundus and medius	Nuchal lig. and cervical fascia	Caudolat. and caud. surface of auricle	Caud. auricular n. from facial nerve	Turn intertragic notch laterally	
Cervicoscutularis (37.2)	*Nuchal lig., parietal bone caud. to intercornual protuberance*	Caud. border of scutiform cartilage	Caud. auricular n. from facial nerve	Raises auricle and tenses scutiform cartilage	Broad muscle plate
Interscutularis (37.3)	*Cornual proc., temporal line*	Medially on scutiform cartilage	Rostral auric. brr. of auriculopalpebral n. from facial n.	Tensor of scutiform cartilage	*Has no connection to contralateral muscle*
Frontoscutularis	Temporal line and zygomatic proc. of frontal bone	Scutiform cartilage	Rostral auric. brr. of auriculopalpebral n. from facial n.	Tensor of scutiform cartilage	Two distinct parts according to origin
Zygomaticoscutularis (37.B)	Zygomatic arch	Rostrally on scutiform cartilage	Rostral auric. brr. of auriculopalpebral n. from facial n.	Tensor of scutiform cartilage	
Scutuloauricularis superficialis et profundus (37.D, E)	Scutiform cartilage	Rostromedial on auricle	Rostral auric. brr. of auriculopalpebral n. from facial n.	Levator and protractor of auricle	Two muscles crossed on scutiform cartilage
Zygomaticoauricularis (37.12)	Zygomatic arch	Auricular concha, at intertragic notch	Rostral auric. brr. of auriculopalpebral n. from facial n.	Turns intertragic notch rostrally	
Parotidoauricularis (37.13)	Parotid fascia	Auricular concha, at intertragic notch	Auriculopalpebral n. from facial nerve	Depressor and retractor of auricle	
Styloauricularis	Cartilage of acoustic meatus	Rostromedial border of auricle	Caud. auricular n. from facial nerve	Muscle of the acoustic meatus	May be absent

MUSCLES OF THE LIPS AND CHEEKS (p. 36)

MUSCLE / FIG.	ORIGIN	TERMINATION	INNERVATION	FUNCTION	REMARKS
Orbicularis oris (37.10)	Surrounds the opening of the mouth, *except the middle of the upper lip*		Buccal brr. of facial nerve	Closes rima oris	*Contralat. fibers do not join in the upper lip*
Buccinator (37.26)	Between coronoid process of mandible and angle of the mouth		Buccal brr. of facial nerve	Muscular substance of cheek; presses food from vestibule into oral cavity proper	Separable into a molar part with rostroventral fiber course, and buccal part with dorsoventral fiber course
Zygomaticus (37.11)	*Parotidomasseteric fascia*	In orbicularis oris at angle of mouth	Auriculopalpebral n. from facial n.	Retractor of angle of mouth	Well developed
Caninus (37.23)	*Rostrally on facial tuber*	*With 3 tendons on lat. rim of nostil*	Buccal brr. of facial nerve	Dilates nostril and raises upper lip	Passes through levator nasolabialis; lies between levator and depressor of upper lip

MUSCLE / FIG.	ORIGIN	TERMINATION	INNERVATION	FUNCTION	REMARKS
Levator labii superioris (37.22)	*Facial tuber*	*Planum nasolabiale dors. and med. to nostril*	Buccal brr. of facial nerve	Levator and retractor of upper lip and planum nasolabiale	Passes through levator nasolabialis; right and left tendons may join between nostrils
Depressor labii superioris (37.24)	*Rostrally on facial tuber*	*Upper lip and planum nasolabiale*	*Buccal brr. of facial nerve*	*Depressor of upper lip and planum nasolabiale*	*Lies ventral to caninus*
Depressor labii inferioris (37.25)	*Caudal alveolar border of mandible*	*Lower lip*	Buccal brr. of facial nerve	Depressor and retractor of lower lip	

MUSCLES OF THE EYELIDS AND NOSE (p. 36)

MUSCLE / FIG.	ORIGIN	TERMINATION	INNERVATION	FUNCTION	REMARKS
Orbicularis oculi (37.4)	The muscular ring around the eye in the eyelids		Auriculopalpebral n. from facial n.	Narrowing and closure of the palpebral fissure	
Levator nasolabialis (37.5)	Frontal bone	*Deep part on nasal proc. of incisive bone and lat. nasal cartilages; supf. part between nostril and upper lip*	Auriculopalpebral n. from facial n.	Levator of upper lip, dilator of nostril	Broad and thin; levator labii superioris and caninus pass between supf. and deep parts
Malaris (37.20)	Lacrimal bone and parotidomasseteric fascia	Cheek; orbicularis oculi near medial angle of eye	Buccal brr. of facial n.	Levator of the cheek	Can be divided into rostral and caudal parts
Frontalis (37.1)	*Base of horn and intercornual protuberance*	*Upper eyelid and frontal region*	*Auriculopalpebral n. from facial n.*	*Levator of upper eyelid and medial angle of eye*	*Much reduced in other domestic mammals*

*The **retractor anguli oculi lat.** is absent and the **levator anguli oculi med.** is replaced in the ox by the frontalis.*

MUSCLES INNERVATED BY THE MANDIBULAR NERVE (p. 38)

SUPERFICIAL MUSCLES OF THE INTERMANDIBULAR REGION

MUSCLE / FIG.	ORIGIN	TERMINATION	INNERVATION	FUNCTION	REMARKS
Digastricus (39.31)	Tendinous on paracondylar process	*Medially on vent. border of mandible rostral to vascular groove*	Caud. belly: digastric br. of facial n.; rostral belly: mylohyoid n. from mandib. n.	Opens the mouth	Two bellies not distinctly divided; connected to contralat. m. by fibers on lingual proc. of hyoid bone
Mylohyoideus (39.25)	*Rostral part from angel of chin to first cheek tooth; caud. part from 3rd to beyond last cheek tooth*	Lingual proc. of hyoid bone	Mylohyoid n. from mandib. nerve	Raises the floor of the mouth and elevates the tongue against the palate	The two parts have different fiber directions

LATERAL MUSCLES OF MASTICATION

MUSCLE / FIG.	ORIGIN	TERMINATION	INNERVATION	FUNCTION	REMARKS
Temporalis (39.17)	Temporal fossa	Coronoid proc. of mandible	Deep temporal nn. from masticatory n. from mandibular n.	Masticatory m.: raises and presses mandible to maxilla, closing the mouth	Relatively poorly developed
Masseter (39.13)			Masseteric n. from masticatory n. from mandibular n.	Masticatory m.: raises and presses mandible to maxilla; closes the mouth; unilat. contraction pulls mandible laterally	Very tendinous
Supf. Part	*Facial tuber*	Angle and caud. border of mandible			
Deep part	*Facial crest; zygomatic arch*	Lat. surface of ramus of mandible			

MEDIAL MUSCLES OF MASTICATION

MUSCLE / FIG.	ORIGIN	TERMINATION	INNERVATION	FUNCTION	REMARKS
Pterygoideus (39.22)	Pterygoid bone and surroundings	Pterygoid fossa medial on ramus of mandible; condylar proc. of mandible	Pterygoid nn. from mandibular n.	Synergists of masseter; unilateral contraction pulls mandible laterally	Brr. of mandibular n. pass between pterygoid mm.
—medialis					
—lateralis					

MUSCLE / FIG.	ORIGIN	TERMINATION	INNERVATION	FUNCTION	REMARKS
EYE MUSCLES: (See pp. 40, 41)					
PHARYNGEAL MUSCLES (p. 46)					
Stylopharyngeus caudalis (47.15)	Medially on prox. half of stylohyoid	*Mainly on thyroid cart.; dorsolat. wall of pharynx*	Glossopharyngeal n.	Only dilator of pharynx; *elevator of larynx*	
MUSCLES OF THE SOFT PALATE (p. 46)					
Tensor veli palatini (47.11)	Muscular proc. of tympanic part of temporal bone, hamulus of pterygoid bone	Tendinous on soft palate, laterally on auditory tube	Mandibular n.	Tensor of soft palate, dilator of auditory tube	
Levator veli palatini (47.12)	Muscular proc. of tympanic part of temporal bone; laterally on auditory tube	Soft palate	Pharyngeal plexus (IX, X)	Levator of soft palate	
Palatinus	Choanal border of palatine bones	Soft palate	Pharyngeal plexus (IX, X)	Shortens the soft palate	*A small strand of muscle (m. uvulae) is present near the palatine arch*
ROSTRAL PHARYNGEAL CONSTRICTORS (p. 46)					
Stylopharyngeus rostralis	*Mediodistal half of stylohyoid*	*Pharyngeal raphe*	*Pharyngeal plexus (IX, X)*	*Constrictor of pharynx*	*Regularly present*
Pterygopharyngeus (47.13)	Pterygoid bone and palatine aponeurosis	Pharyngeal raphe	Pharyngeal plexus (IX, X)	Constrictor and protractor of pharynx	
MIDDLE PHARYNGEAL CONSTRICTOR (p. 46)					
Hyopharyngeus (47.16)	*Thyrohyoid, cerato-hyoid, and stylohyoid*	Pharyngeal raphe	Pharyngeal plexus (IX, X)	Constrictor of pharynx	
CAUDAL PHARYNGEAL CONSTRICTORS (p. 46)					
Thyropharyngeus (47.17)	Thyroid cartilage	Pharyngeal raphe	Pharyngeal plexus (IX, X)	Constrictor of pharynx	
Cricopharyngeus (47.18)	Cricoid cartilage	Pharyngeal raphe	Pharyngeal plexus (IX, X)	Constrictor of pharynx	
LARYNGEAL MUSCLES (Intrinsic muscles of the larynx, p. 46)					
Cricothyroideus	Ventrolaterally on cricoid arch	Caudally on thyroid cartilage	Cran. laryngeal n. (X)	Narrows rima glottidis, tenses vocal cords	
Cricoarytenoideus dorsalis (47.9)	Dorsolaterally on cricoid lamina	Muscular proc. of arytenoid cartilage	Caud. laryngeal n. (X)	Widens rima glottidis	
Cricoarytenoideus lateralis (47.7)	Craniolaterally on cricoid arch	Muscular proc. of arytenoid cartilage	Caud. laryngeal n. (X)	Narrows rima glottidis	
Arytenoideus transversus (47.6)	Arcuate crest rostral to muscular procc. of both arytenoid cartilages		Caud. laryngeal n. (X)	Narrows cartilaginous rima glottidis	Unpaired muscle with a dorsomedian raphe
Thyroarytenoideus (47.8)	*Thyroid cart., base of epiglottis, cricothyroid lig.*	*Muscular and vocal procc. of arytenoid cartilage*	*Caud. Laryngeal n. (X)*	*Narrows rima glottidis*	*Not divided into ventricularis and vocalis*
MUSCLES OF THE TONGUE AND HYOID (radiate from the basihyoid into the tongue, p. 45)					
Lingualis proprius (45.l)	Intrinsic muscle of tongue		Hypoglossal n.	Changes shape of tongue	Longitudinal, trans-verse, and perpendicu-lar fibers

MUSCLE / FIG.	ORIGIN	TERMINATION	INNERVATION	FUNCTION	REMARKS
EXTRINSIC MUSCLES OF TONGUE (pp. 45, 47)					
Styloglossus (47.n)	Stylohyoid	Apex of tongue (streaming in from each side)	Hypoglossal n.	Draws tongue caudodorsally; Unilat. contraction draws it lat.	
Hyoglossus (47.n)	Basihyoid, lingual proc., thyrohyoid	Tongue, dorso-median to apex	Hypoglossal n.	Draws tongue caudoventrally	
Genioglossus	Medially on mandible in angle of chin	Tongue, back to hyoid bone	Hypoglossal n.	Draws tongue rostroventrally	Lingual septum divides right and left mm.
MUSCLES OF HYOID APPARATUS					
M. geniohyoideus	Incisive part of mandible	Lingual process of basihyoid	Hypoglossal n.	Draws hyoid apparatus (and tongue) rostrally	
M. thyreohyoideus	Thyroid cartilage	Thyrohyoid bone	Hypoglossal n.	Draws larynx and thyrohyoid toward each other	
Mylohyoideus (See Superficial muscles of the intermandibular region, pp. 38, 39, 104)					
Styhlohyoideus	Tendinous, from angle of stylohyoid	Fleshy on thyrohyoid	Facial n.	Draws hyoid bone and larynx caudodorsally	The termination is not perforated by digastricus
Occipitohyoideus	Paracondylar process	Caudodorsal end of stylohyoid	Facial n.	Lowers root of tongue and larynx	
Hyoideus transversus	Ceratohyoid	On median raphe, joined to contralateral muscle	Glossopharyngeal n.	Levator of root of tongue	
Ceratohyoideus	Ceratohyoid, epihyoid, and vent. end of stylohyoid	Thyrohyoid	Glossopharyngeal n.	Raises thyrohyoid, drawing larynx rostrodorsally	Fills triangle between cerato- and thyrohyoid
Hyoepiglotticus (45.o)	Basihyoid	Rostral surface of base of epiglottis	Hypoglossal n.	Draws epiglottis rostroventrally	
LONG HYOID MUSCLES (p. 60)					
Sternothyroideus (61.15)	Manubrium sterni	Laterally on thyroid cartilage	Medial br. of vent. br. of C1	Synergist of sternohyoideus and retracts thyroid cart.	Sternothyroideus and -hyoideus have no tendinous intersection, unlike the horse, but are joined in the middle of the neck
Sternohyoideus (61.14)	Manubrium sterni	Basihyoid	Medial br. of vent. br. of C1	Retractor of hyoid bone and tongue	
Omohyoideus (61.13)	*Indirectly by deep cervical fascia from 3rd (4th) cervical vertebra*	Basihyoid	Medial br. of vent. br. of C1	Synergist of sternohyoideus	Thin in the ox; fused with sternohyoideus deep to mandibular gland
CUTANEUS MUSCLES (pp. 37, 60, 66)					
Platysma:					
Cutaneus faciei (37.A)	From supf. fascia of laryngeal region	Angle of mouth	Auriculopalpebral n. (VII)	Tenses and moves skin of face; retracts angle of mouth	
Cutaneus colli	Ventrally on supf. fascia of the neck	Directed cranially to skin	Auriculopalpebral n. (VII)	Tenses and moves skin of ventral neck	Thin and often not demonstrable in the ox

MUSCLE / FIG.	ORIGIN	TERMINATION	INNERVATION	FUNCTION	REMARKS
Cutaneus trunci	Supf. fascia of trunk and thigh on a line from withers to fold of flank; minor tubercle of humerus	Skin over ribs, hypochondrium, and lower flank	Lat. thoracic n.	Tenses and moves skin of the trunk	Joined to omo-brachialis; becomes aponeurotic along a line from fold of flank to dorsal third of last rib. Vent. border covers milk vein
Cutaneus omobrachialis	Supf. fascia of scapular and brachial regions	Skin of scapular and brachial regions	Lat. thoracic n.	Tenses and moves skin of scapular and brachial regions	Thin; partly without connection to cutaneus trunci
Preputialis cranialis	Xiphoid proc. with a portion from ventral border of cutaneus trunci	On the prepuce	Vent. brr. of last thoracic and 1st lumbar nn.	Protractor of the prepuce	Paired; forms with contralat. m. a loop around caud. border of preputial orifice
Preputialis caudalis (80 text fig.)	Fascia lateral and medial to vaginal tunic	On the internal lamina of the prepuce	Vent. brr. of last thoracic and 1st lumbar nn.	Retractor of internal lamina of prepuce	Paired; absent in polled breeds

VERTEBRAL COLUMN MUSCULATURE:
(A) Dorsal (epaxial) vertebral column muscles: (pp. 61, 63, 87)

MUSCLE / FIG.	ORIGIN	TERMINATION	INNERVATION	FUNCTION	REMARKS
Splenius (61.k)	*Spinous procc. of T1–T3 (4); thoraco-lumbar fascia*		Dorsal brr. of corresponding spinal nn.	Extension, elevation, and lat. flexion of head and neck	
—capitis		*Dorsolat. on occipital bone*			
—cervicis		*Wing of atlas and transverse proc. of axis*			
Iliocostalis				Fixation of loin and ribs; extends vert. column and bends it laterally; assists in expiration	
—cervicis (61.o)	Ends as continuation of iliocostalis thoracis on transverse process of C7		Dorsal brr. of corresponding spinal nn.		
—thoracis (61.o')	*Transv. proc. of L1–L4, mainly on L3.*	Angles of ribs and transverse procc. of thoracic vertebrae	Dors. brr. of corresponding spinal nn.		M. fiber bundles cross over up to 7 ribs
—lumborum (61.o'')	*Tendinous from iliac crest*	*Caud. border of last rib*	*Dors. brr. of corresponding spinal nn.*		
M. longissimus			Dors. brr. of corresponding spinal nn.	Fixation and extension of vert. column; raises cranial part of trunk; raises neck and head; unilat. contraction bends neck	
—atlantis et capitis (61.n)	Artic. procc. of C3–T2	Wing of atlas, mastoid proc. of temporal bone, temporal line			
—cervicis (61.n')	Transv. procc. of first 6–7 thor. vertt.	Transv. procc. of last 4 cervical vertebrae			
—thoracis (61.n'')	Spinous procc. of last thor. vertt.	Transv. procc. of C7 (6);			A short thin tongue of gluteus medius lies on the longissimus lumborum
—lumborum (61.n''')	lumbar, and sacral vertt.; iliac crest, and tuber coxae	vert. ends of ribs; transv. procc. of thor. and lumbar vertt.; artic. and mamillary procc. of lumbar vertebrae			
Semispinalis capitis (61.l)	Transv. procc. of T1–T8 (9); artic. procc. of C3–C7; lig. nuchae	Occipital bone; laterally on lig. nuchae	Dorsal brr. of corresponding spinal nerves	Lifting and lat. bending of head and neck. Has great active role in the horn thrust	Thicker dorsomed. biventer cervicis can be distinguished from thinner, ventrolateral, purely fleshy complexus

MUSCLE / FIG.	ORIGIN	TERMINATION	INNERVATION	FUNCTION	REMARKS
Spinalis et semi-spinalis thoracis et cervicis (61.m)	*Spinous procc. of L1 and T (10) 11–T13; supraspinous lig.; transv. procc. of T9–T12 (semispinalis part); spinous proc. of T1*	*Spinous procc. of T1–T6 and C4–C7*	*Dorsal brr. of corresponding spinal nerves*	*Fixation of back and neck; raising and lat. bending of neck; synergist of longissimuss*	*Fleshy semispinalis part is present; it lies on longissimus thoracis from T5–T13 like a cap*
Multifidus		Spinous procc. of the more cran. vertebrae, including axis	Dorsal brr. of corresponding spinal nerves	Fixes and rotates vert. column; raises neck and bends it laterally	The fiber bundles cross over as many as 5 vertebrae
—cervicis	Artic. procc. of C(3) 4–C7				
—thoracis	Transv. prod. of T1; mamillary and artic. procc. of last thoracic and lumbar vertt.				
—lumborum	Sacrum; Cd1	L5 and L6			

Interspinales: *In the ox they are muscular only in the neck. In thoracic and lumbar regions they are replaced by interspinal ligaments.*

MUSCLE / FIG.	ORIGIN	TERMINATION	INNERVATION	FUNCTION	REMARKS
Intertransversarii (87.h)	Artic. procc. of C3–C7 and cran. artic. proc. of T1; transv. procc. of all lumbar and caud. vertebrae	Transv. procc. of C2–C7; transverse procc. and costal tubercles of preceding segments; lumbar segments end on prox. end of last rib; caud. segments on caud. transv. processes	Dorsal and ventral brr. of corresponding spinal nn.	Fixation and lateral bending of vertebral column	*Ventrolat. bundles in neck form intertransversarius longus cervicis, dorsolat. to longus capitis and ending on wing of atlas*
Sacrocaudalis [—coccygeus] dorsalis medialis (87.e)	Between spinous and mamillary procc. of 2–3 last sacral and first caudal vertebrae		Dorsal brr. of corresponding spinal nerves	Raises tail and bends it laterally	Considered the caudal continuation of the multifidus
Sacrocaudalis [—coccygeus] dorsalis lateralis (87.f)	Laterally on the sacrum and transv. proc. of 1st caudal vertebrae	Tendinous on 5th to last caud. vertebrae	Dorsal brr. of corresponding spinal nerves	Raises tail and bends it laterally	Caudal continuation of longissimus

B) Ventral vertebral column muscles (pp. 47, 61, 87)

MUSCLE / FIG.	ORIGIN	TERMINATION	INNERVATION	FUNCTION	REMARKS
Scaleni			Ventral brr. of spinal nn.		
Scalenus dorsalis (61.p)	*Ribs (2) 3–4*	*Transv. procc. of C4–C6*		*When neck is fixed, levator of first ribs; when ribs are fixed, draws neck ventrally or bends it laterally*	*More supf. than dorsal; absent in horse*
Scalenus medius	Cran. border of first rib	*Transv. procc. of C4–C7*		Draws neck laterally	Dorsal to brachial plexus
Scalenus ventralis (61.p')	Cran. border of first rib	Transv. procc. of C3–C7		Bends neck laterally	Ventral to brachial plexus; is very robust
Longus capitis (61.h)	Transv. procc. of C2–C6	Muscular tubercle on base of skull	Ventral brr. of spinal nn.	Flexes head and neck and bends them laterally	Thin triangular muscle
Longus colli	Cervical part: transv. procc. and bodies of C3–C7. Thoracic part: bodies and transv. procc. of C6–C7; bodies of T1–T6	Ventral crest of more cran. vertebrae and vent. tubercle of atlas	Ventral brr. of spinal nn.	Flexor of the neck	Relatively thick; fiber bundles often cross over one segment

MUSCLE / FIG.	ORIGIN	TERMINATION	INNERVATION	FUNCTION	REMARKS
Sacrocaudalis [—coccygeus] ventralis			Ventral brr. of spinal nn.	Draws tail ventrally; unilateral action draws tail lat.	
—medialis (95.l)	Last sacral segment to end of tail (ventral on caud. vertebrae)	Second following hemal proc.			Connected with terminal tendons of sacrocaudalis vent. lateralis
—lateralis (95.k)	Ventrally from S2–S3; transv. procc. of 1st caud. vertebrae	Ventrolat. on caudal vertebrae			Thicker than the med. muscle
Rectus capitis ventralis	Ventral arch of atlas	Base of skull, caud. to longus capitis	Ventral br. of 1st spinal n.	Flexor of the atlanto-occipital joint	More robust than in other domestic animals
Rectus capitits lateralis	Ventral arch and vent. surf. of wing of atlas	Paracondylar process	Ventral br. of 1st spinal n.	Flexor of the atlanto-occipital joint; rotates head	Relatively weak and covered by rectus capitis ventralis

C) DORSAL MUSCLES ACTING ON THE HEAD

MUSCLE / FIG.	ORIGIN	TERMINATION	INNERVATION	FUNCTION	REMARKS
Rectus capitis dorsalis major	Spinous process of axis	Occipital bone, medial to obliquus cap. cran.	Dorsal br. of C1	Levator of the head	
Rectus capitis dorsalis minor	Dorsal arch of atlas	Occipital bone dorsal to foramen magnum	Dorsal br. of C1	Levator of the head	More robust than in carnivores
Obliquus capitis cranialis	Cran. border of wing of atlas and atlantal fossa	Occipital squama, base of jugular proc.	Dorsal br. of C1	Extensor and rotator of head	
Obliquus capitis caudalis	Spinous process and cd. artic. proc. of axis	Cran. border of wing of atlas	Dorsal br. of C2	Rotator of atlas around dens of axis	Very robust

DORSAL TRUNK-LIMB MUSCLES (p. 60)

MUSCLE / FIG.	ORIGIN	TERMINATION	INNERVATION	FUNCTION	REMARKS
Trapezius Pars cervicalis (61.11) Pars thoracica (61.11')	*Dorsally on funiculus nuchae and supra-spinous lig. from C1–T12*	Spine of scapula	Dorsal br. of accessory n.	Fixation of scapula, protractor and abductor of limb	Well developed; cervical and thoracic parts separated by tendinous strip on scapular spine
Omotransversarius (61.8)	Acromion; brachial fascia	Wing of atlas (partly also transverse proc. of axis)	Medial brr. of vent. brr. of cervical nn.	Protractor of limb and lat. flexor of neck	Supf. cervical ln. lies deep to omotransversarius and cleido-brachialis
Rhomboideus —cervicis (61.28) —thoracis (61.28')	*Dorsomedian on funiculus nuchae and supraspinous lig. from C2–T8*	*Medially on scapular cartilage*	Med. brr. of vent. brr. of cervical nn. of thoracic nn.	Fixes, raises, and retracts the limb; raises neck	The rhomboideus capitis is absent as in the horse
Latissimus dorsi (61.12)	Thoracolumbar fascia; *ribs 11 and 12*	*Teres major tuberosity and deep pectoral, coracobrachialis, and long head of triceps*	Thoracodorsal nerve	Retractor of limb, flexor of shoulder joint, protractor of trunk when limb is fixed	Relatively thin; course over the caud. angle of scapula fixes scapula on thoracic wall

VENTRAL TRUNK-LIMB MUSCLES (p. 60)

MUSCLE / FIG.	ORIGIN	TERMINATION	INNERVATION	FUNCTION	REMARKS
Pectorales superficiales			Cran. and caud. pectoral nerves	Connect limb to trunk; adductors, protractors, and retractors of limb	Thinner than in horse; the two muscles are less distinct
Pectoralis transversus (61.25')	*1st to 6th* costal cartilage; ventrally on sternum	Antebrachial fascia, *humerus*			
Pectoralis descendens (61.25)	Manubrium sterni	Crest of major tubercle of humerus and brachial fascia			

MUSCLE / FIG.	ORIGIN	TERMINATION	INNERVATION	FUNCTION	REMARKS
Pectoralis profundus [Pectoralis ascendens] (61.26)	*Sternum from 2nd rib caudally and sternal costal cartilages; tunica flava*	Major and minor tubercles of humerus; *coracoid proc. of scapula*	Cran. and caud. pectoral nerves	Supports trunk; retracts limb; fixes shoulder joint	Unified; no accessory part like that of the dog; gives a flat muscular strap to the supraspinatus
Subclavius (61.26')	*Cartilage of 1st rib*	Clavicular intersection on deep surface of brachiocephalicus	Cran. pectoral nerves		Rudimentary
Serratus ventralis				Most important supporter of trunk, raises neck when limb is fixed, auxiliary inspiratory muscle	The parts are distinctly divided
—cervicis (61.27)	*Transverse procc. of C(3)4–C7*	*Cranially on facies serrata of scapula*	Med. brr. of vent. brr. of cervical nn.		
—thoracis (61.27')	*Ribs 1 to 7, 8, or 9*	*Caudally on facies serrata; subscapular fossa*	Long thoracic nerve		Digitations of origin markedly tendinous
Sternomandibularis (61.5)	Manubrium sterni *and 1st rib*	Rostral border of masseter, mandible, and depressor labii inferioris	Ventral br. of accessory n.	Opens mouth; fixes mandible and pharynx in swallowing	Courses ventral to jugular groove as a thick muscular cord
***Sternomastoideus** (61.4)*	*Manubrium sterni*	*Mastoid proc. of temporal bone; with cleidomastoideus and longus capitis, on muscular tubercle of occipital bone*	*Ventral br. of accessory n.*	*Fixes and draws head and neck ventrally*	*Flat band lat. to trachea; in upper half of neck separates ext. jugular v. from com. carotid a. With sternomandibularis, makes up **sternocephalicus***
Cleidomastoideus (61.6)	Clavicular intersection	Mastoid proc. of temporal bone; and, *with sternomastoideus and longus capitis, on muscular tubercle of occipital bone*	Ventral br. of accessory n.	Protractor of limb; draws head ventrally or laterally	Joins cleidooccipitalis in the middle of neck to form **cleidocephalicus** which joins the cleidobrachialis (p. 4)
***Cleido-occipitalis** (61.7)*	*Clavicular intersection*	*Funiculus nuchae and occipital bone*	*Dorsal br. of accessory n.*	*Protractor of limb, raises head*	*Adjoins cranial border of trapezius*

EXPIRATORY MUSCLES (pp. 61, 63, 67)
Compress thorax by drawing ribs mediocaudally

Serratus dorsalis caudalis (61.r')	Thoracolumbar fascia	Caud. border of *ribs 10–13*	Intercostal nerves	Expirator	Interdigitates with ext. abd. obl. and ext. intercostal mm.
Intercostales interni (67.d)	Fiber bundles run cranioventrally in intercostal spaces		Intercostal nerves	Expirators	
Retractor costae	*Transverse processes of L1–L3*	Caud. border of last rib	Intercostal nerves	Expirator	
Transversus thoracis (63.v)	*Costal cartilages 2–7*	*Sternebrae 2–7; 8th costal cartilage*	Intercostal nerves	Expirator	Right and left halves separated on median line

INSPIRATORY MUSCLES (pp. 61, 63, 67)
Expand thorax by drawing ribs craniolaterally

Serratus dorsalis cranialis (61.r)	Supraspinous ligament	*Cran. border of ribs 5–9*	Intercostal nerves	Inspirator	Weak
Rectus thoracis (67.c)	First rib	Costal cartilages 2–4 (6)	Intercostal nerves	Inspirator	

MUSCLE / FIG.	ORIGIN	TERMINATION	INNERVATION	FUNCTION	REMARKS
Intercostales externi (61.e)	Fiber bundles run caudoventrally in intercostal spaces		Intercostal nerves	Inspirators	Very tendinous fiber tracts; pass into ext. abd. obl. near the last ribs
Levatores costarum	*Transverse and mamillary procc. of T1–T12*	*Cran. border of next rib*	Dorsal brr. of thoracic nn.	Inspirators	10–12 muscles; same fiber direction as ext. intercostals
Diaphragm (63.2–63.5)			Phrenic n.	Inspirator; main respiratory muscle	
Costal part (63.3)	From knee of 8th rib, across the middle of 11th to ventral end of 12th rib	Tendinous center			More steeply inclined than in other dom. Mammals
Sternal part	Xiphoid process	Tendinous center			Clearly divided from the costal part
Lumbar part (63.2)	Ventral surfaces of L1–3 (4)	Tendinous center			Forms right and left crura of diaphragm

The subcostales are not present in the ox.

ABDOMINAL MUSCLES (p. 66)

MUSCLE / FIG.	ORIGIN	TERMINATION	INNERVATION	FUNCTION	REMARKS
External abdominal oblique (67.2)	Costal part: ribs (4) 5–13 *along vent. border of latissimus dorsi.* Lumbar part: last rib, thoracolumbar fascia	Abdominal tendon: linea alba and prepubic tendon. Pelvic tendon: tuber coxae, inguinal lig., and prepubic tendon	Vent. brr. of corresponding intercostal and lumbar nn.	As a whole: contractile sling adaptable to weight and volume of abd. organs; reinforced by strong tunica flava of abdomen	*Inguinal canal:* abd. and pelvic tendons bound ext. ing. ring; pelvic tend. is caud. border of deep ring *Sheath of rectus: abdominal tendon is in ext. lamina*
Internal abdominal oblique (67.10)	*Thoracolumbar fascia; transverse procc. of lumbar vertebrae,* tuber coxae, inguinal ligament	Linea alba and last rib	Vent. brr. of corresponding intercostal and lumbar nn.	Abd. press in urination, defecation, and parturition, with inspiratory position of diaphragm fixed by closed glottis. Flexion of vert. column by rectus abdominis. Auxillary exspirators; *straight strapping:* rectus and transversus; *oblique strapping:* ext. and int. abd. obl.	*Inguinal canal:* cran. border of deep ring; *Sheath of rectus:* aponeurosis is *only* in ext. lamina. Costochondral crus is caudovent. border of paralumbar fossa *Sheath of rectus: int. lamina is formed by transversus alone*
Transversus abdominis (67.7)	Costal part: *last 7–8 costal cartilages;* Lumbar part: transverse process of lumbar vertebrae	Linea alba	Vent. brr. of corresponding intercostal and lumbar nn.		
Rectus abdominis (67.6)	Fourth to ninth costal cartilages	Prepubic tendon, *symphyseal tendon and symphyseal crest*	Vent. brr. of corresponding intercostal and lumbar nn.		Has 5 tendinous intersections; near the 2nd is the "milk well" where the subcutaneous abd. v. perforates the abd. wall to int. thoracic v.

INTERNAL LUMBAR MUSCLES (p. 81)

MUSCLE / FIG.	ORIGIN	TERMINATION	INNERVATION	FUNCTION	REMARKS
Quadratus lumborum (81.g)	Proximoventral on last rib; *T10–T13* and transv. procc. of lumbar vertrebrae	Ventrally on wing of sacrum	Vent. brr. of intercostal and lumbar nn.; lumbar plexus	Stiffens lumbar vert. column and arches it dorsally	All 4 internal lumbar mm. show about the same relations as in horse; very tendinous

MUSCLE / FIG.	ORIGIN	TERMINATION	INNERVATION	FUNCTION	REMARKS
Psoas major (81.e)	Fleshy on cran. border of last rib; body and transverse processes of all lumbar vertebrae	The iliacus and psoas major end together as the iliopsoas on minor trochanter of femur	Vent. brr. of inter-costal and lumbar nn.; lumbar plexus	Protractor of pelvic limb; flexor and supinator of hip joint; stabilizer of vertebral column when limb is fixed	The iliopsoas and psoas minor form the tenderloin (filet)
Iliacus (81.f)	*Ventrally from body of L6*; ventral surface of wing of ilium; wing of sacrum; tendon of psoas minor				
Psoas minor (81.d)	T12–T13, L1, and crura of diaphragm	Psoas minor tubercle of ilium	Vent. brr. of inter-costal and lumbar nn.; lumbar plexus	Rotates pelvis forward at sacroiliac joint when vert. col. is fixed; stabilizes and arches lumbar vertebral column when pelves is fixed	Strong tendon at termination

PERINEAL MUSCLES (p. 94)
Pelvic diaphragm:

Levator ani (95.3)	Spine of ischichium and med. surface of sacrosciatic lig.	External anal sphincter, caudal fascia	Pudendal and caud. rectal nn. from vent. brr. of sacral nerves	Holds anus against contraction of rectum; aids coccygeus	
Coccygeus (95.2)	Spine of ischium and medial surface of sacrosciatic lig.	Transv. procc. of first 3 caud. vertebrae	Pudendal and caud. rectal nn. from vent. brr. of sacral nerves	Unilat. contr. draws tail laterally; bilat. contr. draws tail ventrally	

Muscles of anal region

External anal sphincter (95.12)	Fiber bundles completely encircle anus, cross ventral to anus in perineal body, and continue in constrictor vulvae		Pudendal and caud. rectal nn. from vent. brr. of sacral nerves	Closes the anus	Voluntary striated muscle
Internal anal sphincter	Thickened annular muscle layer of rectum		Caud. rectal nn.	Closes the anus	Involuntary smooth muscle
Rectococcygeus (95.11)	Continuation of dorsal longitudinal muscle of rectum	*Ventromedian on caudal vertebrae 1–3*	Caud. rectal nn. from vent. brr. of sacral nn.	Supports and stabilizes anal canal and rectum	Smooth muscle. Ventral fibers of rectum cross in the perineal body and enter the labia and vestibule

Urogenital muscles (bull, p. 92; cow, p. 87)

Bulbospongiosus (93.6)	Continuation of urethralis caud. to urogenital membrane; median dorsal raphe	Tunica albuginea on sides of bulb of penis	Deep perineal n. from pudendal n. (S2–S4)	Forces the flow of urine, semen, and blood	Very thick; ca. 17 cm long from bulboure-thral gll. to junction of crura penis
Constrictor vestibuli (87.m)	Vent. border of levator ani and fascia on levator	Tendons of rt. and left muscles join vent. to vestibule	Pudendal and caud. rectal nn. from vent. brr. of sacral nerves	Narrows the vestibule of the vagina	Bilateral, embracing the vestibule
Constrictor vulvae (87.n)	External anal sphincter in perineal body	Subcut. in labia; fascia of semimembranosus	Caud. rectal nn. from vent. brr. of S4–S5	Constricts vulva	Striated muscle of labia vulvae
Retractor penis (93.8)	Caud. vertebrae 1 and 2; rectum, ext. anal sphincter, levator ani	1. distal bend of sigmoid flexure 2. on tunica albuginea 15–20 cm. prox. to glans	Deep perineal n. and dorsal n. of penis from pudendal n.; caud. rectal n. from vent. brr. of sacral nerves	Retracts penis by folding sigmoid flexure	Smooth muscle, paired
Retractor clitoridis (87.o)	Caud. vertebrae 2 and 3 or 3 and 4; rectum, ext. anal sphincter, levator ani	Body of clitoris, vestibule, fascia of semimembranosus	Pudendal and caud. rectal nn. from vent. brr. of sacral nn.	Retracts clitoris	Smooth muscle, paired
Ischiocavernosus (93.7)	Medial surface of tuber ischiadicum	Body of penis or clitoris at junction of crura	Deep perineal n. from pudendal n. (vent. brr. of S2–S4)	Rhythmic pumping of blood into corpus cavernosum in erection	Broad, paired muscle covering crura; rudimentary in the cow

2. LYMPHATIC SYSTEM

LYMPHOCENTER LYMPH NODE	LOCATION	AFFERENTS FROM	EFFERENTS TO	REMARKS
PAROTID LYMPHOCENTER (p. 38)				
Parotid ln. (39.12)	Ventrolat. to temporomandib. jt.; between rostral border of parotid gl. and masseter	Skin and mm. of whole dors. part of head, skull bones, parotid gl.; ext. ear, eyelids, lacrimal app., rostral half of nasal cavity, hard palate, chin	Lat. retropharyngeal ln.	6–9 cm long. Regularly incised in meat inspection
MANDIBULAR LYMPHOCENTER (P. 38)				
Mandibular ln. (39.10)	Ventr. to mandible midway between rostr. border of masseter and angle of mandible; covered by sternomandibularis	Skin of head, facial and masticatory mm., rostr. nasal cavity, oral and nasal mucosa, paranasal sinuses, tongue mm., pharynx, larynx, salivary gl.	Lat. retropharyngeal ln.	3–4.5 cm long, palpable. Regularly incised in meat inspection
Pterygoid ln.	On rostral border of ramus of mandible; med. to med. pterygoid m.	Hard palate	Mandibular ln.	Inconstant
RETROPHARYNGEAL LYMPHOCENTER (p. 38)				
Lat. retropharyngeal ln. (39.11)	Under the wing of atlas; covered by dorsal end of mandib. gland	Skin of head-neck union, lips, salivary gll., buccal mucosa, mandib. mucosa in diastema, masticatory mm., tongue and parts of hyoid mm., mandible, part of thymus, nearby neck mm., ear mm.	The efferents join to form tracheal trunk	4–5 cm long, smooth, oval; palpable if enlarged; may be associated with 1–3 small ln. Regularly incised in meat inspection
Med. retropharyngeal ln. (49.a)	Between caudodors. wall of pharynx and longus capitis; med. to stylohyoideus	Tongue, hyoid mm., oral mucosa, palate, tonsils, maxillary and palatine sinuses, mandible, caudal half of nasal cavity, larynx and pharynx, mandibular and sublingual gll., longus capitis	Lat. retropharyngeal ln.	3–6 cm long, oval, surrounded by fat; rarely double; palpable from pharynx. Regularly incised in meat inspection
Rostral hyoid ln.	Lat. to thyrohyoid	Apex of tongue	Lat. and med. retropharyngeal lnn.	Inconstant; 1–1.5 cm in diameter
Caud. hyoid ln.	Lat. to angle of stylohyhoid	Mandible	Lat. retropharyngeal ln.	Inconstant; 1–1.5 cm in diameter
SUPERFICIAL CERVICAL LYMPHOCENTER (p. 60)				
Supf. cervical ln. (61.9 and 67.a)	In the groove cranial to supraspinatus above shoulder jt., covered by omotransversarius and cleido-occipitalis	Skin of neck, thoracic limb, thoracic wall back to level of 12th rib. Shoulder girdle mm. and mm. dors. to scapula, antebrachial fasciae, manus	Left side: thoracic duct or left tracheal trunk. Rt. side: rt. tracheal trunk	7–9 cm long, 1–2 cm thick, palpable; Examined in suspected cases in meat inspection
DEEP CERVICAL LYMPHOCENTER (p. 60)				
Deep cervical lnn.:				To be considered in suspected cases in meat inspection. 4–6 lnn., 1–2.5 cm each; rarely absent
Cran. deep cerv. lnn. (61.22)	From thyroid gl. to 7th tracheal ring	Ventr. cervical mm., flexors of neck, thyroid gl., larynx and pharynx, cervical trachea and esophagus, cervical thymus	Left side: thoracic duct or end of tracheal trunk, may go directly to angle between bijugular trunk and subclavian v. Right side: caud. part of right tracheal trunk	
Middle deep cerv. lnn. (61.23)	In the middle 1/3 of neck, on the right of the trachea and on the left of esophagus			1–7 lnn., 0.5–3 cm long
Caud. deep cerv. lnn. (61.24)	On the trachea just cran. to the 1st rib			2–4 separate lnn.

LYMPHOCENTER LYMPH NODE	LOCATION	AFFERENTS FROM	EFFERENTS TO	REMARKS
Costocervical ln.	Cran. to costocerv. trunk craniomed. to 1st rib	Supraspinatus, infraspinatus, dors. shoulder girdle mm. extensors of neck and back, flexors of neck, omohyoideus, pleura, trachea	Left side: thoracic duct and caud. deep cerv. lnn. or cran. mediastinal lnn. or angle between bijugular tr. and subclavian v. Right side: rt. tracheal trunk or vas efferens of supf. cerv. ln.	1.5–3 cm long, often merged with caud. deep cerv. lnn. Adjoins common carotid a. ventrally, esophagus and trachea medially. To be considered in suspected cases in meat inspection

AXILLARY LYMPHOCENTER (p. 6)

LYMPHOCENTER LYMPH NODE	LOCATION	AFFERENTS FROM	EFFERENTS TO	REMARKS
Proper axillary ln.	6–10 cm caud. to shoulder jt. at level of 2nd intercostal space, med. to teres major	Mm. of shoulder and brachium, parts of shoulder girdle mm., cutaneous omobrachialis, bones of thoracic limb down to the carpus	Axillary lnn. of 1st rib, caud. deep cervical lnn.	2.5–3.5 cm long single ln. To be considered in suspected cases in meat inspection
Axillary lnn. of 1st rib	On the lat. surface of the rib and 1st intercostal space; covered by the lat. part of deep pectoral m.	Pectoral mm., transversus thoracis, serratus ventr., scalenus, shoulder and brachial mm., bones of thoracic limb down to carpus	Caud. deep cervical lnn. or on the left side to thoracic duct; on the rt. side to rt. tracheal trunk	2–3 separate lnn. To be considered in suspected cases in meat inspection
Accessory axillary ln.	At the level of the 4th rib		Proper axillary ln.	Inconstant small single ln.
Infraspinatus ln.	On the caudal border of that m., covered by the cran. border of latissimus dorsi	Latissimus dorsi	Proper axillary ln.	0.5–1 cm long; occurs very rarely

DORSAL THORACIC LYMPHOCENTER (p. 62)

LYMPHOCENTER LYMPH NODE	LOCATION	AFFERENTS FROM	EFFERENTS TO	REMARKS
Thoracic aortic lnn. (63.11)	Dorsolat. to aorta and med. to sympathetic trunk. Right side: dorsal to thoracic duct. Left side: ventr. to left azygos v. (p. 65)	Subscapularis, shoulder girdle mm., thoracic mm. extensors of back, diaphragm, heart, possibly spleen, pleura, and peritoneum, mediastinum, ribs	Right side: thoracic duct; left side: caud. lnn. through caud. media-stinal lnn.; cran. lnn. through cran. mediastinal lnn. or directly into the angle between bijugular tr. and subclavian v.	1–3.5 cm long, number of lnn. varies. To be considered in suspected cases in meat inspection
Intercostal lnn. (63.10)	Subpleural at level of heads of the ribs, lat. to sympathetic trunk	Mm. of lat. and dorsal thoracic wall, extensors of the back, longus colli, subscapularis, ext. abd. oblique, pleura, parts of perito-neum, ribs, thoracic vertebrae	Right side: IC spaces 1–3 to cran. and middle mediastinal lnn. Left side: IC spaces 1–2 (3) to costocerv. lnn. IC spaces 3–4 to cran. mediastinal lnn. All other IC to thoracic aortic lnn.	0.4–2 cm long; 1, rarely 2 or 0 lnn. in each IC space

VENTRAL THORACIC LYMPHOCENTER (p. 62)

LYMPHOCENTER LYMPH NODE	LOCATION	AFFERENTS FROM	EFFERENTS TO	REMARKS
Cran. sternal ln. (63.17)	Dors. to manubrium sterni, ventr. to int. thoracic a. and v. at 1st IC space	Sternum, costal cartilage, trans-versus thoracis, mm. of thoracic wall, pleura, pericardium	Caud. mediastinal lnn. or tracheal tr. or the end of thoracic duct	Usually paired, 1.5–2.5 cm long. To be considered in suspected cases in meat inspection
Caud. sternal lnn.	Ventr. to transversus thoracis along int. thoracic a. and v. other lnn. dors. to transversus thor. just cran. to attachment of diaphragm	Diaphragm, pericardium, pleura, peritoneum, ribs, sternum, mm. of thoracic wall, ventr. mm. of shoulder girdle, abd. mm., liver	Cran. sternal ln.	1–5 lnn. on both sides of median line, and 2–5 lnn. just cran. to attachment of diaphragm on sternum. To be considered in suspected inspection

LYMPHOCENTER LYMPH NODE	LOCATION	AFFERENTS FROM	EFFERENTS TO	REMARKS
MEDIASTINAL LYMPHOCENTER (p. 62)				
Cranial mediastinal lnn. (63.14)	Right and left variable in cran. mediastinum, on aortic arch, brachiocephalic tr., trachea, and esophagus	Thoracic esophagus and trachea, thymus, lungs, pericardium, heart, pleura	On the left, to thoracic duct; on the right, to the end of the right tracheal trunk	Regularly incised in meat inspection
Middle mediastinal lnn. (63.12)	On dors. and right surfaces of esophagus over the heart	Thoracic esophagus and trachea, lungs	Thoracic duct or right cran. mediastinal lnn. or a vas efferens of caud. mediastinal lnn.	2–5 lnn., each 0.5–5 cm long, visible only on the right. Regularly incised in meat inspection
Caudal mediastinal lnn. (63.13)	In caud. mediastinum; dors. to esophagus, extending to diaphragm	Lung, thoracic esophagus, pericardium, diaphragm, mediastinum, peritoneum, spleen, and liver	Thoracic duct, occasionally to left tracheobronchial ln.	A very long (15–20 cm) ln., sometimes divided; possible cause of irritation of vagal trunks. Regularly incised in meat inspection
Phrenic ln.	On thoracic side of for. venae cavae	Diaphragm, mediastinum	Caud. mediastinal lnn.	1–4 small lnn. Inconstant
BRONCHIAL LYMPHOCENTER (p. 62)				
Left tracheobronchial ln. (63.24)	Caud. to lig. arteriosum, between arch of aorta and left pulmonary a.	Thoracic esophagus, bifurcation of trachea, heart	Caud. and cran. mediastinal lnn., thoracic duct	2.5–3.5 cm long. Regularly incised in meat inspection
Right tracheobronchial ln. (63.25)	Between apical and middle lobes on lat. surface of rt. main bronchus	Lung; pulmonary lnn.	Middle mediastinal lnn.	1–3 cm long. Present in 75 % of cattle. Regularly incised in meat inspection (supervisor's node)
Middle tracheobronchial ln. (63.27)	Dorsal to the bifurcation of the trachea	Lung	Right tracheobronchial ln.	0.75–1 cm long; present in 50 % of cattle. Regularly incised in meat inspection
Cran. tracheobronchial ln. (63.21)	On right side of trachea, cran. to origin of tracheal bronchus	Lung; pulmonary lnn.	Cran. mediastinal lnn.	2–5 cm long. Regularly incised in meat inspection
Pulmonary lnn. (63.28)	Around both main bronchi, covered by lung tissue	Lung, except right apical lobe	Right and left tracheobronchial lnn., more rarely, caud. mediastinal lnn.	1 or 2 ln., 0.5–1.5 cm in size; present in 50 % of cattle

LYMPHOCENTER LYMPH NODE	LOCATION	AFFERENTS FROM	EFFERENTS TO	REMARKS
LUMBAR LYMPHOCENTER (p. 82)				
Aortic lumbar lnn. (83.8)	Dors. and ventr. to aorta and caud. vena cava, ventr. to lumbar vertt.	Hypaxial lumbar mm., extensors of the back, thoracolumbar fascia, lumbar vertebrae, peritoneum, kidneys, adrenal gl.	Lumbar trunk	12–15 small lnn. to be considered in suspected cases in meat inspection
Proper lumbar lnn. (76.G)	Near the intervert. foramina of lumbar vertebrae	Extensors of back, (latissimus dorsi), abdominal mm.	Aortic lumbar lnn.	Separate, about 0.5 cm; on one side or bilateral or absent
Renal lnn. (83.9)	Close to renal a. and v.	Kidneys, adrenal gll.	Cysterna chyli	Not sharply distinct from aortic lumbar lnn. Regularly examined in meat inspection
CELIAC LYMPHOCENTER (p. 72, 74)				
Celiac lnn. (77.A)	On celiac a.	Spleen	Visceral trunk or directly into cisterna chyli	Cannot be sharply delimited from nearby lnn.
Splenic (or atrial) lnn. (73.E)	Between atrium ruminis and left crus of diaphragm, dorsocranial to the spleen	Spleen, rumen, reticulum; lymph from all other gastric lnn.	Variable, usually gastric trunk	1–7 lnn. Regularly examined in meat inspection
Right ruminal lnn. (73.D)	Subserous, in right longitudinal groove of rumen	Rumen	Splenic lnn. or gastric trunk	1–4 more lnn. in the cran. groove of rumen
Left ruminal lnn. (73.C)	Subserous in left longitudinal groove	Rumen	Cran. ruminal lnn., partly to right ruminal lnn.	1–2 inconstant, 1–2 cm long lnn.
Cran. ruminal lnn.	In the cran. groove of rumen	Rumen	Right ruminal lnn., splenic lnn.	2–8 lnn., 0.5–1.5 cm each
Reticular lnn. (73.F)	On the diaphragmatic and visceral surfaces of the reticulum	Reticulum	Splenic lnn., rarely directly into the gastric trunk	1–7 small, 0.5–1.5 cm lnn.
Omasal lnn.	On the visceral surface of the omasum	Omasum	Splenic lnn.	6–12 lnn., 0.5–4 cm each
Ruminoabomasal lnn. (73.B)	On the left, cranially on rumen and greater curvature of abomasum	Rumen, omasum, abomasum	Reticuloabomasal lnn. or reticular lnn.	2–7 lnn., 0.5–4 cm long
Reticuloabomasal lnn. (73.A)	On the left, between reticulum, abomasum, and atrium ruminis	Rumen, reticulum, and abomasum	Reticular lnn.	2–8 lnn., 0.5–4 cm long
Dors. abomasal lnn. (73.G)	Near the lesser curvature of abomasum	Duodenum, omasum, abomasum	Hepatic lnn.	3–6 lnn., 0.5–4 cm each
Ventr. abomasal lnn. (73.H)	Near the greater curvature of the abomasum, in the greater omentum	Duodenum, abomasum	Hepatic lnn.	1–4 lnn., inconstant
Hepatic lnn. (75.23)	Porta hepatis	Liver, pancreas, duodenum	Hepatic trunk	6–15 lnn., 1–7 cm long. Regularly incised in meat inspection
Accessory hepatic lnn. (74.29)	On dors. border of liver, near the caud. vena cava	Liver	Hepatic trunk	Several small lnn.

116

LYMPHOCENTER LYMPH NODE	LOCATION	AFFERENTS FROM	EFFERENTS TO	REMARKS
Pancreaticoduodenal lnn.	On visceral surf. of pancreas near portal v., between pancr. and duod., and between pancr. and transverse colon	Pancreas, duodenum, nearby parts of colon	Intestinal trunk	Varying number of small lnn. Regularly incised in meat inspection

CRANIAL MESENTERIC LYMPHOCENTER (p. 76)

LYMPHOCENTER LYMPH NODE	LOCATION	AFFERENTS FROM	EFFERENTS TO	REMARKS
Cran. mesenteric lnn. (77.A)	At the origin of cran. mesenteric a.	Spleen	Visceral trunk or directly into cisterna chyli	Not clearly separate from celiac and nearby lnn.
Jejunal lnn. (77.E)	In the mesojejunum along the collateral br. of cran. mesenteric a., near jejunum, outside spiral colon	Jejunum, ileum	Intestinal trunk and colic lnn.	10–50 lnn., each 0.5–12 cm long. Regularly considered in meat inspection
Cecal lnn. (77.D)	In ileocecal fold	Ileum, cecum	Colic lnn. or directly to the intestinal trunk	1–3 lnn., 0.5–2 cm long, inconstant. Regularly examined in meat inspection
Colic lnn. (77.C)	1. Between limbs of the prox. loop 2. Between prox. and distal loops dorsocran. to the spiral loop 3. On the right surf. of the spiral loop	Ascending colon, ileum, cecum	Intestinal trunk	1. 1–6 lnn. 2. 1–4 lnn. 3. 7–30 lnn., only 0.5–4 cm each. Regularly considered in meat inspection

CAUDAL MESENTERIC LYMPHOCENTER (p. 76)

LYMPHOCENTER LYMPH NODE	LOCATION	AFFERENTS FROM	EFFERENTS TO	REMARKS
Caud. Mesenteric lnn. (77.B)	On the sides of the descending colon	Descending colon	Lumbar trunk	Routinely examined in meat inspection

ILIOSACRAL LYMPHOCENTER (p. 82)

LYMPHOCENTER LYMPH NODE	LOCATION	AFFERENTS FROM	EFFERENTS TO	REMARKS
Medial iliac lnn. (83.4)	At the termination of aorta and origin of deep circumflex iliac a.	Hip jt., hypaxial lumbar mm., pelvic and femoral mm., testis and spermatic cord; or ovary, uterine tube, uterus, bladder, kidneys, female urethra	Lumbar trunk	1–4 lnn. 0.5–5 cm long. Considered in suspected cases in meat inspection
Lat. iliac ln. (83.12)	At the bifurcation of deep circumflex iliac a. and v.	Pelvic bones, fascia lata, abd. mm., deep gluteal m., peritoneum; subiliac and coxal lnn.	Lumbar trunk, med. iliac lnn., in part iliofemoral ln.	1–2 lnn., 1.25–2.5 cm long, may be absent. Considered in suspected cases in meat inspection
Sacral lnn. (83.5)	In the angle between right and left int. iliac aa.	Iliopsoas, gluteal mm., and mm. of tail, intrapelvic urogenital organs, including their mm.	Med. iliac lnn., iliofemoral ln. or directly into lumbar trunk	A second, inconstant group lies on the internal surf. of the sacrosciatic lig. at the level of the lesser sciatic foramen
Anorectal lnn. (76.K)	On the anus and rectum	Descending colon, rectum, anus	Med. iliac lnn.	12–17 lnn. 0.5–3 cm long

ILIOFEMORAL LYMPHOCENTER (p. 20 and 82)

LYMPHOCENTER LYMPH NODE	LOCATION	AFFERENTS FROM	EFFERENTS TO	REMARKS
Iliofemoral ln. (83.5)	In the angle between ext. iliac and deep circumflex iliac vessels	Femoral and crural mm., abd. mm., bones and joints of pelvis and pelvic limb down to the hock, intra-abdominal urogenital organs	Med. iliac lnn., lumbar trunk	3.5–9.5 cm long. Considered in suspected cases in meat inspection

LYMPHOCENTER LYMPH NODE	LOCATION	AFFERENTS FROM	EFFERENTS TO	REMARKS
SUPERFICIAL INGUINAL LYMPHOCENTER (p. 90 and 92)				
Supf. inguinal lnn.			Iliofemoral ln.	
Scrotal lnn. (93.9)	Caud. to spermatic cord, dorsolat. to penis at level of pecten pubis	Scrotum, prepuce, penis, skin of thigh, crus, and stifle		Considered in meat inspection
Mammary lnn. (91.B)	Med. to caud. border of lat. laminae of suspensory apparatus of udder	Udder, vulva, vestibule, clitoris, skin of thigh, crus, and stifle		1–3 lnn., 6–10 cm long; palpable caudally between the thighs, dorsal to the caud. quarters. Regularly examined in meat inspection
Subiliac ln. (67.5)	At cran. border of tensor fasciae latae above the level of the stifle	Skin of abd. wall, pelvis and hind limb, prepuce	Iliofemoral lnn., med. iliac lnn., in part, coxal ln.	6–11 cm long, palpable; to be considered in suspected cases in meat inspection
Coxal ln.	Med. to tensor fasciae latae at the tuber coxae	Fascia lata, quadriceps femoris	Lat. iliac ln. or med. iliac lnn.	1.5–2 cm long; inconstant
SCIATIC LYMPHOCENTER (p. 20)				
Sciatic ln. (17.B)	On the sacrosciatic lig. dors. to lesser sciatic for. or in the foramen	Skin of the pelvic region and tail, gluteal mm., hip jt., rectum, anus, urogenital organs at pelvic outlet	Sacral lnn.	2.5–3.5 cm long. To be considered in suspected cases in meat inspection
Gluteal ln. (17.A)	On the sacrosciatic lig. at the greater sciatic foramen	Pelvic bones, hip jt., deep gluteal m., thoracolumbar fascia	Sacral lnn.	1 or 2 lnn., up to 1 cm each; inconstant
Tuberal ln. (19.B)	On the med. surface of the tuber ischiadicum and on the attachment of the sacrosciatic lig.	Skin of pelvic region and tail, gluteobiceps	Sciatic ln., rarely sacral lnn.	2–3 cm long, inconstant
POPLITEAL LYMPHOCENTER (p. 20)				
Deep popliteal ln. (17.C)	In the space between gluteobiceps and semitendinosus and the heads of the gastrocnemius	Pes, crus, and caud. thigh mm.	Iliofemoral and sacral lnn.	3–4.5 cm long. To be examined in suspected cases in meat inspection. A supf. popliteal ln. is absent in ruminants.

3. PERIPHERAL NERVOUS SYSTEM

NERVE	INNVERVATION	REMARKS
SPINAL NERVE		Leaves the vertebral canal through an intervertebral for. (exceptions C1; C2; S1–S5)
• Dorsal branch (nd)		
•• Lateral branch (ndl)	Skin of dors. third of lat. surf. of trunk	Sensory; except cervical nn.: motor
•• Medial branch (ndm)	Epaxial mm. of trunk	Motor; except cervical nn.: sensory
• Ventral branch (nv)		
•• Lateral branch (nvl)	Skin of ventr. body wall and limbs	Except nerves of plexuses
•• Medial branch (nvm)	Hypaxial trunk mm. and mm. of limbs	Except nerves of plexuses
I. CERVICAL NERVES: C1–C8 (p. 57, 61)		C1 leaves the vert. canal through the lat. vert. for. of atlas; C2 through the lat. vert. for. of axis
• Dorsal branches		C3d–C6d form the dorsal cervical plexus
•• Lateral branches	Cervical part of the dorsal mm. of the trunk	Motor
•• Medial branches	Skin of dorsolat. part of neck	Sensory; C2dm, as the **major occipital n.,** innervates the skin of the nape
• Ventral branches		
•• Lateral branches	Skin of lat. and ventr. cervical region; mm. cutanei colli, facies and labiorum	C2vl, as the **transverse cervical n.** innervates the cutaneous mm. on the head and neck, and as the **great auricular n.** supplies sensation to lat. parts of the auricle; brr. of C5vl as the **supraclavicular nn.** innervate the skin over the cranial thorax and shoulder joint
•• Medial branches	Long hyoid mm. and hypaxial mm. Mm. omotransversarius, rhomboideus, and serratus ventralis cervicis	C4 and C5 form the ventr. cervical plexus; brr. of C5v to C7v course through the thoracic inlet as the **phrenic n.** to the diaphragm; C6v, C7v, and C8v, together with T1v and T2v form the brachial plexus
II. THORACIC NERVES: T1–T13 (p. 61, 67)		
• Dorsal branches		
•• Lateral branches	Skin over the dorsal thoracic wall down to parts of the lateral thoracic and abdominal wall	Also known as the first cutaneous branch
•• Medial branches	Thoracic part of the epaxial muscles of the trunk	See Muscle Tables (Vertebral column Musculature: epaxial muscles)
• Ventral branches	Internal and external intercostal muscles	Course ventrally under the pleura (except for the last n.) as **intercostal nn.** in the costal groove
•• Lateral branches	Musculature of the lateral thoracic and abdominal wall	
••• Lateral cutaneous branches	Skin of the lateral thoracic and abdominal wall	Second cutaneous br.; lat. cut. brr. of T1v–T3v and a br. of lat. thoracic n. form the **intercostobrachial n.** It innervates the cutaneous omobrachialis and skin over the triceps.
•• Medial branches	Musculature and skin of the ventr. thoracic and abdominal wall	In the region of the sternal ribs they innervate the internal intercostal mm. and transversus thoracis; in the region of the asternal ribs, the ext. and int. oblique, rectus, and transversus abd. mm. T13v, as the **costoabdominal n.,** innervates parts of the psoas mm. and the quadratus lumborum
••• Ventral cutaneous branches	Skin lat. and ventr. to the sternum, and of the abdomen to the udder or prepuce	Also known as the third cutaneous branch

NERVE	INNVERVATION	REMARKS
III. LUMBAR NERVES: L1–L6 (p. 85)		
• Dorsal branches		
•• Lateral branches		
••• Lat. and med. cutaneous branches	Skin on the lat. abd. wall down to the level of the patella; and lumbar and cran. gluteal regions	Important in anesthesia of the paralumbar fossa; also include **cran. clunial nn.**
•• Medial branches	Lumbar part of the epaxial mm.	
• Ventral branches		Form the roots of the lumbar plexus (see p. 122)
•• Lateral branches	Skin and muscles of the lateral and ventral	
•• Medial branches	abdominal wall and pelvic limb	
IV. SACRAL NERVES: S1–S5 (p. 85)		
• Dorsal branches		Leave vert. canal through dorsal sacral foramina
•• Lateral branches	Skin of caud. gluteal region and thigh	Known as the **middle clunial nn.**
•• Medial branches	Caud. parts of multifidus and dorsal muscles of the tail	
• Ventral branches	Muscles of the pelvic limb	Leave vert. canal through ventral sacral foramina
•• Lateral branches		
•• Medial branches		Form the roots of the sacral plexus (see p. 123)
V. CAUDAL [COCCYGEAL] NERVES: Cd1–Cd5		Form the cauda equina (see p. 57.18)
• Dorsal branches	Dorsal sacrocaudal mm., intertransversarii; skin of dorsal surface of tail	Form the dorsal caudal plexus
• Ventral branches	Med. and lat. ventral sacrocaudal mm. and intertransversarii; skin of ventral surface of tail	Form the ventral caudal plexus

BRACHIAL PLEXUS

Ventr. brr. of the 6th to 8th cervical nn. and the 1st and 2nd thoracic nn. form the roots of the plexus, which pass between the scalenus mm. to the craniomedial side of the shoulder joint. Supplies the thoracic limb, parts of the shoulder girdle mm., and the thoracic wall.

Suprascapular nn. 5.8	Supraspinatus and infraspinatus	Fibers from C6v and C7v; it passes directly over the cran. border of the scapula from med. to lat.
Subscapular n. 5.4	Subscapularis	Fibers mostly from C7v, additionally from C8v
Axillary n. 5.13		Fibers mostly from C7v and C8v; main parts pass between subscapularis and teres major to the lat. side of the thoracic limb
• Muscular branches	Shoulder joint; caud. parts of the subscapularis; teres major, teres minor, deltoideus	
• Cran. cutaneous antebrachial n.	Skin over the shoulder to the craniolateral surface of the middle of the antebrachium	

NERVE	INNVERVATION	REMARKS
Musculocutaneous nerve (5.9)		Fibers from C6v–C8v; forms the ansa axillaris with the median n.
• Proximal muscular br. (5.b)	Coracobrachialis and biceps brachii	Crosses deep to coracobrachialis en route to biceps
• Distal muscular branch (5.d)	Brachialis	
• Med. cutaneus antebrachial n. (5.31)	Skin on the med. side of the forearm; cran. surface of elbow joint capsule	Communicates prox. to carpus with supf. br. of radial n.
Radial nerve (5.15)		Fibers from C7v, C8v, and T1v; passes between the med. and long heads of triceps to the lat. side and over the lat. supracondular crest of the humerus, where it may be crushed, causing radial paralysis
• Muscular branches	Triceps brachii, tensor fasciae antebrachii, anconeus; distal parts of brachialis	
• Caud. lat. cutaneus brachial n.	Lat. parts of brachial skin	
• Deep branch (5.20)		
•• Muscular branches	Extensor carpi radialis, ext. carpi ulnaris, ext. digitalis communis, ext. digitalis lat., ext. carpi obliquus	
• Superficial branch (5.32)		Communicates prox. to carpus with med. cut. antebrachial n. of musculocutaneous n.
•• Lat. cut. antebrachial nerve (5.33)	Skin on lat. side of forearm almost down to carpus	
•• Dorsal common digital n. II (7.34)		
••• Axial dors. digital n. II	Dorsomed. region of med. dewclaw	
••• Abaxial dors. digital n. III	Skin of digit III to dorsomed. bulbar and coronary regions; digital joints	The nerve may be connected at the level of the fetlock jt. with the corresponding palmar nerve
•• Dorsal common digital n. III		
••• Axial dors. digital nn. III and IV	Skin of digits III and IV in the dors. coronary regions; digital joints	Each n. receives an interdigital communicating br. from the corresponding palmar nn.
Median nerve (7.29)		Fibers from C8–T2; forms the ansa axillaris with the musculocutaneous n.; gives sensory brr. to the med. pouch of the elbow jt.; runs with the median a. deep to the pronator teres and flexor carpi rad. to the carpus; passes through the carpal canal on the med. border of the deep belly of the supf. digital flexor (without dividing into med. and lat. palmar nn., unlike horse)
• Muscular branches	Pronator teres, flexor carpi radialis, humeral and radial heads of deep digital flexor, interflexorii	
• Palmar common digital n. II (7.18)		
•• Axial palmar digital n. II	Mediopalmar region of med. dewclaw	
•• Abaxial palmar digital n. III	Skin of digit III on mediopalmar bulbar and coronary regions to the apex of the digit; digital joints	The nerve may be connected at the level of the fetlock jt. with the corresponding dorsal nerve
• Communicating branch (7.f)	To palmar common digital n. IV, of the ulnar n.	
• Palmar common digital n. III (7.17)	Usually double; the brr. may unite at the beginning of the interdigital space to form a common trunk (see p. 10)	
•• Axial palmar digital nn. III and IV	Skin of the axial palmar digital regions of digits III and IV to the apices of the digits; digital joints	Each n. gives off an interdigital communicating br. to the corresponding dorsal nerve

NERVE	INNVERVATION	REMARKS
Ulnar nerve (5.10)		Fibers from C8v–T2v; runs caud. to brachial a. and v., medially on the brachium over the med. head of the triceps (covered by the tensor fasciae antebrachii) to the caud. surface of the elbow jt. and into the groove between the ulnaris lat. and flexor carpi ulnaris; gives off sensory fibers to elbow and carpal joints
• Caud. cut. antebrachial nerve (5.24)	Skin on the caudomed. and caudolat. sides of the forearm and carpus	
• Muscular branches	Flexor carpi ulnaris, supf. digital flexor, humeral and ulnar heads of deep digital flexor	
• Dorsal branch (5.43)		Passes laterally over the carpus and in the metacarpus becomes the dorsal common digital n. IV
•• Dorsal common digital n. IV		
••• Axial dors. digital n. V	Laterodorsal region of lat. dewclaw	
••• Abaxial dors. digital n. IV	Skin of digit IV to the laterodorsal coronary and bulbar regions; digital joints	At the level of the fetlock jt. the n. may be connected to the corresponding palmar n.
• Palmar branch (7.14)		Passes over the carpus lateral to the tendons of the supf. digital flexor
•• Deep branch	Interosseus III and IV	The deep branch is given off from the palmar br. distal to the carpus
•• Superficial branch		Passes distally lat. to the flexor tendons, receives the communicating br. from the median n., and becomes palmar common digital n. IV
••• Palmar common digital n. IV		Has a short course.
•••• Axial palmar digital n. V (9.22)	Lateropalmar region of the lat. dewclaw	
•••• Abaxial palmar digital n. IV (9.24)	Skin of digit IV on the lateropalmar coronary and bulbar regions to the apex of the digit; digital joints	At the level of the fetlock jt. the n. may be connected to the corresponding dorsal n.
Cran. and caud. pectoral nerves (61.t and 61.u)	Supf. and deep pectoral mm. and subclavius	Fibers from the cran. roots of the plexus
Long thoracic nerve (61.v)	Serratus ventralis thoracis	Fibers mainly from C7v and C8v
Lateral thoracic nerve (61.w)	Cutaneus trunci and, together with intercostal nn., skin on ventral thorax and abdomen	Fibers from C8v–T2v; see also intercostobrachial n. under **THORACIC NN.** (p. 119)
Thoracodorsal nerve (5.3)	Latissimus dorsi	Fibers from C7v and mainly from C8v
LUMBAR PLEXUS	Ventral brr. of L2–L6 form the roots of the plexus	Forms, with the sacral plexus, the lumbosacral plexus
Iliohypogastric nerve (67.8)		Fibers from L1v; no communication with other spinal nn., therefore not a plexus n.
• Lateral ventral branch	Ext. and int. abdominal oblique mm., transversus abdominis	Perforates the abd. mm. and ends in the lat. and ventr. cutaneous brr.
•• Lateral cutaneous br.	Skin of the flank back to the craniolateral surface of stifle	
•• Ventral cutaneous br.	Skin on the ventr. abdominal wall, prepuce or udder, skin on medial surface of thigh	
• Medial ventral br.	Caud. parts of all abd. mm.; peritoneum cran. to inguinal region	Courses subperitoneally to the vicinity of the internal inguinal ring

NERVE	INNVERVATION	REMARKS
Ilioinguinal nerve (67.9)		Fibers from L2v and L3v
• Lateral ventral branch	See also iliohypogastric n.	Perforates the abdominal wall
•• Lateral cutaneous branch	Skin of paralumbar fossa, over the cran. surface of thigh to lat. surface of stifle	The field of innervation adjoins that of the iliohypogastric n. caudally
•• Ventral cutaneous branch	See iliohypogastric n.	
• Medial ventral branch	Peritoneum of the inguinal region, skin of the prepuce or udder	Perforates transversus, rectus, and aponeuroses of oblique abd. muscles
Genitofemoral n. (91.c)		Fibers from L2v–L4v, crosses the deep circumflex iliac a. and v. Extremely variable
• Genital branch (81.11 and 81.19)	Cremaster, tunica vaginalis, skin of the prepuce or udder	Passes through the caudomedial angle of the supf. inguinal ring with the ext. pudendal a. and v.
• Femoral branch	Skin on the med. surface of thigh and the prepuce or udder	Passes through the lacuna vasorum
Lateral cutaneous femoral n. (67.11)	Psoas major, skin of the fold of the flank, cranial, and in part medial, surfaces of thigh; stifle joint	Fibers from L3v and L4v; accompanies caud. branch of deep circumflex iliac a. and v.; after perforating the abd. wall runs at first medial, then craniolat. on the thigh down to the stifle
Femoral n. (21.f)		Fibers from L4v–L6v; passes between psoas minor and cran. head of sartorius and iliopsoas through lacuna musculorum; gives off saphenous n. here
• Muscular branches	Sartorius, quadriceps femoris	
• Saphenous n. (21.11)		Runs with femoral a. and v. in the femoral triangle; sensory to stifle jt.; supplies the pectineus part of the pectineus (et adductor longus)
•• Muscular branches	Sartorius, pectineus (et adductor longus), gracilis; sensory to stifle joint	
•• Cutaneous branches	Skin of med. surface of limb down to hock	
Obturator n. (21.n)	Pectineus (et adductor longus), gracilis, adductor magnus (et brevis); obturator externus (with intrapelvic part)	Fibers from L4v–L6v, but also from S1; runs in obturator groove to obturator for.; supplies adductor longus part of pectineus (et adductor longus)
SACRAL PLEXUS		Roots from sacral nerves
Cranial gluteal n. (17.2)	Middle, deep, and accesory gluteal mm., tensor fasciae latae	Fibers from L6v–S2v; branches off cranially from lumbosacral trunk
Caudal gluteal n. (17.16)	Gluteobiceps	Fibers from L6v–S2v; branches off caudally from lumbosacral trunk
Caudal cutaneous femoral nerve (21.i)	Skin on the gluteal region and caudal thigh	Fibers from S1v and S2v; arises from lumbosacral tr. caud. to caud. gluteal n.; runs outside sacrosciatic lig. and divides at minor sciatic for.; med. br. enters for. and joins pudendal n; lat. (cutaneous) br. may be absent
Caudal clunial nn.	Skin of the gluteal region	May be replaced by the prox. and dist. brr. of the pudendal n.
Sciatic n. (17.17)		Fibers from L5v–S2v; direct continuation of lumbosacral trunk; emerges through major sciatic for. to lat. surface of sacrosciatic lig., passes over the deep gluteal, then between the sciatic spine and major trochanter over the hip joint
• Muscular branches	Deep gluteal, gemelli, quadratus femoris	

NERVE	INNERVATION	REMARKS
• Common peroneal n. (17.6)		Runs over lat. head of gastrocnemius, passes under peroneus longus, runs between that and the lat. dig. extensor and divides in the middle of the crus into supf. and deep peroneal nn.
•• Lat. cutaneous sural n. (17.21)	Skin lat. to the stifle and crus	Perforates the terminal tendon of the biceps femoris
•• Supf. peroneal n. (17.14)		Originates from the common peroneal n. in the middle of the crus
••• Cutaneous branches	Skin on the dorsolat. surface of the metatarsus	
••• Dorsal common dig. n. IV (23.6)		Origin from supf. peroneal n., usually in the crus, crosses deep to the cran. br. of the lat. saphenous v. and runs down the metatarsus
•••• Axial dors. dig. n. V (23.14) and Abaxial dors. dig. n. IV (23.15)	Distributed like corresponding nn. on the manus which originate from the ulnar n. (see p. 9)	
••• Dorsal common dig. n. II (23.4)		Smaller terminal br. of supf. peroneal n.; divides distal to prox. third of metatarsus
•••• Axial dors. dig. n. II (23.12) and Abax. dors. dig. n. III (23.13)	Distributed like corresponding nn. on the manus which originate from the radial n. (see p. 9)	
••• Dorsal common dig. n. III (23.7)		Larger terminal br. of supf. peroneal n. in prox. third of metatarsus; runs to the interdigital space, exchanges communicating brr. with dors. metatarsal n. III (see. p. 11)
•••• Axial dors. dig. nn. III (23.21) and IV (23.22)	Skin of digits III and IV to the dorsal coronary region, digital joints	
•• Deep peroneal n. (17.9)		Origin from com. peroneal n. in middle of crus; runs on lat. border of extensor digit. longus, deep to the extensor retinacula, to the flexion surface of the tarsus
••• Muscular brr.	Tibialis cran., long, lat., and short extensors, peroneus tertius, peroneus longus	
••• Dorsal metatarsal n. III (23.1)		Runs on the metatarsus with vessels of the same name in the dors. mtt. groove to the interdigital space; after exchanging communicating brr. with dors. com. dig. n. III, ends in communicating brr. to each plantar axial digital n.
• Tibial nerve (17.19)		Passes between the two heads of the gastrocnemius and divides at the dist. end of the crus into med. and lat. plantar nn.
•• Prox. muscular brr.	Semitendinosus and semimembranosus and ischial head of biceps femoris	
•• Caud. cutaneous sural n. (17.19')	Skin on caudolat. surface of crus down to hock	Supplies lat. part of capsule of stifle joint; runs with lat. saphenous v. and passes distally on the lat. side of the common calcanean tendon
•• Dist. muscular brr.	Popliteus, extensors of the hock, and flexors of the digits	
•• Medial plantar n. (19.14)		Runs with supf. brr. of the med. plantar a. and v. on the med. border of the deep flexor tendon to the distal third of the metatarsus, where it divides
••• Plantar common digital n. II (23.9)		
•••• Axial plant. dig. n. II (23.11) and Abax. plant. dig. n. III (23.17)	Distributed like the corresponding palmar nn. on the manus which come from the median n. (see p. 9)	
••• Plantar common digital n. III (23.8)		Runs over the med. br. of the supf. dig. flexor tendon to the interdigital space; may be double or divide and reunite
•••• Axial plant dig. nn. III (23.20) and IV (23.19)	Like the corresponding palmar nn. on the manus, except that each receives a communicating br. from the union of the supf. and deep dors. nn. (see. p. 11)	
•• Lateral plantar n. (19.13)		Crosses deep to the long plantar lig. of the tarsus to the lat. border of the interosseus

NERVE	INNERVATION	REMARKS
••• Deep branch	Interossei III and IV	
••• Plant. common dig. n. IV		
•••• Axial plant. dig. n. V and Abax. plant. dig. n. IV	Like the corresponding palmar nn. of the manus which come from the ulnar n.	
Branch to coccygeus **Branch to levator ani (95.17)**	Corresponding muscles	Fibers from S3 and S4, possibly also from the pudendal n. or caudal rectal nerves
Pudendal nerve (95.9)	Rectum, internal and external genital organs	S2–S4; accompanies int. pudendal a. and v. caudally on pelvic floor and over ischial arch
• Proximal cutaneous branch	Skin on semitendinosus	Emerges through biceps just cran. to dors. process of tuber ischiadicum or through sacrotuberous lig.
• Distal cutaneous branch	Skin on semimembranosus	Emerges from ischiorectal fossa
•• Supf. perineal brr.	Skin of perineum	
••• Dorsal scrotal nn. or dors. labial nn.	Scrotum or labia and skin of caud. surface of udder	
• Deep perineal n.	Perineal muscles, vagina, vulva, major vestibular gl., skin of perineum	Communicating br. with caud. rectal nn.
• Dorsal n. of penis or clitoris	Penis or clitoris	
• Preputial and scrotal branch or mammary branch	Prepuce and scrotum or udder	The mammary br. is closely associated with the convoluted ventral labial v.
Caudal rectal nerves (97.17)		Fibers from S4, S5; communicate with deep perineal n.
• Muscular branches	Caud. part of rectum, ext. anal sphincter, retractor penis (clitoridis), coccygeus, levator ani, constrictor vestibuli	
• Cutaneous branches	Skin of anal region	

CONTRIBUTIONS TO CLINICAL-FUNCTIONAL ANATOMY

THORACIC LIMB

C. STANEK

2 Fractures of the **humerus** occur after a fall on the lateral aspect of the shoulder region. Cows may fall due to sexual activity on slippery surfaces. Young cattle may fracture the humerus when rushing en masse through a narrow doorway. These, most frequently, are long spiral fractures associated with lesions of the radial nerve. Any paralysis of the radial nerve in cattle must be examined for a fracture of the humerus. The clinical presentation is characteristic: the digital joints cannot be extended and the extremity is unable to bear weight. The animal shows a flexed posture and is unable to protract the limb. This condition may cause injuries to the dorsal aspect of the digit and the fetlock and often animals fall because of failing to protract the limb. Radial paralysis may also be caused by improper use of ropes when casting cattle into lateral recumbency, e.g. for surgery or claw trimming.

Fractures of the **radius** are rare, most often they occur in the distal half of the bone.

12 The **carpal joint** is a composite hinge joint normally opposed at 180 degrees. Flexion is the major movement with additional limited ab- and adduction. The main movement occurs in the radio-carpal joint (**Fig. 12.2**).

The carpal joint in cattle is heavily stressed when the animal is in ventral recumbence as well as when lying down or rising. Cattle get up with their hind legs first, subsequently resting on their carpal joints for a moment; in cases of painful processes, they can remain for extended periods in this position. If the cubicle is too short, an animal may crawl backwards on its carpal joints. This results in an increased occurrence of lesions on the dorsal aspect of the carpal joint starting initially with hairless, hyperkeratotic areas, with the possibility of developing into a bursa, which can become infected and inflamed, reaching the size of a man's head.

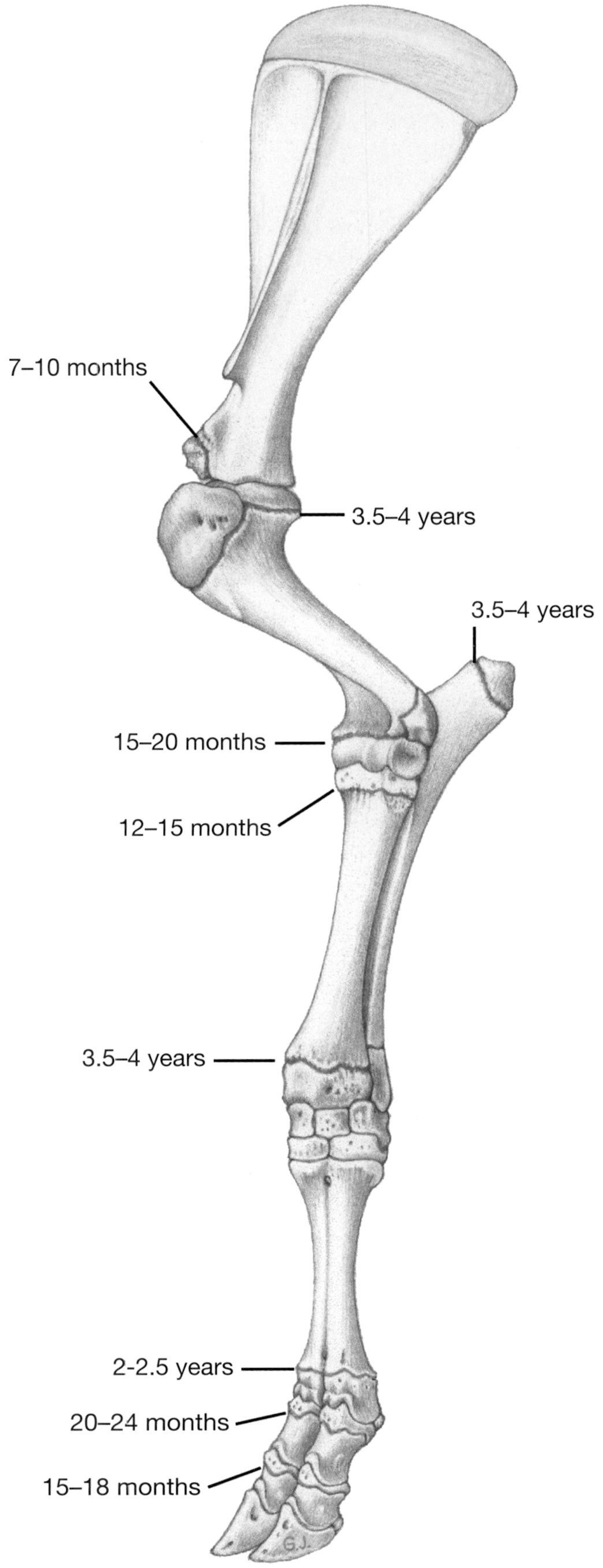

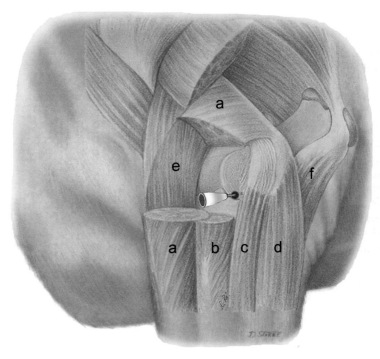

Fig. 12.1 Intra-articluar injection of the elbow joint. (a) extensor carpi radialis muscle, (b) common digital extensor muscle, (c) lateral digital extensor muscle, (d) extensor carpi ulnaris muscle, (e) brachialis muscle, (f) deep digital flexor muscle.

7–10 months

3.5–4 years

3.5–4 years

15–20 months

12–15 months

3.5–4 years

2-2.5 years

20–24 months

15–18 months

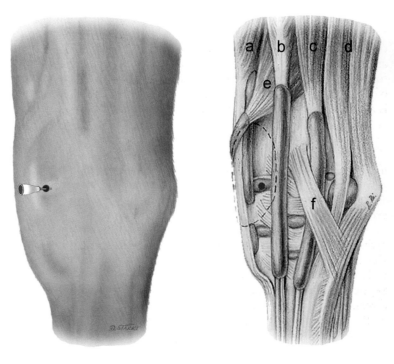

Fig. 2 Closure of physeal lines in the apophyses and epiphyses of the thoracic limb.

Fig. 12.2 Intra-articluar injection of the carpal joint. (a) extensor carpi radialis muscle, (b) common digital extensor muscle, (c) lateral digital extensor muscle, (d) extensor carpi ulnaris muscle, (e) abductor pollicis longus mucle, (f) lateral collateral ligament of the carpal joint.

Typically, the inflammation of this bursa – **precarpal bursitis** – causes only mild lameness. An invasion of the infection into a tendon sheath or the carpal joint occurs rarely. During surgical intervention on the precarpal bursa, penetration of the synovial structures has to be carefully avoided.
Septic arthritis of the carpal joint is mainly metastatic in origin. Clinical symptoms include limited mechanical mobility (reduced flexion) and severe pain during flexion. An increased filling of the joint is often visible during inspection as an increased filling of the palmar joint recess proximal to the accessory carpal bone.

Fetlock region
The following structures are clinically relevant in this region:
- fetlock joint,
- digital flexor sheath,
- dew claws.

The extensor tendons in this region are rarely affected by any disease.
The **fetlock joint** is a composite joint. The proximal articular surface of the joint is complemented by **two tear-drop-shaped sesamoid bones**, which are embedded into the distal branches of the **medial interosseus muscle**. One extensor branch runs dorsally from each sesamoid bone, blending into the extensor tendon. This extensor branch hardly ever causes clinical problems. The sesamoid bones are oriented almost vertically with their cartilaginous articular surface in the loaded digit. They consequently transfer little weight to the respective extremity but rather prevent a caudal shift of the metacarpal/metatarsal bone. On the proximal joint surface of each proximal phalanx is a shallow sagittal groove. Corresponding to this groove is a sagittally oriented, not very prominent, ridge on the respective metacarpal condyle. These two corresponding structures provide rotational stability to the fetlock joint. This rotational stability is not pronounced resulting in a low incidence of fetlock fractures in cattle. The sesamoid bones are connected by a cartilaginous bridge, which provides a section of the wall of the tendon sheath. This sliding bridge acts as a pivot enabling the flexor tendons to bend while surrounded by the digital tendon sheath. Below the fetlock, the tendon sheath is constrained by the annular ligaments of the pastern. An abscess to the foot will cause pus to rise above the level of the fetlock filling the groove between the metacarpus and the flexor tendons. Lancing this abscess should only be undertaken under regional anesthesia.
The fetlock joint of the 3rd and 4th digits have their own independent joint recess. Both joint cavities, however, communicate via a slit comparable to the opening of the joint sacs in the area of the **incisura intercapitalis**. This opening is sufficiently wide to permit the spread of infection from one fetlock joint to that of the neighboring digit. However, this opening is too small to flush both joints efficiently from one side. Needle penetration of the fetlock joint is possible from the dorsal plane as well as from palmar/plantar side. For dorsal access to the joint, one palpates the angle formed by the bulging dorsal margin of the joint surface of the proximal phalanx and the rounded joint surface of the metacarpus. Injection is performed at this site by inserting the needle abaxially in the direction of the axial surface beneath the extensor tendon. The **plantar recess is approached** through the boundaries of a triangle made up of the caudal margin of the metacarpal bone, the proximal boundary of the abaxial sesamoid bone and the contour of the abaxial course of the interosseus muscle. The fetlock joint is flexed and the needle is inserted approx. 2 cm into the centre of this triangle in an axiodistal direction (**Fig. 12.3**). [50]
The fetlock joint is mainly of clinical interest as a site of septic arthritis, i.e. arthritis caused by a variety of infectious agents such as *Actinomyces pyogenes* or *E. coli*, etc. In addition, acute aseptic arthritis can be result of dislocation or other traumatic injury. Degenerative processes – arthroses – can be identified radiographically in older bulls or cows.
Septic arthritis can develop in different ways: either caused by direct, penetrating trauma, e.g. a fork stab, a cut or, very rarely in cattle, iatrogenically. Any wound close to the fetlock has to be examined very carefully for the presence of a perforation. In case of doubt, fluid should be injected into the joint through a site away from the wound. If the joint capsule is breeched, fluid will be observed leaking from the wound. Furthermore, infection of the joint can occur via invasion of sepsis from the adjacent tissues into the joint. This occurs if infection from a tendon sheath invades the

fetlock joint. Introduction of pathogens into the fetlock joint can also occur from the blood or lymphatic vessels (see tarsal joint). In older cattle most often only one joint is affected (monarthritis), whereas in calves quite often several, mostly larger joints are involved (polyarthritis). A septic arthritis is characterized clinically by marked swelling and periarticular inflammation, severe pain during flexion or extension, and severe (supporting leg) lameness. An increased filling of the joint cavity, palpable in the region of the joint recesses, is only present in the early stages.
Lameness and swelling are less prominent in **aseptic traumatic arthritis**; certain movements corresponding to the main damaged structure (e.g. a collateral ligament) are painful; skin lesions are not present.
Arthroses in the old bull are characterized by a marked induration of the periarticular structures; the skeletal elements are difficult to palpate. Evaluation of joint mobility as well as provocation of a pain reaction is not an option for practical reasons. In most cases, several joints are affected.
The **dew claws** are in an exposed position caudal to the fetlock joint. They are attached to the main digit via connective tissue. They are subject to traumatic injury or can be torn off when caught in a gate. Subsequent suppuration can develop at the base of the dew claw. Changes in the skin surrounding the dew claws may be caused by digital dermatitis.

Biomechanics of the digital joints (interphalangeal joints)
The **fetlock joint** is hyperextended when the animal is at rest. When the limb is elevated, the fetlock flexes and during protraction there is some degree of flexion. The bones are kept in position by the collateral ligaments and the sagittal crest on Mc/Mt III and IV in opposition to the corresponding groove on the articular surface of the proximal phalanx. This arrangement allows only minor rotational and lateral movement. The sagittal crest represents a locking mechanism, which is effective only under full load. The sagittal crests are parallel to one another, restricting any abduction.
The **pastern joint** (distal interphalangeal joint) is described in literature as a saddle joint. It is undisputable that the distal joint surface of the middle phalanx has the shape of a saddle. However, the concavity of the proximal joint of the middle phalanx largely corresponds to the convex surface of the distal surface of the proximal phalanx. Especially under maximum load, large movements are only possible as a flexion and extension around a transverse axis. This transverse axis is not oriented in a 90° angle to the axial wall of the claw capsule but encloses an angle of approx. 82°. The intra-articular crest that is essential for linear tracking runs in a dorso-axial to palmaroabaxial direction. Simultaneously, the middle phalanges of the two digits move slightly apart.
Unilateral load, e.g. of the abaxial portion, leads to a minor lateral shift of the middle phalanx relative to the proximal phalanx. The tough collateral ligaments prevent the joint from opening; the sagittal crest and the corresponding groove prohibit a significant lateral shift.

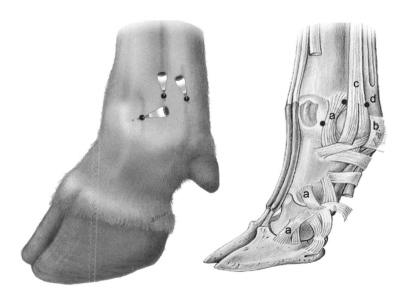

Fig. 12.3 Intra-articular injection of the fetlock joint. (a) abaxial collateral ligaments, (b) palmar annular ligament, (c) 4th interosseus muscle, (d) superficial digital flexor muscle.

Supported by the convexity of the articular surface, the lateral shift converts to flexion. When the pastern joint is flexed, the proximal phalanx articulates with the palmar/plantar part of its joint surface, which is more convex than the relatively flat central region of the articular surface of the middle phalanx. A passive rotation and shifting are possible in this position. In combination with the eccentric parts of the collateral ligaments, a situation is created where unilateral forces (in terms of an ab- or adduction) during the initial phase of locomotion cause a minor lateral shift. Subsequently, flexion occurs then, finally, rotation movements are neutralized. Therefore, rotation or abduction is automatically corrected towards the normal by the elastic function of the collateral ligaments and the distal portion of the superficial flexor tendon (close to its insertion). Radiography indicates that the digital axis between the proximal and dorsal phalanges, at rest, is slightly hyperextended. This means that the long axes of the proximal and middle phalanx establish an angle of approx. 165°. Loading of the digits with approx. 2300 N causes further hyperextension of the pastern joint by 8–15°. This construction represents one of the major suspensory mechanisms of the bovine digit. Under load, the pastern joint shows a tendency to hyperextend still further, this is however prevented by the flexor tendons. The transmission of this inhibiting force occurs via the two annular ligaments as well as the flexor tendons, which insert into the two middle and distal phalanges. During hyperextension, the branches of the interosseus muscle running to the dorsal aspect of the digit are stressed. At the same time, tension is exerted by the flexor tendons on the plantar/palmar aspect of the pastern joint. Flexion of the digit during lifting the foot results in a much greater flexion of the pastern joint. The overall flexion of the digit is accomplished not only by flexion of the distal interphalangeal joint but also by flexion of the pastern joint. Hyperextension of the pastern joint is prevented by the extensor process of the middle phalanx acting as a controlling mechanism. In contrast to the horse, traumatic lesions of the extensor process do not play a role in cattle.

Unlike the pastern joint, the **pedal joint** can be strongly flexed. For this movement, the synchronizing effect of two structures is of importance: the terminal part of the deep flexor tendon attaching to the **flexor tubercle** and the elastic ligament running from the deep flexor tendon to the middle phalanx. The fiber bundles running from the terminal part of the superficial flexor tendon to the distal part of the proximal phalanx synchronize in a similar manner. The extensor process of the distal phalanx prevents hyperextension. Contrary to in the horse, traumatic lesions of the extensor process are irrelevant in cattle.

The main directions of movement in the pedal joint are flexion and extension. However, in the pedal joint the joint axis is not precisely transversely oriented. In relation to the dorsoventral orientation of the cannon bone, the joint axis runs in an abaxioproximal axiodistal direction. The longitudinally oriented crest on the articular surface of the pedal bone (distal phalanx) is not parallel to the axial wall of the hoof capsule. Its orientation is from palmar and slightly abaxial to dorsoaxial. The palmar surface of the joint makes an angle of approx. 15°, while towards the extensor process it reaches an angle of 30° or more. If the middle phalanx is considered a fixed system and the pedal bone a mobile system, the distal phalanx undergoes a screw-like torsion during flexion of the claw joint. During movement of this joint, there is a widening of the interdigital space and due to the increase in angle towards the extensor process there is also a spreading of the claws. If forces in terms of an ab- or adduction act on the claw (unilateral load on the outer or inner part of the solar surface), a torque is generated due to the different shape and height of the articular surfaces, that results in a tendency to rotate. This is neutralized by the ligamentous structures.

In summary, the following actions occur in the digital bones under maximal load of the cannon bone (during the peak of the supporting phase): the hyperextension is increased in the fetlock joint and there is limited flexion in the pastern joint (an almost direct transfer of forces is possible in the pastern joint up to an angle of 165° to 170°). As a result of flexion, a certain degree of resilience occurs in combination with strain of the flexor tendons. The pedal joint (distal interphalangeal joint) is a saddle joint in which the articular surface of the pedal bone is approximately congruent with the surface of the middle phalanx. Joint ligaments and tendons enable (in addition to the dominating flexion and extension) a lateral shift and rotation, which are required for the spreading of the claws during maximum load and uncoiling (pushing off) of the foot.

PELVIC LIMB

C. Stanek

14 **Fractures of the thigh** (femur) are relatively common in cattle with most cases occurring in new-born calves. Calves suffer both fractures of the epiphysis as well fractures of the distal shaft of the femur (**Fig. 14**). When taking a history, it is necessary to inquire from the farmer if there was forced extraction of the calf either in anterior or breech presentation. In anterior presentation with inappropriate adduction of the limb, the femur can become locked in the bony pelvis and can fracture when it is compressed. In breech presentations, the stifle can jam in the pelvis and the **femur frac-**

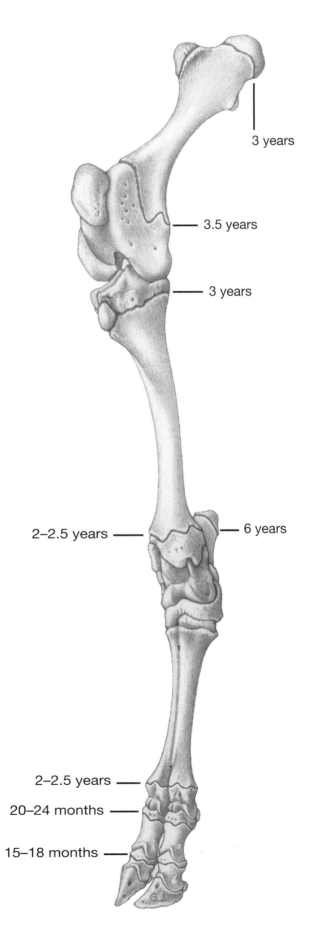

Fig. 14 Closure of physeal lines in the apophyses and epiphyses of the pelvic limb.

tures during forced extraction. Fracture of the epiphysis of the head of the femur occurs in newborn calves under forced extraction as well as with fighting among young cattle. The head of the femur is sheared off. The head of the femur usually remains in the acetabulum, however, the femur moves proximally. The **major trochanter** is clearly palpable. During the clinical examination, abnormal mobility in the hip is noticeable when the extremity is moved forwards or backwards. **Considerable crepitation** can be felt and restricted abduction and pain occurs during this manipulation. **Dislocation of the hip** must be considered as a point of differential diagnosis.

The **distal epiphysis of the tibia** is frequently the site of fractures in calves and/or young animals with or without dislocation. Also septic osteomyelitis caused by different pathogens, particularly those from navel infections, are quite common. The **third and fourth metatarsal bones** are already completely fused in the newborn calf. Only the distal condyles of the 3rd and 4th digits remain separate for life. The metatarsus is involved in diseases of the digital tendon sheaths and the fetlock joint. Other clinically significant disorders are:

- fractures of the metatarsus (metacarpus),
- injuries to different severities of trauma to tendons, blood vessels and nerves,
- other injuries that will lead to the formation of bony sequestra.

Palpating the pulse in the arterial blood flow in cases of an infection is difficult in the hind limb. In severe cases, the pulse can be palpated in the 3rd **dorsal metatarsal artery** at a point dorsoaxial directly beneath the tarsometatarsal joint.

In the metatarsal region, it is possible to perform regional anesthesia of the digits. It is possible to access five and/or six localizations by which local anesthetic may perfuse nerves running to the digits. The method is technically challenging because of the inconsistent distribution of the nerves. Restraining an animal in order to perform this procedure is difficult. This technique is even more difficult if the tissues are swollen and inflamed. Because of these difficulties, most workers prefer to use **intravenous regional anesthesia** which only involves the intravenous injection of anesthetic at one site. This method desensitizes the entire region distal to the tourniquet. [39]

The **metatarsus and metacarpus** are the bones most frequently fractured in cattle. All age groups may be involved and there is no particular specific risk predisposition. Depending on localization, differentiation of a fracture of the diaphysis, metaphysis or epiphysis can be made. When using calving chains, comminuted fractures of the diaphysis or metaphysis are unfortunate sequelae. Fractures of the epiphyses are the most common fracture type until closure of the epiphyses at about two and a half years. These fractures are classified according to SALTER and HARRIS. Crepitation is often absent in these types of fracture. Fractures of the shaft occur in all age groups. Long diagonal fractures increase the risk of a "complicated fracture", making the prognosis much worse. The reason for this is that there is no protection from muscles and sharp fragments of bone can easily penetrate the skin. Generally, cattle are good fracture patients because they rapidly form strong calluses and are disinclined to move.

In the **metacarpal region**, relatively often, injuries differing in severity involve tendons, blood vessels and nerves. The regions usually affected are those where the tendons of the 3rd and 4th digit have not yet separated. Causes for these injuries are fragments of glass, metal sheets, mower blades, barbed wire, etc. Because of the large number of arteries in the distal extremity, necrosis of the digit rarely occurs if only one vessel is cut. Severe blood loss may be unimportant even if the cuts are deep. In septic processes in the interdigital space, such as infectious **interdigital necrosis**, ultrasonography is valuable in identifying thrombosis of superficial and deep veins. Affected animals often show inflammatory reactions and poor wound healing. During the evaluation of metacarpal wounds, it is important in adult cattle, in particular, to discover which tendons have been cut and to what degree. If only the superficial flexor tendon has been cut, it will heal without major problems if the wound is managed properly. When the deep flexor tendon has also been cut, the **fetlock will drop** and the **toe will turn up** during the weight-bearing phase. The interosseus muscle in cattle has a high portion of muscle fibers. Unlike the horse, this muscle alone cannot support the fetlock, therefore, if the flexor tendons are cut it will eventually rupture even if a supporting cast has been applied. Cuts affecting both flex-

or tendons, even under the most fastidious care have a bad prognosis. Suturing of tendons is not recommended as suturing in a contaminated environment under a heavy load is contraindicated. **Cuts of the extensor tendons** often heal spontaneously by second intention and functional losses are not to be expected.

Cuts in the metatarsal region may expose large areas of bone. Bone death can occur as the inevitable result of wound infection under field conditions together with the over use of strong disinfectants. A sequestrum is formed and becomes encapsulated by connective tissue which is attached to periosteal exostoses. Each fistula in the metatarsal region failing to heal should be examined for the presence of a sequestrum. This usually requires radiological investigation.

16 **Injections into the muscles of the caudal thigh** (hamstring muscles) can result in large foci of infection. These may cause paralysis of different nerves depending on the level of the lesion. If the **tibial nerve** is involved dropping of the hock and some knuckling of the fetlock will occur, skin sensibility is reduced or absent. When the lesion affects the **fibular (peroneal) nerve** marked knuckling of the fetlock will be seen. Both of these problems have been seen as the consequence of pressure damage during birth (even normal births). If the lesion is located in the gluteal region, the sciatic nerve may be involved and complete collapse of the limb will occur.

In cattle lying in lateral recumbency for any length of time, localized pressure causes problems with blood perfusion. A so-called compartment syndrome develops in the lateral thigh muscles, especially in the region of the lateral condyle or epicondyle. In such animals, inflammation of an adventitious synovial bursa may be observed as well as generalized edema. This clinical picture is called **perigonitis**. This can fairly often be associated with an infection of the local muscles (biceps femoris muscle, vastus lateralis muscle), which can in turn lead to extensive muscle necrosis.

Due to trauma in the trochanteric region (e.g. by hitting themselves on hard objects), cattle can develop an (usually) **aseptic bursitis** in the **trochanteric bursa of the biceps femoris** lying on the caudal edge of the greater trochanter. The **trochanteric bursa of the gluteus muscle** can also become inflamed.

Rupture of the peroneus (fibularis) tertius muscle can also occur in cattle. It usually happens in adult animals with an anamnesis of slipping or the use of ropes to lift the hind leg. Affected animals show an obvious instability of the hock (buckling) in the weight-bearing phase. During the swing phase, the stifle is flexed normally but the hock remains extended and the toes are dragged. Palpation of the cranial lower leg muscles reveals swelling and pain. It is typical of this condition that the leg can be extended far back caudally, during which the hock can be opened to an angle of 180° and the skin over the Achilles tendon is typically corrugated.

18 **Paralysis of the obturator nerve** is mainly seen in cows *post partum*. During expulsion of the calf, the obturator nerves are in danger of being compressed where they run over the shaft of the ilium. If there is unilateral nerve damage, the cow exhibits a difficult gait with an abducted forwards motion of the limb. If there is bilateral damage, the cow lies down with its hind legs doing the splits. It is impossible for the standing animal to correct its stance if it stands with its legs straddled. Paralysis of the obturator nerve can occur in isolation or in combination with an often extensive **rupture of the adductor muscles**. Rupture of the adductors can also occur independently as a consequence of an animal slipping with sudden marked abduction of the limbs. Typically, with such a rupture, edema or blood can be palpated in the affected muscle group. **Pelvic fractures** or **disruption of the pubic symphysis** can cause similar symptoms.

The prognosis for lacerations and (partial) tendon rupture in the region of the **Achilles tendon** – including the superficial digital flexor tendon – should be assessed critically with respect to the loss of function. The region of the calcaneal tract and the groove lateral to it is vulnerable to lacerations, while partial or total ruptures can occur at various points in the gastrocnemius muscle: the muscle belly, the musculotendinous junction or the insertion into the calcaneus. The clinical picture is characterized by a severe lameness, severe dropping of the hock combined with knuckling of the fetlock when weight is placed on the limb and swelling in the region of the lesion. Animals with a complete bilateral tendon rupture bear weight on their metatarsi (plantigrade position); the hocks touch the ground and the animal moves forward sitting on its haunches.

22 The common digital flexor tendon sheath extends from the distal third of the metacarpus/metatarsus to the coronary band of the bulbs of the heels. Running through this sheath are the superficial digital flexor tendon to its insertion on PII with weaker fibers inserting on PI and the deep digital flexor tendon to its insertion on the **flexor tubercle of the pedal bone** and via the elastic ligament on the distal part of the middle phalanx. The separation of these two flexor tendons into the flexor tendons of the third and fourth digits occurs just prior before they enter the tendon sheath. The tendon sheathes in the third and fourth digits do not normally communicate with each other. Proximally (in the lower third of the metacarpus/metatarsus), they are only separated by the thin wall of a tendon sheath, which may not be incised during surgery.

The **superficial digital flexor tendon (SDFT)** and **deep digital flexor tendons (DDFT)** cross each other in the fetlock flexor tendon sheath. At the distal end of the metacarpus/metatarsus lies the palmar/plantar SDFT. Together with a branch of the **interosseus muscle**, it forms a tube, the flexor sleeve (manica flexoria), which encloses the DDFT. Distal to the sesamoid bones, this tube opens up and phases out in the two terminations of the SDFT. Analogous to the complicated organization of the tendons, the cavity system of the fetlock flexor tendon sheath is also complex. Proximally, there is an outer compartment and inside the tendon sheath there is an inner compartment. These two compartments only communicate with each other in the communal distal compartment. Effective irrigation of the compartment system is difficult to impossible. The standard **puncture point** lies abaxially over the tendon sheath, where a concavity is palpable between the tendons and the interosseus muscle when the fetlock is flexed. The tendon sheath recesses function as a surge tank and are where the synovial fluid for the tendon sheath is produced. In addition, displacement of the SDFT and DDFT during flexion of the fetlock is compensated for by a telescopic displacement of the sheath (**Fig. 22.1**).

The most common disease affecting the digital flexor tendon sheath and the tendons running through it is **septic tendovaginitis**. This condition is a complication of primary septic processes (such as **pododermatitis circumscripta**, infection of the abaxial white line or infectious interdigital phlegmone). Perforations, e.g. due to a hay fork, can lead to **infection of the tendon sheath**. The predilection sites are the heel bulb and the region just above the dew claws. Lacerations or injuries following accidentally catching the foot in a gate or chains, with secondary opening of the tendon sheath also occur. In addition to the primary symptoms, diagnostic signs of septic tendovaginitis are reduced weight-bearing with a slightly flexed fetlock and a medium to severe supporting leg lameness in addition to a phlegmonous swelling in the heel bulb and at the back of the metacarpus/metatarsus. The possibility of the tendon sheath being open should always be considered with lacerations in this region.

Tendon sheaths are formed everywhere in the body where tendons undergo a change in direction with a relatively large displacement over a fixed point (which needs not always be a bony prominence). The displacement of the tendons is made easier by the synovial fluid containing high-molecular hyaluronic acid present within the sheath. The tendons within the tendon sheath consist of tightly packed fibril bundles with a small amount of loose connective tissue. The nutrition of tendons over a distance of 15 cm or more is achieved by a number of mechanisms: initially by diffusion out of the synovial fluid; then through vessels, which run from the transfer points of the tendon sheath, mainly on the surface of the tendon; and through vessels which run over the short mesotenon to the tendon; and finally via vessels which run via the short vincula to the tendon. A long continuous mesotenon is missing both in cattle and horses. The blood vessel supply to the SDFT and DDFT is independent of each other with respect to the tendon sheath. The SDFT is more strongly vascularized than the DDFT. The blood vessels on the tendon itself avoid those parts of the tendon that are affected by the pressure forces in the region of the sesamoid bones. The existence of a movement-independent blood pump – continual movement of the blood in the region of the fine blood vessels during tensing of the fibers – can be assumed. With septic tendovaginitis, there is a massive disturbance of the tendon's nutrient supply due to changes in the synovial fluid (leucocytes and degeneration) and the extensive fibrin production typical of cattle. The re-establishment of the nutrient supply using antimicrobial therapy and irrigation is urgently indicated. Partial resection of tendons within the tendon sheath is very problematical due to the microstructure of their vascular system.

Intravenous regional anesthesia is recommended for **surgery in the region of the metacarpus/metatarsus** (**Fig. 22.2**). A tourniquet is placed proximally on metacarpals/metatarsals III and IV. Preferably, the local anesthetic should be injected into the cranial branch of the saphenous vein, though in principle every larger vein lying distal to the tourniquet can be used. If the operation is to be done on the proximal metacarpus/metatarsus or in the region of the tarsus, the tourniquet can also be placed in the region of the calcaneal

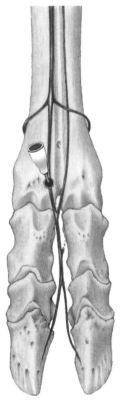

Fig. 22.1 Common digital flexor tendon sheath (1). Contrast radiograph, lateral view. (Courtesy of Prof. C. Stanek, Clinic for orthopedics in ungulates, Vetmeduni Vienna.)

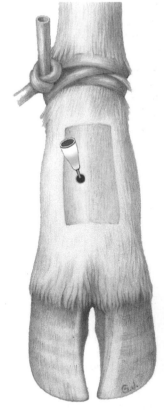

Fig 22.2 Intravenous regional anesthesia.

groove over the Achilles tendon and the associated muscles. In such cases, the calcaneal groove must be padded out with coarse calico bandages so that the blood vessels running in this region are also occluded.

CLAW

C. MÜLLING, C. STANEK

24 The interdigital space between the main claws (3rd and 4th digit) of a limb is bridged by the **interdigital skin**, which lacks hair and has a thick cornified layer. The biomechanical connection between the two digits is established by the distal interdigital cruciate ligaments, which connect the palmar/plantar aspect of the middle phalanx with the sesamoid bone and the pedal bone of the opposite side (**Fig. 24.1**). Their abaxial and axial attachments keep the digital fat cushion and the deep flexor tendon in their position. They act as restraining ligaments, which are progressively stretched during weight bearing, preventing the digits from excessive spreading. The space between the digits is filled by a large fat cushion, which is surrounded by a connective tissue capsule. The ligaments are embedded in this fat tissue, which acts as a shock-absorbing cushion between the digital bones (**Fig. 24.1**). The interdigital space is a site of predilection for infection and mechanical irritation. Hygienic problems and moisture prepare the pathway for bacterial invasion via the damaged skin barrier. Infection and inflammation of deeper living tissues are the consequence. Infections which invade the loose interdigital tissues may spread rapidly and may cause inflammation with a fast pressure increase in the interdigital compartment. Severe pain and lameness are the consequences. An example of this is interdigital phlegmone. Hyperkeratosis occurs frequently in the interdigital space due to mechanical stress.

A specific disease of the interdigital region is **interdigital hyperplasia (limax)**, which is a bulging hypertrophy of scar tissue subsequent to chronic irritation of the interdigital skin, found mainly in heavy cows and breeding bulls. Another very important disease is **infectious interdigital necrosis**, a necrotic inflammation caused by lack of hygiene in the environment (unhygienic housing conditions), moisture, etc. This disease may occur as an endemic problem. It is caused by bacteria and characterized by a rapidly progressing and spreading necrosis which affects large parts of the interdigital skin. This infection has the tendency to invade joints or tendon sheaths as well as to cause metastatic infection of inner organs and other joints. Traumatic lesions of the interdigital skin are most often cuts and may be related to details of the husbandry system, such as free metal edges, scrapers, etc.

An infectious disease of the claws of worldwide significance/importance is **digital dermatitis (strawberry foot rot – Mortellaro's disease; Fig. 24.2)**. The typical round, reddish and elevated lesions occur in the palmar/plantar pastern region at the junction between skin and bulb. This is primarily a disease of the skin (dermatitis), which secondarily affects the interdigital region and may spread into the claw causing destruction of the horn capsule. The classical acute lesions are erosions measuring several centimeters in diameter, colored red, with a surface resembling a strawberry surrounded by a white hyperkeratotic margin and the hair standing up. These lesions develop into chronic stages, which are dominated by proliferative as well as hyper- and parakeratotic processes, that typically lead to filamentous warts (hairy wart disease – papillomatous digital dermatitis). The chronic stages, in turn, may develop into acute stages later on. Once animals have been infected they represent a permanent infectious threat to the herd.

The **dew claws** have a very limited clinical relevance. Occasionally, a primary exungulation or a local phlegmone may occur if the animal slips across an edge or resists restraint in a trimming tilt table. Approx. 1.5 centimeters away from the margin of the horn capsule of the medial as well as of the lateral dew claw, runs a subcutaneous digital vein (axial and abaxial palmar/plantar proper digital arteries III and IV), which is suitable for intravenous regional anesthesia and intravenous antibiotic treatment.

26 The bovine claw serves as an interface between the animal and its environment. Its performance is genetically determined and limited. The interaction between the structural elements of the claw, the animal's metabolism and the environment result in responses that range from adaptive changes to massive damage to the tissues. The following structural elements are of crucial importance for proper functioning of the claw: 1. the subcutaneous digital cushions and the digital ligaments; 2. the dermis, including the suspensory apparatus of the pedal bone; 3. the dermal vascular system; 4. the demo-epidermal junction; and 5. the epidermis with its living horn-producing part and the horn capsule made of dead cornified epidermal cells.

The **subcutaneous digital cushions (Fig. 24.1)** are highly efficient shock absorbers. In functional synergy with the soft elastic horn of the bulb, they absorb forces during the initial ground contact during weight bearing, distributing them equally within the tissues. The composition of the fats in these cushions changes with age and physiological state of the animal. The fat content is significantly higher in cows than in heifers. The amount of fat tissue is lower in animals with sole ulcers compared animals with sound claws. In dairy cows with ketosis, the lipid mobilization causes alterations in the fat composition of the cushions leading to a decrease of their shock-absorbing capacity.

The dermo-epidermal **suspensory apparatus** of the pedal bone in the wall region consists of systems of collagen fibers and epidermal cell clusters. Both are arranged in lamellae and suspend the pedal bone from the inner aspect of the epidermal claw capsule. Quality and integrity of the collagen fibers are of crucial importance for

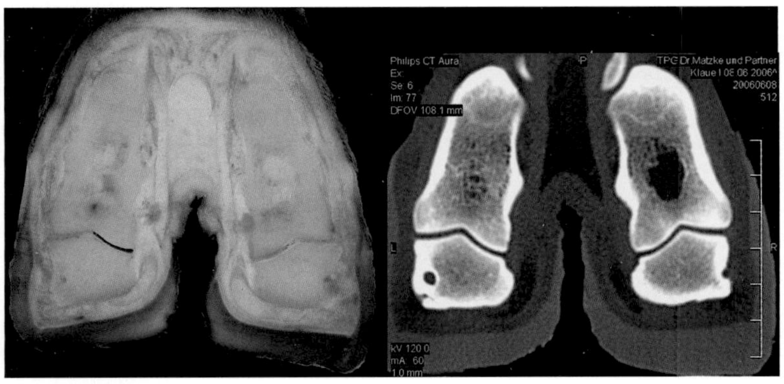

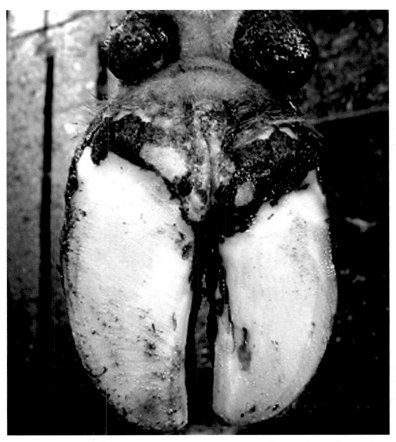

Fig. 24.1 Cross section through the distal limb at the level of the distal phalanx (pedal bone) and corresponding CT image. The following structures are visible: interdigital ligaments; interdigital fat cushion; distal, middle and proximal phalanx; digital fat cushions beneath the pedal bone and the interdigital space. (Courtesy of Prof. C. Mülling.)

Fig. 24.2 Digital dermatitis: Characteristic acute lesion (strawberry foot rot) in the skin of the pastern region above the coronary band of the claw (typical localization). (Courtesy of Prof. C. Mülling.)

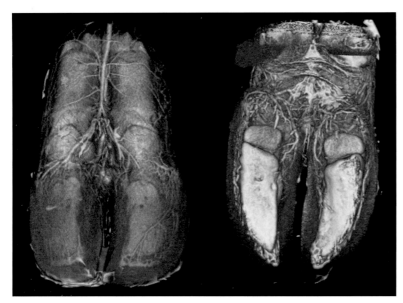

Fig. 26.1 Vascular system of the claw: Computer-aided reconstruction based on a series of CT images that were obtained subsequent to injection of contrast medium. (Courtesy of Prof. C. Mülling.)

The **horn capsule** (claw capsule) protects the enclosed bones, tendons, pedal joint and the different modified parts of the **cutis** and **subcutis** from physical (mechanical and thermal), chemical and microbial influences from the environment. The claw capsule enables the transfer of forces from the skeleton of the limb to the ground (and vice versa) that is essential for locomotion. It also provides partial absorption of the ground reaction forces during landing and weight bearing. The **horn-producing epidermis** is structurally and functionally closely tied with the **dermo-epidermal junction zone**. The avascular epidermis receives its supply of nutrients and oxygen via this zone. Molecular signals are exchanged regulating epidermal proliferation and differentiation, thus controlling the quantity and quality of the claw horn produced. The process of horn formation in the living layers of the epidermis is influenced by numerous factors originating from metabolic disorders and systemic disease.

The shape and size of the claws vary between the front and hind legs. In the hind limb, the outer (lateral) claws are larger; on the front limb, the outer claws are smaller than the inner claws. This allows identification of front and hind limb claws as well as differentiation of the lateral and medial claws. The thickness of the horn sole depends on the rate of horn production and on wear, as well as on the frequency of hoof trimming. In adult cattle, the thickness of the sole should be a minimum of 5 mm in the apical region and 8 mm in the heel. The sole should be trimmed slightly thicker on rough abrasive floors.

The **claw capsule** completely encloses the pedal bone, the distal sesamoid bone and the most distal part of the middle phalanx. All three bones make up the pedal joint. The distal **sesamoid bone** complements the joint surface of the pedal bone towards the palmar/plantar side; when loaded it will sink relative to the pedal bone. This sinking is controlled by the ligaments of the sesamoid bone as well as by the broad tongue-shaped insertion of the deep flexor tendon. Near to the bone, chondroid tissue (fibrous cartilage) is present in the deep flexor tendon. This is a clear indication that this part of the tendon is exposed to pressure forces when loaded. The blood supply to the deep flexor tendon in this region originates from the deep vascular network distal to the bone.

If this vascular network is damaged by a septic process or surgery, the supply to the deeper structures is disrupted. Complete removal is strongly recommended in cases of a clinical problem that requires resection of the deep flexor tendon. Between the deep flexor tendon and the distal sesamoid bone lies the **podotrochlear bursa**, which usually does not communicate with either the pedal joint or the distal pouches of the common digital flexor tendon sheath. The bursa is, however, separated from the pedal joint by only the relatively thin impar ligament and the also very thin palmar section of the joint capsule. During inflammation, these structures may be destroyed and spreading of the infection into the bursa may occur.

Puncture of the pedal joint is performed dorsally. The dorsal joint recess is punctured by inserting the needle 1.5 cm proximal to the coronary band, axial at the dorsoaxial margin of the middle phalanx or alternatively 3 cm abaxial to it. The needle is directed distally and slightly abaxially or axially, respectively. In addition, there is also a palmar access to the joint lateral to the deep flexor tendon.

Infectious and noninfectious diseases of the claw and the neighboring skin can be differentiated depending on their etiology and pathogenesis. They have a multifactorial etiology in common, i.e. several to multiple factors in a specific interaction are responsible for their development.

Infectious claw diseases are caused by bacterial infection; they are contagious and may spread rapidly after introduction of an infected animal into a herd. Environmental factors such as husbandry-related poor hygiene and continuous exposure to moisture weaken or damage the horn barrier. Ubiquitous and partly keratolytic bacteria and fungi prepare the pathway and lead in synergy with specific pathogens such as treponemes in digital dermatitis to infection and inflammation of the deeper tissue layers.

Laminitis plays a major role among the **non-infectious claw diseases**. A syndrome called **subclinical laminitis** (SCL), also more recently referred to as claw horn disruption (CHD) weakens the integrity of the claw tissues and increases their susceptibility to secondary diseases such as ulcers and white line disease. SCL has a multifactorial etiology and a complex pathophysiology. SCL is caused by a variety of risk factors that are intrinsically tied to modern intensive housing of dairy cows. Feeding management, cow comfort, genetic selection, poor peripartal management as well as

maintaining a stable position of the pedal bone inside of the horn capsule and for a physiological transfer of forces during locomotion. During the peripartal period and with the onset of lactation, the properties of the collagen connective tissue change, the stability of the suspensory apparatus is reduced and dislocations of the pedal bone may occur. Bruising of the dermis and damage to the horn-producing epidermis ranging from hemorrhages to sole ulcers is one of the consequences. Research has shown direct correlations between the housing of cows in loose stall systems with cubicles and concrete slatted floor and structural alterations of the collage fiber systems of the suspensory apparatus. Collagen-degrading enzymes, so called matrix metalloproteinases (MMPs) are activated by this type of housing system. MMPs and potentially damaging regulatory cascades within the claw tissues may also become activated by a variety of cytokines, mediators, endotoxins and metabolic byproducts, but also simply by mechanical action such as chronic overload.

The elements of the **suspensory and supporting apparatus of the pedal bone (suspensory apparatus and subcutaneous digital cushions)** as well as the **ligaments** between the digits and the coronary cushion function in a coordinated manner. In functional synergism, they stabilize the position of the pedal bone inside of the horn capsule. The junction zone between the hard and soft horn of the sole in the bulb-heel region has initial contact with the ground during footing. When the soft elastic horn of the bulb and the subcutaneous digital cushions beneath are loaded, they are compressed and act as efficient shock absorbers, at the same time they transfer pressure laterally onto the wall.

The proximal and, in particular, the distal **interdigital cruciate ligaments** limit and stop the spreading of the claws during progressive loading of the foot during locomotion; this is referred to as the **claw mechanism**. The suspensory apparatus in the dorsal wall region is loaded when the apical region of the toe is in contact with the ground. During the final phase of weight bearing, the pedal bone is pushed dorsally towards the wall of the claw capsule. Simultaneously, the dorsal part of the wall of the horn capsule is pushed slightly inwards due to the tension of the suspensory apparatus. The pressure that is generated in the coronary region is absorbed by the prominent coronary cushion, which is compressed absorbing and distributing the pressure equally. This coronary cushion most likely plays a similar role when pushing the foot off the ground.

The **dermal vascular system (Fig. 26.1) plays an important role** during the development (pathogenesis) of claw diseases. Recent research has demonstrated that microcirculation and the regional patterns of perfusion are highly adaptable to metabolic and mechanical challenges. The vascular system adapts to these challenges by structural remodeling. The precise links between metabolic problems and local changes in the vascular system remain to be discovered. Existing knowledge clearly accentuates the need to take metabolic as well as environmental factors into consideration in developing preventive strategies to reduce the incidence of claw disease in dairy herds.

the knowledge and skills of the farmer are among the more important risk factors. Traditionally, the assumption was that the pathogenesis of subclinical laminitis is mainly associated with nutrition and metabolism. Up to now, neither a link between a metabolic disorder and local tissue damage has been established nor has the question been resolved as to whether laminitis of the bovine claw is an inflammation at all. Nowadays, we have a plethora of results, evidence and indications that bovine SCL and the secondary claw diseases are rather associated with housing, cow comfort, claw trimming and the cow management during the transition period around parturition.

A variety of secondary claw diseases, in particular ulcers, white line diseases and hemorrhages (**Fig 26.2**) occur in addition to the typical deformations of the claw capsule as a consequence of the damage of claw tissues. These diseases may; however; also develop independently of any underlying subclinical laminitis.

The **Rusterholz ulcer (specific traumatic sole ulcer, pododermatitis circumscripta; Fig 26.3)** occurs on the sole axial at the junction between the heel and bulb on the outer claw of the hind limbs; significantly less frequently on the inner claw of the front limbs. Causative factors are (in addition to primary diseases such as laminitis) poor claw trimming, malposition of limbs due to the housing system and biomechanical factors. Pressure exerted by the flexor tubercle on the dermis and horn-producing epidermis plays

a role as well as exostosis on the flexor tubercle as a result of a periostitis (**Fig 26.4**). If only the dermis is infected, the lesion is referred to as an uncomplicated Rusterholz ulcer. In complicate ulcers, the deeper structures are also involved. The infection progresses usually in a well-defined sequence:

Uncomplicated Rusterholz ulcer > invasion of the infection into the deep flexor tendon (necrosis of the deep flexor tendon) > invasion of the podotrochlear bursa (septic bursitis) > invasion of the flexor tubercle may also occur (osteomyelitis of the flexor tubercle) >invasion of the distal sesamoid bone (osteomyelitis and necrosis of the sesamoid bone) > invasion of the infection into the pedal joint (septic arthritis of the pedal joint).

Depending on the cause, the infection may also spread into the common digital flexor tendon sheath; a septic tendovaginitis is the result. These clinical presentations can be differentiated using clinical diagnostics and diagnostic imaging. They can be treated using different surgical techniques, such as arthrodesis. For a prognostic evaluation of a claw infection, the proper identification of the structures involved is essential.

White line disease or **white line infection** begins in most cases at the abaxial part of the white line (zona alba). The soft horn of the white line is progressively destroyed by mechanical and chemical influences. This process advances towards the dermis and, once the protective horn barrier is disrupted, causes infection of the dermis, a pododermatitis circumscripta. The inflammation may, however, ascend within the lamellar system of the wall towards the periople and finally penetrate just above the claw capsule. In this situation, a canal running from the white line up to the perioplic region can be probed. Infection may spread laterally and invade the deep flexor tendon or the pedal joint.

Toe ulcers occur in the most apical region of the sole (tip of the toe). Most of the affected animals suffer from a subclinical laminitis. An ulcer develops at the typical site caused by the sinking and/or rotation of the pedal bone. The disturbance of blood perfusion present in laminitis aggravates the condition and support the development of infection. Toe ulcers may also occur subsequent to incorrect claw trimming resulting in a thin sole. They are more frequent in certain housing systems with rough abrasive flooring and poor cubicle comfort. The infection may spread into the tip of the pedal bone as a complication. This can be distinguished from an uncomplicated toe ulcer as an osteomyelitis of the tip of the pedal bone.

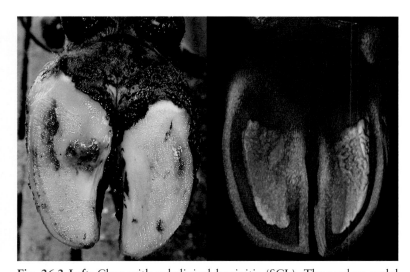

Fig. 26.2 **Left:** Claw with subclinical laminitis (SCL). The sunken pedal bone has caused bruising of the dermis and subsequent blood infiltration of the claw horn (hemorrhage). The hemorrhages are located in the typical Rusterholz site beneath the abaxial plantar margin of the pedal bone.
Right: The computer-aided reconstruction shows the position of the pedal bones surrounded by dermis inside the horn shoe of the claw. Changes in position during subclinical laminitis cause tissue damage which depending on its severity becomes visible as a hemorrhage or ultimately results in a complete perforation of the claw capsule, a sole ulcer. (Courtesy of Prof. C. Mülling.)

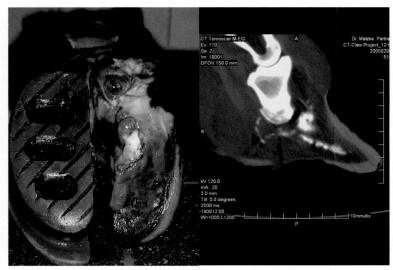

Fig. 26.3 Claw ulcers: A Rusterholz ulcer and an ulcer in the heel region in a lateral hind claw. The ulcer has been already treated and weight has been removed from the diseased claw by glueing a rubber block under the sound medial claw. The CT scan shows the ulcerated claw: prolapsed dermis in the ulcer and massive osteolysis of the pedal bone. (Courtesy of C. Prof. Mülling.)

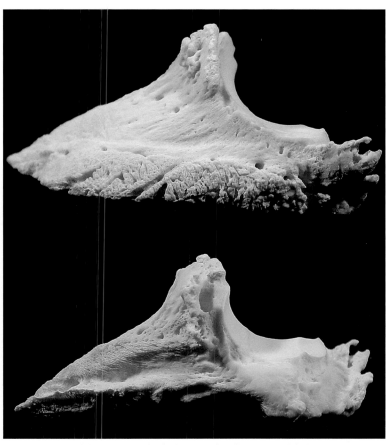

Fig. 26.4 Pedal bone (distal phalanx) of a five-year-old dairy cow. Top: abaxial view, bottom: axial view. Formation of exostoses on the flexor tubercle and the bottom part of the abaxial aspect of the phalanx where the collagen fibers of the suspensory apparatus are anchored in the bone. (Courtesy of Prof. C. Mülling.)

Total or partial **exungulation** (separation of the horn capsule from the underlying dermis) may occur if a claw gets caught between two bars or a cleft or crack in the floor. The massive primary trauma causes a partial or complete loss of the horn capsule. Such accidents may involve dislocation of the pedal joint or fracture of the pedal bone. In most cases, surgical amputation of the claw will be required.

Septic arthritis of the pedal joint most commonly occurs associated with a complicated Rusterholz ulcer or subsequent to an infection of the white line. It also may occur as a result of an infection spreading from the interdigital region (infectious interdigital necrosis). Metastatic infections are uncommon. The symptoms characteristic of septic arthritis include edema and inflammation in the coronary band, swelling, and red discoloration of the interdigital region, severe pain during flexion and extension of the joint, and a severe supporting leg lameness. An increased filling of the joint recess is palpable only in the initial stages. A breakout of the infection in the dorsal coronary region, axial and abaxial to the tendon is pathognomonic for septic arthritis. The joint cavity can be explored with a probe via the fistula canal.

Fractures of the pedal bone occur relatively often; groups at high risk are cows in estrus and bulls during breeding. The fracture is most often an intra-articular transverse fracture of the flexor tubercle with moderate dislocation of the palmar/plantar part of the bone. A (pathological) fracture may also occur subsequent to an osteomyelitis.

JOINTS OF THE PELVIC LIMB

C. STANEK

28 The **pelvis** forms a ring-like bony connection between the hind legs and the rump. The forces necessary for the locomotion of the animal are transferred via the small **sacroiliac joint** from the pelvic ring to the sacrum and so to the vertebral column. Lesions affecting this joint and its supporting ligaments occur peripartum in cows. Downer cow syndrome can occur in animals with bilateral luxation. From both visual and manual examination, it is obvious in such cases that the sacrum is sunk between the wings of the ilium. The geometry of the pelvis enables certain bony points to be palpated: **iliac crest, sacral tuber, ischial tuber** and the fused spinous processes of the sacrum. With equal weight bearing, these bony points should lie symmetrically. A misalignment may be due not only to changes in pelvic geometry, but also in the (usually caudal) vertebral column. During every rectal examination, the veterinarian should check the relationship of the bones of the pelvis to each other (see **Fig. 78.1**). The assessment of pelvic symmetry on rectal examination is especially difficult in the **downer cow**. The search for secondary symptoms of a fracture or displacement (e.g. a step-like displacement of certain bones), localization of fragments, fracture hematomas, swellings, callus formation or a displaced femoral head, are of great significance in some cases of hip luxation. When palpating the spinous processes in the lumbar and sacral region, it should be ensured that the space between the spinous processes of the last lumbar vertebra and of the first sacral vertebra (site for CSF collection) is as large as that between the final sacral vertebra and the first tail vertebra (site for epidural anesthesia). This should not be misinterpreted as being due to a (sub-)luxation or a fracture.

The pelvic ring with its bony components (ilium, pubis and ischium) augmented by the sacrum forms a rigid bony circle, which can be fractured. Pelvic fractures are frequently observed not only in parturient cows but also after falls to one side (the femoral head pushes the acetabulum medially). Pelvic fractures also may be the result of assisted calving. Another biomechanical cause of pelvic fractures, and particularly of **fractures of the body of the ilium**, is falling on the **iliac crest (tuber coxae)**. A rigid ring usually breaks at two or more sites at the same time; for example, a combination of a fracture of the body of the ilium with a pubis fracture. Fractures of the body of the ilium are usually long oblique fractures with sharp fragments. In such cases, there is a danger of acute fatal hemorrhaging if the **internal iliac artery or vein** or their branches are torn. The **sciatic nerve** can also be damaged or enclosed in a fracture. This results in severe nerve deficits. Pubic symphysis disruption should also be considered in postpartum downer cows.

A special form of pelvic fracture is the **fracture of the iliac crest (tuber coxae)**, when the stability of the pelvis is not affected. It occurs when the animal runs into door jams, stall posts or such like. This type of fracture can also be unilateral. During clinical investigation, the unilateral hand's-width ventral displacement of the tuber is obvious. The cow appears to be asymmetrical, but shows little handicap in its gait. In certain cases, skin lesions may occur with subsequent infection and the formation of a sequestrum. Every non-healing wound around the iliac crest should be evaluated for the presence of a sequestrum.

The **hip joint** itself with its joint capsule, ligaments and associated bones cannot be palpated externally. Only the **major trochanter** can be vaguely felt. At its cranial edge is the site for **intra-articular injection**. The assessment of the hip's mobility and the presence of pain is problematic in growing and adult cattle.

Two other diseases of the hip joint are (1) **hip dysplasia**, which can be seen in the first months of life in quick-growing beef breeds, usually bilaterally. Affected animals exhibit a wiggling gait with short steps and ground contact is with the dorsal part of the digits. Diagnosis can only be achieved using radiography. (2) **Hip luxation** arising unilaterally as a consequence of a heavy fall. The femoral head can be luxated in various directions, though most frequently, the luxation is dorsocranially (supraglenoidal luxation). With this type of luxation, the trochanter appears to be displaced dorsally on palpation. Affected cattle exhibit severe lameness in association with a secondary patella fixation: the leg is rotated outwards and abducted and moved forwards in extension. Complete hip luxation is always associated with a total **rupture of the joint capsule** including its fibrocartilaginous part and rupture of the **femoral head ligament**. The leg appears to be shorter on the affected side.

Degenerative joint disease of the hip joint (arthrosis) can occur but is mainly recognized post mortem and is found mostly in old animals, but cows nowadays rarely reach an age in which the occurrence of **coxarthrosis** is to be expected.

The **knee joint** (stifle joint) is perhaps the most complex joint in an animal's body. It consists of the medial and lateral **femorotibial joints** as well as the **femoropatellar joint**. All three sections of the joint communicate with each other through preformed openings. In an infection, it can be assumed that all three sections are affected, which makes effective irrigation difficult. For diagnostic puncture, it is enough to tap the medial femorotibial joint cranial to the internal lateral ligament (palpable). The femoropatellar joint distal to the patella can also be used in the calf (**Fig. 28.1**).

The stifle joint is not subjected to trauma very frequently in domestic cattle due to their phlegmatic locomotion and its position protected by the rump. One exception is in animals, which ride on other animals during heat or during (attempted) mating. This can lead to rupture of the cruciate ligaments, particularly of the cranial cruciate. This ligament is about the width of the small finger in adult cattle, and so great force is needed for it to rupture. Clinically, the animals exhibit a severe lameness of the supporting leg. The leg is moved forwards without any change in the angle of the knee joint. In addition, there is a severe swelling of the whole knee, making it difficult to determine the individual structures. With a complete **rupture of the cranial cruciate ligament**, there is a subsequent subluxation of the tibia cranially associated with instability of the whole knee. This displacement often cannot be easily palpated; at best, the **tibial tuberosity** is markedly prominent. Even incomplete ruptures lead initially to a severe lameness. Mainly a secondary functional stiffness of the knee develops in association with a severe arthrosis, cartilage defects in the joint and a severe periostial reaction at the onset of the joint capsule. Radiographically in some cases, small fracture fragments can be visible in the region of the **intercondyloid eminence** in addition to the subluxation. The total extent of the damage to the cartilage, intra-articular ligaments and menisCuses can only be assessed arthroscopically.

Inflammation of the stifle joint, aseptic gonitis or even **septic gonitis** can be present without rupture of the knee ligaments. Swelling of the stifle is then most obvious on both sides of the middle straight patella ligament. By pushing the joint capsule onto the articular surface of the femoral condyles, information can be gleaned about any thickening of the joint capsule.

While the stifle is extended, the **patella** glides upwards over the groove in the articular surface formed by the two condyles. With overextension – often in association with knee dysplasia – the patella (or better said the medial parapatellar fibrocartilage) can catch on the hook-like upper end of the medial condyle. As a conse-

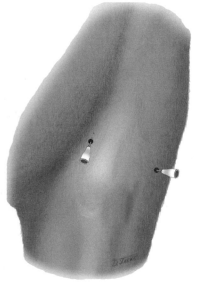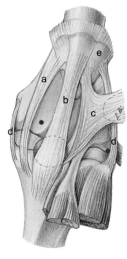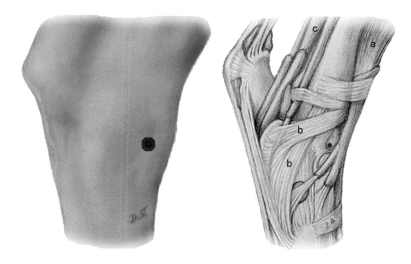

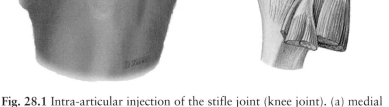

Fig. 28.1 Intra-articular injection of the stifle joint (knee joint). (a) medial patellar ligament, (b) middle patellar ligament, (c) lateral patellar ligament, (d) medial and lateral collateral ligaments, (e) patella.

Fig. 28.2 Intra-articular injection of the hock joint (tarsal joint). (a) peroneus (fibularis) tertius muscle, (b) short and long medial collateral ligament of the tarsus, (c) lateral digital flexor muscle.

quence, the stifle joint is fixed in extension and via the ligaments the hock is also extended, while the toe joints are flexed. Clinically, there can be an intermittent (the patella is spontaneously caught and released) or a fixed proximal **patella luxation** (the patella remains caught in the position in which it is in contact with the femur). This disease was frequent when cattle were employed as draft animals; however, nowadays it is very rare. **Patella luxation** in conjunction with severe tissue rupture can be (rarely) caused by massive trauma. Congenital (usually lateral) displacement (ectopia) of the patella can also occur. Affected calves sit on their haunches. As a rule, their very small patellae can only be diagnosed radiographically, lying laterally at the level of the popliteal space.

The skin around the **hock region** is close to the underlying bone on the inner, caudal and outer sides of the limb. It is virtually immovable, which can be confirmed by palpating this area. The subcutis contains virtually no fatty tissue to act as a cushion. When the animal lies in sternal recumbency with its hocks flexed, the lateral aspect of the lower hock is exposed. Unsuitable lying conditions (such as rough floors, forced lying on the edge of a stall, lack of bedding, wet bedding, etc.) initially adversely affect the skin and then the subcutis. Housed cattle often have a well-defined lateral **hygroma** at the level of the proximal III and IV metatarsal bones and the small tarsal bone. The hygroma is about the size of a hand and is prominent as it consists of a hairless region with obviously hyperkeratotic skin. Hygromas, as a rule, do not cause any clinical problems.

The formation of a subcutaneous bursa can also occur on the hock. In some cases, the skin may become necrotic, especially under adverse hygienic and mechanical conditions. The necrosis can also reach the size of a hand. There is leathery, usually dark, necrotic skin in the centre of the lesion, which is tightly fixed to the underlying bone, surrounded by a wall of connective tissue. If infection is present, a child's head-sized subcutaneous bursa can be formed lying from the proximal metatarsus to the calcaneus. The bursa has an obvious capsule and often purulent contents. This **tarsal periarthritis** is mainly only associated with a mild degree of lameness, unless the infection has progressed to the underlying joints, which luckily only rarely happens. During veterinary procedures (e.g. curettage, insertion of a drain, etc.) care must be taken not to open the compartments of the hock joint.

The **tarsocrural joint** is openly conjoined with the proximal intertarsal joint. Similarly, the **tarsometatarsal joint** communicates with the small **distal intertarsal joint**. There is no open communication between the tarsocrural articulation and the tarsometatarsal articulation. The filling of the tarsocrural joint and the quality of the joint contents can be assessed by palpating the recesses. Two plantar recesses can be found laterally and medially in every angle formed by the extreme distal caudal edge of the tibia and the cranial edge of the calcaneus. To palpate the dorsal recess, the veterinarian orientates himself/herself on the distal end of the respective malleolus – laterally from the lateral malleolus (which cannot be felt on palpation) to the cranial edge of the tibia and to the border of the

joint cavity where the talus can be felt. If the hock, or more concretely the tarsocrural joint, has excessive fluid in it, it is called a **puffy hock** (serous tarsitis). There is an increased filling of the joint's recesses of the tarsocrural joint and the contents of the synovial cavity can be pushed backwards and forwards. The most common causes of increased joint fluid are not only aseptic or septic inflammation of the joint (arthritis), but also traumatic joint hemorrhage. Occasionally, there can be a heritable predisposition for joint hemorrhages. Infections of the hock joint occur mainly metastatically, i.e. the infectious agents reach the joint capsule via the blood or lymph, often from distant primary loci such as a navel or gut infection, pyometritis, pyelonephritis or necrosis of the tail root. The infectious agents are then secondarily transferred to the joint lumen. In such cases, there is naturally no local point of entry on the skin. Severe swelling of the joint with periarticular inflammation and severe to extreme lameness associated with general malaise are a clear indication of septic arthritis.

One of the most important diagnostic steps when there is a suspicion of septic arthritis is **arthrocentesis** with subsequent investigation of the synovial fluid. The optimal site for arthrocentesis is the dorsomedial recess, although all the other recesses can be used. For an effective therapeutic irrigation of the complex hock joint, at least two diagonal recesses – from cranial to caudal – must be punctured (**Fig. 28.2**).

Infections around the tarsometatarsal articulation are usually metastatic. The most obvious symptoms are the massive palpation and percussion pain of the bone in the affected area. In older cows, especially very old animals, massive arthritic exostosis can be palpated in the region of the taut sections of the hock joint. This is called "bovine spavin". These exostoses are especially obvious on radiographs.

Lacerations in the region of the hock can occur both on its cranial and plantar aspects. It is often difficult on the cranial aspect of the hock to determine whether only the tendon sheaths have been damaged or whether the joint sacculations have also been opened (barbed wire injuries, etc.). This question can be cleared up with a high degree of certainty with heterotopic arthrocentesis – tapping of a joint recess at a distance from the laceration, assessment of the synovial fluid, irrigation of the joint with lactated Ringer's solution and the search for emergence of the irrigation fluid from the wound. With lacerations on the plantar aspect of the hock, assessing the position of the fetlock and digits will reveal which structures are capable of bearing weight and which have been completely severed.

Another very exposed structure is the **calcaneal tuber** which is the insertion point of the Achilles tendon (tendon of the gastrocnemius muscle) together with a section of the biceps femoris muscle. The tendon of the superficial digital flexor muscle (SDFT) is thickened in this area where the bone (calcaneus) is covered by a fibrocartilaginous cap. Between the calcaneal cap and the calcaneal tuber lies a large bursa, the **subtendinous calcaneal bursa** (retrocalcaneal bursa), which has small lateral sacculations that allow a certain

135

degree of displacement of the calcaneal cap. Between the spoon-shaped calcaneal cap and the similarly shaped skin, there is a subcutaneous bursa in many animals (an acquired bursa), **the subcutaneous calcaneal bursa** (Achilles bursa). This is often contiguous with the subtendinous bursa. Infection of these structures can occur with poor housing, rough floors, sharp stall edges, wooden splinters in the bedding, and in a few cases with directly perforating wounds. This is followed by a usually chronic inflammation that initially affects the subcutaneous bursa (bursitis of the subcutaneous bursa of the Achilles tendon). This is manifested by a discrete firm enlargement of the bursa up to the size of a tennis ball. Usually no fluctuation can be palpated and lameness is slight. The infection may then extend to the calcaneal aponeurosis and the subtendinous bursa (bursitis of the subtendinous bursa of the Achilles tendon). This leads to the animal constantly favoring the affected leg and to a medium lameness. In rare cases, the infection can extend to the bone, leading to an osteomyelitis in the region of the tuber calcanei resulting in severe lameness. Radiography and ultrasonography of the tendons and bursae are indicated in reaching a diagnosis.

HEAD

R. BERG, K. MÜLLER

32 **Actinomycosis** (lumpy jaw) is a sporadically occurring osteomyelitis that preferentially affects the **mandible or maxilla**. The disease is caused by the bacterium *Actinomyces bovis* in combination with other bacterial species. *Actinomyces bovis* invades the tissues through lesions of the buccal mucosa or the dental alveoli, preferentially at a time when the permanent teeth are erupting. Having passed the mucosal barrier, the bacteria reach the spongiosa by a hematogenous or lymphogenous route. While the surface of the bone bulges due to periostal reaction, the inner parts undergo osteolytic cavitation, giving the bone a sponge-like appearance (**Fig. 32**). In the lower jaw, the infection mainly affects the **body of the mandible,** whereas in the upper jaw the preferential site is the **alveolar process.** Cattle suffering from actinomycosis display difficulties in mastication. In the later stages of the disease, fistulas develop on the surface of the skin adjacent to the diseased part of the bone exuding a purulent discharge. Whenever rarefaction of the bone causes fractures of the jaw, the disease will have a fatal outcome.

34 In adult cattle, the **frontal sinus** extends up to the occipital bone and into the corneal process (**Fig. 34**). In cattle, inflammation of the paranasal sinuses (sinusitis, empyema) most often affects the frontal sinus and only sporadically the **maxillary sinus.** Frontal sinusitis often forms a complication of open fractures of the cornual process or the disease occurs following dehorning of adult cattle. The clinical symptoms include unilateral purulent nasal discharge.

Percussion of the frontal bone reveals a dull tone on the affected side and elicits a pain reaction. In the later stages of the disease, due to empyema of the sinus, the frontal bone bulges out giving the forehead an asymmetrical appearance. The frontal sinus can be drained by dehorning or by punching out a bony fragment of the frontal bone by trepanation. The trepanation site of the frontal sinus is located just above a horizontal line running between the temporal corners of the eyes, halfway between the vertical midline of the forehead and its outer edges. The trepanation site of the maxillary sinus is located halfway between a line drawn between the nasal corner of the eye and the tuber malare.

36 **Anesthesia of the auriculopalpebral nerve** does not result in analgesia of the eye but in a paralysis of the orbicularis oculi muscle. This form of anesthesia, however, facilitates the examination of the eye by inhibiting spasms of the eyelids. The branches of the nerve are blocked at a site lying rostrally to the base of the ear at the dorsal edge of the zygomatic arch.

Large volumes of fluids can be administered to cattle by **intravenous drip infusion** into one of the veins draining the outer ear (**Fig. 36**). For this purpose, an indwelling catheter is inserted into the lateral auricular vein (branch of the caudal auricular vein) or the rostral auricular vein; both vessels are located on the outer surface of the ear flap. Intravenous drip infusions over a period of more than 48 hours can be achieved.

The **arteries of the outer ear** are suitable for the sampling of arterial blood for blood gas analysis. In the calf as well as in the adult animal, arterial blood can be obtained by puncture of the caudal auricular branch located on the edge of the outer surface of the ear flap. [28]

38 The **masseter muscle** and the **pterygoideus muscles** have to be incised at meat inspection in order to detect cestode larvae, particularly those from Cysticercus. The course of the **parotid duct** corresponds to a line running from the facial vascular notch to the tuber faciale.

Palpation of the **mandibular lymph node** is part of the clinical examination in cattle. This lymph node is accessible next to the facial vascular notch underneath the tendon of the sternomandibularis muscle. The lymph node has to be distinguished from the rostral part of the mandibular salivary gland which is located in the same region. The mandibular lymph node is inconsistently accessible to palpation. It drains a region of the head ventral to a line connecting the medial canthus of both eyes. [21]

The **medial retropharyngeal lymph nodes** drain the pharyngeal region. Dysphagia or dyspnea may occur as a consequence of the swelling of these lymph nodes in the course of inflammatory diseases located in the pharyngeal region. In healthy animals, the medial retropharyngeal lymph nodes are not accessible to palpation. They can be approached from the retromandibular fossa on either side by trying to bring the finger tips of both hands closely together in a region just dorsal to the larynx. If the lymph nodes are

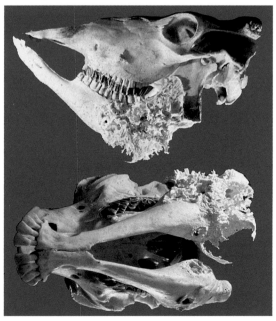

Fig 32 Actinomycosis of the mandible. Bulging and osteolytic cavitation of the bone. (Courtesy of Ruminants and Swine Clinic, FU Berlin.)

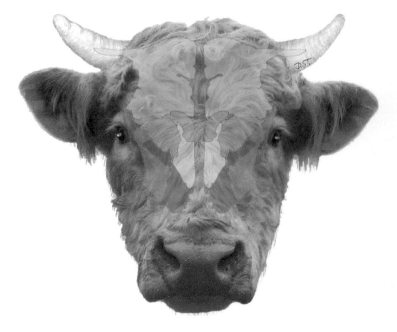

Fig. 34 Projection of the paranasal sinuses onto the surface of the head. (See also figure on page 35.)

unaffected, the examiner will be able to bring the finger tips of both hands in close proximity and no pain reaction will be elicited (**Fig. 38**). If these lymph nodes are enlarged, however, it will be impossible to bring the finger tips close to each other. In addition, palpation will elicit a pain reaction such that the animal will try to escape examination. The retropharyngeal lymph nodes have to be examined during meat inspection. The **lateral retropharyngeal lymph nodes** are easily accessible for palpation (**Fig. 38**).

40 The **conjunctivae** are accessible for clinical examination (**Fig. 40**). In healthy cattle, these mucous membranes have a pale pink color and a shiny appearance due to a thin layer of moisture on their smooth surface. As the conjunctiva lacks pigmentation, it is more suitable for the evaluation of the peripheral circulation than the pigmented and hairy skin.

Local surface anesthesia of the eye is performed by dripping a suitable local anesthetic into the conjunctival sac.

Flushing and exploration of the nasolacrimal duct. Exploration of the drainage system of the nasolacrimal duct can be achieved by cannulation or flushing of the duct through its nasal orifice. The nasal orifice of the lacrimal duct, which is arranged in pairs, is located on the medioventral surface of the alar fold. It has a smaller diameter in cattle than in horses. The orifice is accessible by deflecting the wing of the nose dorsolaterally and passing a cannula into the opening. Subsequently, flushing of the duct will result in draining of the fluid via the lacrimal opening. The nasolacrimal duct has a length of 12 to 15 mm and a diameter of 3 to 4 mm. In some cattle, the lacrimal duct is discontinuous. In these cases, there is an opening halfway up the nasal meatus from which the fluid drains into the nasal cavity.

Anesthesia of the orbital nerves according to PETERSON. The sensory innervation of the eye and orbita is supplied by the ophthalmic nerve, whereas the motor innervation is provided by the trochlear, abducens and oculomotor nerves. In cattle, local anesthesia of the eye and the orbita are performed to induce akinesia and analgesia for ophthalmological examination or surgical intervention. The most frequent indication is the evisceration of the orbita for the treatment of squamous cell carcinoma (cancer eye). Either anesthesia according to PETERSON or retrobulbar anesthesia is suitable. The anesthesia according to PETERSON aims to deposit a local anesthetic in close proximity to the foramen orbitorotundum, a characteristic feature in cattle. It arises from a fusion of the orbital fissure and the foramen rotundum. An injection needle of approximately 12 centimeter length is introduced into the caudal angle between the frontal process and the temporal process of the zygomatic bone and is pushed forward along the rostral edge of the coronoid process of the mandible in order to anesthetize the oculomotor, trochlear, ophthalmic, maxillary and abducens nerves. All these nerves leave the cranial cavity through the foramen orbitorotundum, which is located 7 cm beneath the puncture site of the skin. The success of the anesthesia of the orbital nerves according to PETERSON essentially depends on a precise deposition of the local anesthetic. The fact that this anesthesia is relatively unreliable somewhat limits its use.

The **cornual branch of the zygomaticotemporal nerve** (**cornual nerve**) should be anesthetized before dehorning cattle. This nerve supplies the skin at the base of the horn. The site for anesthesia is located directly underneath the temporal line halfway between the ear and the eye. Lying in close proximity to the orbita, the nerve is located fairly deeply, covered by the frontoscutularis muscle and fat tissue. Close to the horn, the nerve is only covered by skin and by the frontalis muscle. Insufficient anesthesia may occur due to difficulties in precisely localizing the nerve for anesthesia when it runs deeply in the tissues or because of an abnormal length of the infratrochlear and supraorbital nerves. In such cases, anesthesia is achieved by subcutaneous infiltration with local anesthetic at the base of the horn. There are no indications for a nerve supply to the horn base from the cervical nerves.

Anesthesia of the ophthalmic nerve is performed prior to surgical intervention of the eyeball and the orbita. Complete analgesia is achieved by blocking the nerve at the foramen orbitorotundum, where the nerve emerges from the cranial cavity. Following insertion of the needle in the medial canthus of the eye using the caudal lacrimal process as an orientation, the needle is pushed further in to the foramen orbitorotundum in the direction of the lateral condyle of the opposite side.

44 The surface of **the muzzle** in cattle is pervaded by grooves and furrows (sulci), elevations (areae) and small dimples (faveolae). Each individual has a characteristic arrangement of these surface formations that does not change throughout its whole life. After covering the muzzle with ink, a print of the muzzle can be obtained on paper, which is subsequently scanned and stored electronically in order to identify individual cattle.

Insertion of a nasogastric tube. A soft nasogastric tube is passed via the nostril along the ventral nasal meatus via the pharynx and the

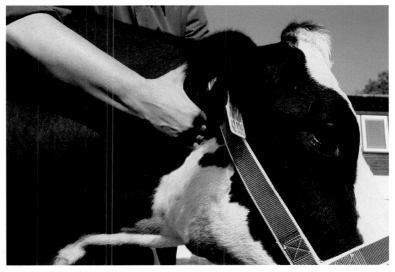

Fig. 38 Palpation of the lateral retropharyngeal lymph nodes. (Courtesy of Ruminants and Swine Clinic, FU Berlin.)

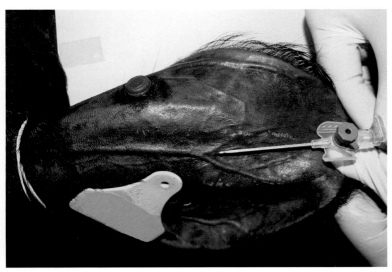

Fig. 36 Intravenous drip infusion into the auricular vein. (Courtesy of Ruminants and Swine Clinic, FU Berlin.)

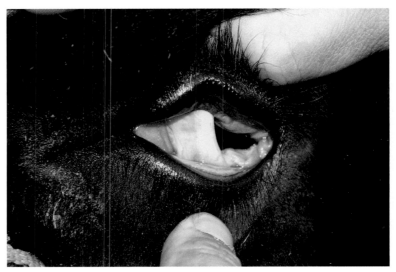

Fig. 40 Examination of the conjunctivae. (Courtesy of Ruminants and Swine Clinic, FU Berlin.)

esophagus into the rumen. Nasogastric intubation is indicated for administration of liquid therapeutic drugs directly into the rumen, letting off gas in bloated animals and the removal of fluids from the distended rumen as well as for removal of an obstruction of the esophagus.

In cattle practice, the **nostrils (nares)** offer access for various instruments. The nostrils in cattle are narrower than in the horse and the alar sulcus gives them a comma-shaped appearance. As cattle – in contrast to horses – do not have a nasal diverticulum, the insertion of the nasogastric tube into the ventral nasal meatus is easier than in the horse.

The **nasal mucous membrane** can be inspected during the clinical examination. In healthy cattle, this mucous membrane has a pale pink color and a shiny appearance due to a thin layer of moisture on its smooth surface. As the mucous membrane is lacking pigmentation and has a thin epithelial lining, it is more suitable for the evaluation of the peripheral circulation than the pigmented and hairy skin.

Regulations for the protection of health standards and workplace safety require the insertion of **nose rings** in bulls older than 12 months. A special type of forceps is used for this purpose. The nose ring has to be inserted in the soft cartilage-free rostral part of the nasal septum, where the mucous membranes of the opposing nasal ducts are attached to each other. Insertion of a nose ring in the cartilaginous part of the nasal septum has to be avoided as it would result in wound complications and cause severe pain.

The **oral cavity** in cattle is larger and shorter than in the horse. All of the oral cavity as well as the pharynx and the proximal part of the esophagus are accessible to manual palpation. The manual exploration of the oral cavity, however, needs proper restraint of the animal and insertion of a mouth gag beforehand. The mucous membrane of the oral cavity, including the ventral aspect of the tongue and the hard palate, has a smooth surface, a shiny appearance and a pale pink color. As the mucous membrane is lacking hair and pigmentation and has a thin lining epithelium it is more suitable for clinical evaluation compared to the pigmented and hairy skin.

Actinobacillosis (wooden tongue) is a soft-tissue infection in cattle resulting in a chronic granulomatous inflammation. The disease is caused by a normal inhabitant of the oral cavity, the bacterium *Actinobacillus lignieresi*. This bacterium uses small lesions of the mucosa, preferentially located at the **lingual fossa** at the base of the tongue, to enter its deeper layers and to cause a chronic granulomatous inflammation. In the later stages of the disease, a characteristic finely granulated pus drains to the exterior. Histological examination of the pus reveals club-like rosettes with a central core of bacteria (fungal druses). Affected animals show profuse salivation and difficulties in food uptake and mastication. With time, fibrous tissue is formed in response to the infection, which causes a hardening (induration) of the tongue (wooden tongue). Due to the latter alterations, the organ enlarges and gradually loses its function. In severe cases, the tongue even protrudes from the mouth (**Fig. 44**). [11]

Paralysis of the tongue is very rarely caused by local damage to the hypoglossus nerve, but most likely is a symptom of various central nervous disorders (encephalitis) or intoxications. A classical symptom of botulism in cattle is tongue paralysis. The tongue can be easily drawn out of the mouth of an affected animal, which subsequently has difficulties or is even unable to draw back the tongue into its mouth. In addition, space-occupying masses in the brain (e.g. tumors, abscessation) can cause paralysis of the tongue.

46 **Traumatization or perforation of the pharynx** may be caused by the uptake of foreign bodies with sharp edges or coarse plant materials carrying thorns. Furthermore, lesions of the pharynx have been reported following inappropriate use of instruments, mainly oral dosing equipment including esophageal or stomach tubes made from metal, or even magnets or boli that were administered orally. Cattle with lesions of the pharynx show dysphagia and profuse salivation. The pharynx is swollen and painful. Perforations of the pharynx may result in abscessation and/or accumulation of air or even gas in the area of the **Viborg triangle**, the latter being produced by anaerobic bacteria invading the tissues through the lesions. [2]

Inflammation of the larynx (laryngitis) occurs in calves and young adults. The bacterium *Fusobacterium necrophorum* plays a key role in its pathogenesis. The disease is clinically characterized by dyspnoea and a snoring respiratory sound (stridor). The bacterium invades the tissues through lesions of the mucosa, which might have been caused by an upper airway infection or trauma due to coarse plant materials. The bacterium causes a typical necrosis. The clinical examination of cattle dyspnoea and snoring includes inspection of the larynx from the oral cavity using a tubular speculum or by insertion of an endoscope via the ventral nasal meatus. The lesions, however, may not be visible because they can be located on the aspect of the **arytenoid cartilage** which is not accessible to visual inspection from the nasal or oral cavities. In chronic cases, cauliflower-like granulation tissue is formed in response to the infection. The centre of the lesion consists of a necrosis which often extends to the sparsely vascularized cartilage. *Fusobacterium necrophorum* can metastasize into the lungs by being aspirated or into the rumen by being swallowed or into various organs via the blood stream. [17]

48 The facial artery, the facial vein and the parotid duct run across the **facial vascular notch** in a rostrocaudal direction (artery, vein, and duct – AVD). In cattle other than in the horse, the facial vein is accompanied by two nerves. Rostral to the vein runs the communicating branch between the ventral and dorsal buccal nerve and caudal to the vein runs the parotid branch of the buccal nerve. The pulse can be evaluated by palpation of the facial artery in the groove at the rostral border of the masseter muscle above the ventral margin of the mandible (**Fig. 48**).

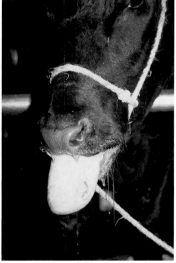

Fig. 44 Soft tissue actinomycosis (wooden tongue). (Courtesy of Ruminants and Swine Clinic, FU Berlin.)

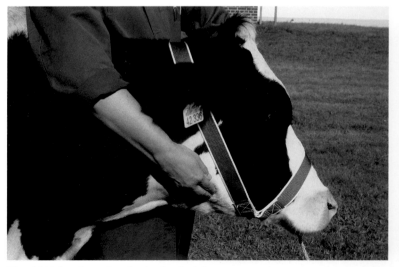

Fig. 48 Palpation of pulse in the facial artery running across the notch for the facial vessels (incisura vasorum facialium). (Courtesy of Ruminants and Swine Clinic, FU Berlin.)

CRANIAL NERVES

S. Buda, R. Berg

52 Lesions of individual cranial nerves or their nuclei as they occur, for example, in *Listeria* encephalitis can be diagnosed based on the resulting functional loss in the region supplied by the respective nerve (**Fig. 52**).

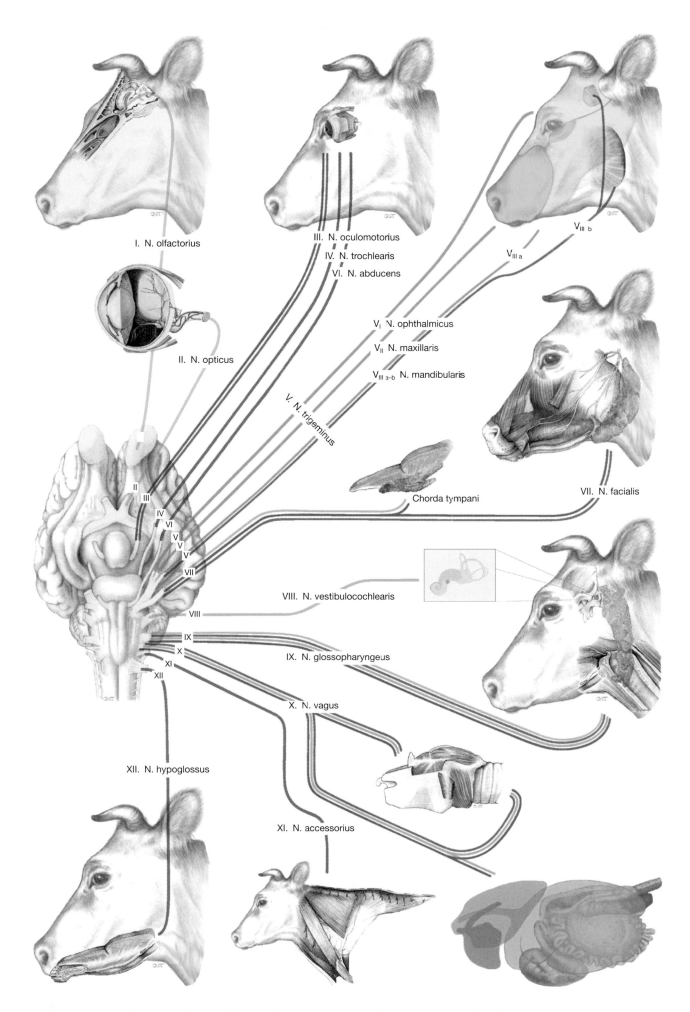

I. N. olfactorius

II. N. opticus

III. N. oculomotorius

IV. N. trochlearis

VI. N. abducens

V$_I$ N. ophthalmicus

V$_{II}$ N. maxillaris

V$_{III\ a-b}$ N. mandibularis

V. N. trigeminus

V$_{III\ b}$

V$_{III\ a}$

Chorda tympani

VII. N. facialis

VIII. N. vestibulocochlearis

IX. N. glossopharyngeus

X. N. vagus

XII. N. hypoglossus

XI. N. accessorius

II
III
IV
VI
V
V
V
VII
VIII
IX
X
XI
XII

Fig 52 Cranial nerves. Mapping of the cranial nerve fibers to the regions they supply (see also pages 52–55).

NECK AND THORACIC WALL

R. BERG, K. MÜLLER

58 Atlanto-occipital cerebrospinal fluid tap (Fig. 58). Cerebrospinal fluid can be obtained in cattle from a bulge of the subarachnoidal space which forms the caudal extension of the cerebellomedullary cistern (term used by clinicians = Cisterna magna). The puncture site is located in the **atlanto-occipital space**, which – with the head kept in a normal position – has a length of 2 to 3 cm in its longitudinal axis and of 2.5 to 3 cm in its transverse axis. The distance from the surface of the skin to the centre of the subarachnoidal space is 8.5 cm in adult cattle. Puncture at the atlanto-occipital site allows for the collection of larger volumes of cerebrospinal fluid.

Rib biopsy can be performed in order to obtain serial samples to evaluate the mineral status of a herd. Sampling is performed with the animal in lateral recumbency from the 2nd or 3rd rib.

Bone marrow biopsies can be obtained from the 2nd or 3rd rib following local anesthesia with the animal in lateral recumbency. These biopsies can be used for the evaluation of the status of the different cell lineages within the bone marrow (thrombopoesis, erythropoesis, and leucopoesis).

Diseases of the **subcutaneous presternal bursa**, which is located in the midline and at the cranial edge of the sternum, are caused by bruises or infections. When affected, the bursa can gain the dimensions of a tennis ball or even a man's head.

The **dewlap** is a suitable site for subcutaneous injection. It is a large skin flap at the end of the neck, which extends from the brisket up to the space between the front limbs.

Bone marrow biopsies can also be obtained from the sternum by **sternal puncture**. The puncture site is located at the level of the 2nd sternebra on the intersection of a vertical axis through the shoulder joint and a horizontal axis through the elbow joint. With the animal in a standing position, the respective sternal segment can be identified with the help of the corresponding rib. In cattle with a body mass ranging from 350 to 450 kg, the puncture site is located approximately 10 cm caudal to the cranial edge of the sternum.

60 Intracutaneous injections in the neck are preferentially done at sites which are easily accessible and not exposed to external influences. The lateral area of the neck is suitable and is used, for example, for the intracutaneous tuberculin test.

Intramuscular injections in cattle are preferably administered into the muscles of the neck, as these are not highly valuable parts of the carcass and drugs are absorbed faster than in other muscle groups (anconeus muscle, gluteus muscle, semimembranosus muscle, semitendinosus muscle). The injection site is located in the **trapezius muscle** a few inches cranial to the scapula. Injections into the **nuchal ligament** have to be avoided as they may cause severe complications.

Larger volumes of drugs should be administered intravenously preferentially into the **external jugular vein** as this vessel can easily be accessed in an animal which is properly restrained. In addition, the diameter of this vessel allows insertion of larger sized needles as well as indwelling catheters used for continuous drip infusions (**Fig. 60**). Improper placement of the needle as well as intravenous administration of irritating solutions could result in severe complications due to inflammation of the jugular vein or its surrounding tissues. The inflammatory reaction may either be restricted to the outer wall of the vessel (periphlebitis), or to its inner lining. The lat-

ter condition bears the risk of thrombus formation (thrombophlebitis) and the detachment of emboli that are subsequently disseminated to other organs of the body. [43] [34]

The most common disease of the **esophagus** in cattle is **esophageal obstruction**. This disease occurs whenever ingestion of solid materials (such as apples, potatoes or beets which have been insufficiently chewed) leads to a partial or complete obstruction of the esophageal lumen. There are three different sites within the esophagus where obstructions are usually observed, due to the fact that at these sites the diameter of the esophageal lumen is smaller than in the other parts of the esophagus. These predilection sites are located in the cranial part of the esophagus just above the larynx, at the thoracic inlet and at the base of the heart. Whenever the esophageal lumen is obstructed by a foreign body, water and food that are swallowed cannot pass the obstruction and will be regurgitated shortly afterwards. If the esophagus is completely obstructed, ruminal fermentation gases will not be removed via the esophagus and bloating (ruminal tympany) will be the consequence. The obstruction has to be removed as soon as possible. Foreign bodies can either be extracted manually or by use of different instruments such as semi-stiff tubes fitted with a loop at one end. Alternatively, the foreign body can be pushed down the esophagus into the rumen. Even after the successful removal of a foreign body, complications may arise from necrosis of the esophageal wall at the obstruction site due to local ischemia. The latter could finally result in perforation or stricture of the esophagus. The passage of food into and gases through the esophagus can also be impaired due to space-occupying masses lying outside the esophagus causing compression and obstruction of its lumen. In addition, inflammatory processes or other alterations of the esophagus such as diverticula and dilatations (megaesophagus) interfere with the various functions of the esophagus including rumination and ructuation. Paralysis of the esophagus with marked dilatation is a characteristic finding in botulism in cattle or may occur as a consequence of lesions affecting the brain stem. [22]

Sporadically, a tumor of the **thymus** (**thymus lymphosarcoma**) may occur in young cattle. In such cases, a space-occupying mass is located in the ventral part of the neck and extending into the thoracic cavity. This can be evaluated by swinging the mass back and forth with one hand and at the same time checking with the other hand if the mass extends into the thoracic cavity. Due to its fatal prognosis, thymic lymphosarcoma has to be differentiated from traumatic hemorrhages in the cervical muscles which sporadically occur if animals have been trapped in a neck rail or gate. On ultrasonography, the thymic lymphosarcoma is seen as a dense mass compared to the more sponge-like appearance in case of a hemorrhage. Space-occupying masses in the neck and the anterior part of the thoracic cavity may result in congestion of the jugular vein, ruminal tympany due to pressure on the esophagus and in irritation of the vagus nerve, leading to disturbances of the rumen motility.

The **superficial cervical lymph node** is clinically important. It is located just cranial and dorsal to the shoulder joint underneath the omotransversarius muscle, lateral to the deep muscles of the neck. The lymph node can be located and evaluated by putting the flat hand on the lateral neck with the finger tips pointing towards the supraspinatus muscle. Moving the fingers cranially, the lymph node can be palpated in the prescapular groove sliding under the finger tips.

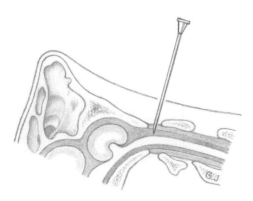

Fig. 58 CSF tap. Atlanto-occipital puncture to collect cerebrospinal fluid (CSF).

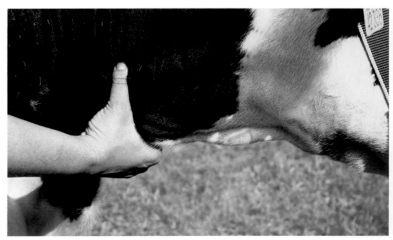

Fig 60 Pressing on the external jugular vein to engorge it. (Courtesy of Ruminants and Swine Clinic, FU Berlin.)

THORACIC CAVITY

K. Müller, R. Berg

[62] Congenital diaphragmatic hernia with prolapse of abdominal organs into the thoracic cavity occurs rarely in neonatal calves. Acquired traumatic hernias are more common than the congenital form of the disease. In neonatal calves, the characteristic symptoms of a diaphragmatic hernia are colic and dyspnoea. In adult cattle, parts of the reticulum may herniate through a tear in the diaphragm that is most often located in close proximity to the esophageal hiatus. The symptoms in this form of diaphragmatic hernia include recurrent ruminal bloat, regurgitation of rumen contents and weight loss due to anorexia.

A myopathy of the diaphragm (inherited diaphragmatic muscle dystrophy) occurs in the adult animals of certain breeds (Dutch Meuse Rhine Yssel cattle) and in some Holstein Friesian cow lines. This myopathy is an autosomal recessive hereditary disease. The disorder affects the synthesis of a distinct heat shock protein and leads to a degeneration of the diaphragmatic muscles. The clinical symptoms are characterized by a dysfunction of rumination and ructuation, dyspnoea and anorexia. [44]

The line of pleural reflection at the insertion of the diaphragm, where the costal pleura reverts and continues as the diaphragmatic pleura, forms the caudal end of the pleural cavity. This line is important for diagnostic procedures and surgical manipulations. It runs in a zigzag pattern from the bone-cartilage junction of the 7th and 8th ribs, crosses the middle of the 11th rib and ends at the vertebra associated with the 11th rib at the lateral edge of the extensors of the back.

Thoracocentesis is the puncture of the thoracic cavity, whereas pleurocentesis is the puncture of the pleural cavity to either collect fluid from the pleural space for diagnostic reasons or to drain the pleural cavity in case of a wet pleuritis. The puncture sites are located in the 6th or 7th intercostal space, ventral to the costochondral joint. Puncture of the intercostal arteries could lead to life-threatening hemorrhages into the pleural cavity.

Perforating lesions of the rib cage (due to rib fractures or a thrust from a horn) and perforations of the pleural lining due to rupture of bullous emphysema (a complication of pneumonia) could cause a leakage of air into the pleural cavity (pneumothorax). Due to the fact that – in contrast to the horse – perforations of the mediastinum, so-called fenestrae, are absent in cattle pleural effusions usually remain limited to one side of the thorax. A pneumothorax is clinically characterized by decreased or absent lung sounds at auscultation and a subtympanic percussion tone over the lung field. In the case of lung emphysema, air sporadically leaks along the fasciae of the muscles of the back and accumulates in the subcutis of a region between the shoulder blades causing subcutaneous emphysema.

Compared to other mammalian species, the lungs in cattle have a relatively small volume and respiratory surface in proportion to the body mass. In contrast to the dog and the horse, the lungs of cattle are characterized by a high grade of segmentation with four lung lobes (cranial, middle, caudal, and accessory) on the right and two (cranial and caudal) on the left. Each of the individual segments of the bovine lung is ventilated by a bronchus that branches in a dichotomous manner within one segment. In cases of obstruction of the main bronchus, no collateral ventilation exists. In the horse, in contrast, alveoli that are ventilated by different main bronchi have pores that maintain ventilation whenever a complete obstruction is present in one bronchus.

The density of the lung capillaries supplying a group of alveoli is lower in cattle than in other domestic mammals. The muscular tunic of the pulmonary vein is thick, allowing it to react to perivascular nerve activity. The amount of connective tissue is larger in the bovine lung compared to other species, which results in a higher resistance and lower elasticity of the lungs of cattle. As a consequence, cattle have to make greater efforts in respiration and have higher respiratory rates at rest. Due to the high grade of segmentation and the absence of collateral ventilation, the bovine lung is prone to atelectasis when there is impaired ventilation. The morphological and physiological characteristics of the bovine lung as well as the fact that the development of the lung is not finished until 12 months of age predispose cattle to respiratory disease.

The respiratory sounds that can be heard at auscultation in the healthy individual originate from turbulences in the air flow, which arise mainly at the branching of the tracheobronchial tree. The sound is subsequently transmitted to the thoracic wall. In the bronchioli with a diameter less than 2 mm, the type of airflow has been proven to be laminar, which means that in the healthy organism no respiratory sounds originate from the smaller bronchioli or the alveoli. Auscultation of the lung is always carried out on both sides and should include the entire aspects of both lung fields and the trachea. The quality of the respiratory sounds differs depending on the site of auscultation. In contrast to the thoracic wall, where the respiratory sounds are attenuated by the air-filled lung tissues and the abdominal wall, there is hardly any loss in intensity of the sounds originating from the bronchi if auscultation is performed in the ventral part of the neck directly above the trachea.

According to Hagen-Poiseuille's law, the resistance to airflow is inversely proportional to the diameter of the airways. The velocity of the air flow is faster in the larger bronchi than in the smaller airways in the periphery of the lung. The intensity and frequency of respiratory sounds decrease towards the periphery. In addition, the air-filled lung tissues also cause an increasing attenuation of breathing sounds to the periphery. Recordings of the respiratory sounds have demonstrated a loud crescendo-decrescendo sound at inspiration, followed by a sound with a lower intensity and frequencies at expiration (Fig. 62.1A). When interpreting the respiratory sounds, different factors have to be taken into consideration. Among these are the site of auscultation, the thickness of the thoracic wall, the respiratory frequency and the age of the animal. In order to be able to recognize "abnormal" respiratory sounds in a diseased animal, the examiner has to rely on his/her past experience obtained from healthy animals differing in age, body condition and respiratory frequency. If sounds that are audible at auscultation of a sick animal reveal an increased intensity and higher frequencies than experienced in a healthy animal, the respiratory sounds are characterized as having an "enhanced respiratory sound". However, in cases where there is a diminished intensity of respiratory sounds compared to past experience the sounds are termed "attenuated". Auscultation of the lung can reveal the following alterations: respiratory sounds are completely absent, diminished, enhanced or clearly bronchial. Altered respiratory sounds can be restricted to certain regions of the lung but also can be present over the whole lung field. The cause of absent or diminished respiratory sounds can be located within or outside the lung. If the ventilation of the part of the lung that is accessible to auscultation is impaired or absent due to partial or complete blockages of the airflow, respiratory sounds are weakened or even absent. Impaired ventilation of parts of the lung can be related to the accumulation of exudate within the bronchial lumen or caused by occlusions of bronchi due to space-occupying masses (Fig. 62.1D) which compress the bronchus from outside.

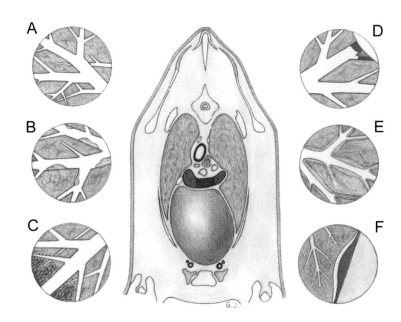

Fig 62.1 Causes for abnormal respiratory sounds during auscultation of the lung: (A) normal respiratory sound in a healthy lung, (B) accumulation of viscous secretion in the bronchi, (C) lung tissue of increased density in pneumonia, (D) obstruction of bronchi and atelectasis of lung tissue, (E) narrowed bronchial lumen due to bronchial constriction or swelling of the mucous membrane, (F) thickened parietal pleura in pleuritis. Cross section at the level of the 5th thoracic vertebra.

In ruminants with pneumonia, the inhaled air is directed to the unaffected areas of the lung while the airflow to the pneumonic parts of the lung is reduced due to bronchospasm. Lung emphysema is characterized by abnormal amounts of air present in the lung tissues. In such cases, respiratory sounds are weakened at auscultation. In addition, fine fizzing sounds (as if opening a bottle of carbonized sparkling water) can result from alveolar emphysema, whereas bullous emphysema causes a rustling sound comparable to the sound generated by crumpling up a piece of wrapping paper. Subcutaneous emphysema or pleural thickening and local effusions outside the lung may weaken the lung sounds (**Fig. 62.1F**). Sometimes friction sounds are audible, which originate from exudates with a high viscosity that cover the parietal and visceral pleura. Splashing sounds, in contrast, originate from the accumulation of large amounts of fluid within the pleural cavity. Accumulation of air within the pleural cavity would either cause diminished or – in case of a total collapse of the lung – even absent breath sounds (**Fig 62.1D**). Increased breath sounds are audible whenever higher velocities of the air flow are present; e. g., as a consequence of increased respiratory frequencies, narrowing of the airways caused by either bronchospasm, or edema of the bronchial mucous membranes, or accumulation of exudate within the bronchial lumen. Loud harsh breath sounds – so called bronchogenic sounds – are caused by extensive pulmonary consolidation and atelectasis in the lung lobes that are still ventilated. In these cases, the sounds that are elicited at the bronchial branchings – due to the decreased or even total lack of air within the lung tissues – are transmitted to the body wall with only a slight loss in intensity. In these cases, the sound that is audible over the affected part of the lung is similar to "listening at the open end of a bronchus" (**Fig. 62.1C**). Crackles and wheezes are abnormal sounds which are caused by the movement of secretion within the lumen of bronchi and bronchioli (**Fig. 62.1B**). The quality of the sounds is determined by the viscosity of the exudate. Buzzing, purring or whistling sounds are audible when highly viscous secretion forms threads within the bronchial lumen. Bubbling sounds, in contrast, are caused by air bubbles that are generated in liquid exudates.

Acoustic percussion of the thorax is either performed manually (digito-digital) or by using a special metal plate (plessimeter) and a percussion hammer. This non-invasive technique is performed to determine the borders of the lung percussion field and to detect alterations in the lung tissues and the thorax. The borders of the lung percussion field are determined by the detection of changes in the resonant sounds elicited by taps delivered with the hammer on the plessimeter. Areas of increased dullness or increased resonance can be delineated. Organs which are located in close proximity to the lung cause dull percussion sounds compared to the air-filled lung tissues. Crossing the assumed limits of the percussion field in a vertical direction will deliver the greatest differences in percussion sounds, making it easier to detect the border lines (**Fig. 62.2**). As the dorsal blind sac of the rumen contains gas, it is difficult to determine the caudal border of the left lung percussion field. The comparative percussion is performed to detect dull or hyper-resonant areas within the lung percussion field. Areas with a dull resonance within the lung percussion field indicate consolidated lung tissues, space-occupying masses or pleural or pericardial effusions. A hyper-resonant sound during percussion of the thorax could indicate abnormal amounts of air within the lung (emphysema) or the thoracic cavity (pneumothorax). [22]

In cattle, **bronchoscopy** is limited to animal hospitals or specialized practices. The equipment suitable for use in adult cattle consists of an endoscope with a length of 170 cm. The endoscope is passed through the ventral nasal meatus and reaches the larynx in the adult animal at a distance of about 35 to 40 cm from the nasal orifice. At a distance of approximately 90 to 110 cm, the **tracheal bronchus** is visible leaving the trachea on the right side. It ventilates the right cranial lobe and the cranial part of the middle lobe of the right lung. The bifurcation of the trachea is located approximately 10 cm distally from the tracheal bronchus. The trachea divides into the two main bronchi, the principal bronchi. The right principal bronchus splits into one lobar bronchus for the right middle lobe and in one for the right caudal lobe. A branch of the left principal bronchus ventilates the left cranial lobe. Subsequently, the principal bronchi each split into four dorsal and four ventral bronchi that ventilate the caudal lobe.

The main lymph nodes of the lung are the tracheobronchial lymph nodes. The following lymph nodes are examined at meat inspection:
1. **Left tracheobronchal lymph node** (between the aortic arch and left pulmonary artery)
2. **Cranial tracheobronchal lymph node** (located on the right side of the trachea at the base of the tracheal bronchus)
3. **Middle tracheobronchal lymph node** (dorsal to the tracheal bifurcation)
4. **Right tracheobronchal lymph node** (lateral to the right principal bronchus)

The **caudal mediastinal lymph nodes** are not only important for meat inspection but also from a clinical point of view. These lymph nodes are located in the fat tissue between the esophagus and aorta. The caudal mediastinal lymph node has a length of approximately 15 cm or larger. The mediastinal lymph nodes drain the esophagus, the pericardium, the dorsolateral thoracic wall, the lungs including the pleura, the diaphragm, parts of the peritoneum as well as the liver and the spleen. In animals suffering from chronic pneumonia, the latter group of lymph nodes – if enlarged – can give rise to vagal dysfunction resulting in ruminal tympany with accumulation of gas in the dorsal blind sac.

64 **Congenital malformations of the heart** are present in 1 % of newborn calves. Typical malformations are: ectopia cordis (the heart is located outside the thorax and is only covered by skin), atrial septum defects (persistent oval foramen) and ventricular septal defects. The latter defects are often accompanied by additional mal-

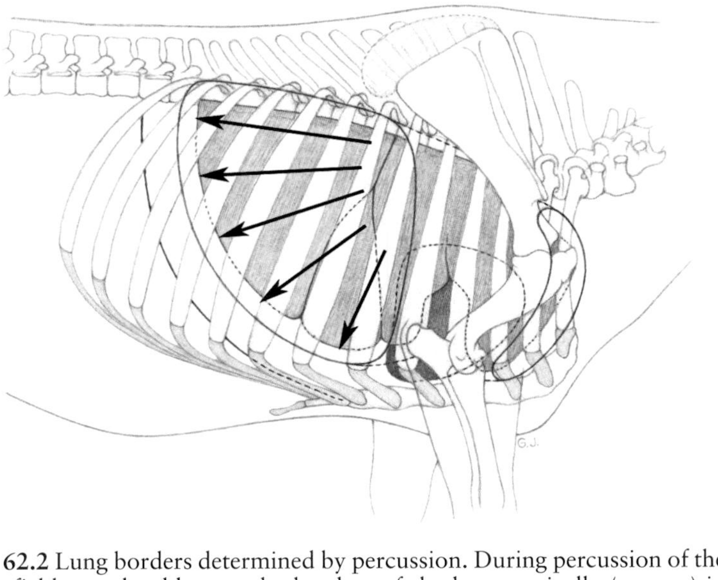

Fig. 62.2 Lung borders determined by percussion. During percussion of the lung field one should cross the borders of the lung vertically (arrows) in order to obtain maximum differences in sound quality between two subsequent sites of percussion (inside and outside of the lung field). Areas outlined in blue: cranial and caudal border of the lung field; red dotted line: silhouette of lung lobes; red line: insertion of the diaphragm.

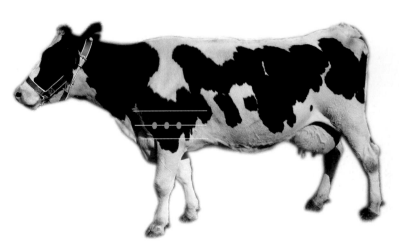

Fig. 64.1 Landmarks for localization of the puncta maxima during auscultation of the heart. For detailed explanation, see text. (Courtesy of Ruminants and Swine Clinic, FU Berlin.)

formations which resemble the Tetralogy of Fallot or the Eisenmenger Complex and the patent Ductus arteriosus observed in humans.

In cattle, **the cardiac impulse (Ictus cordis)** can be palpated on the left thoracic wall by sliding the hand flat underneath the elbow and the anconeus muscle at the level of the 4th or 5th intercostal space. In contrast to humans, the Ictus cordis in cattle is not caused by an apex beat, but by vibrations that originate from the cardiac wall. For this reason, this phenomenon is more accurately termed cardiac impulse and not apex beat. [21] [37]

Auscultation of the heart forms a key element of the clinical examination of the circulatory apparatus. During auscultation, the normal heart sounds are evaluated as well as the frequency, rhythm and intensity of the beats. Furthermore, the clinician should seek for heart murmurs which could be associated with cardiac disease. Auscultation should start on the left side of the thoracic wall and proceed on the right side. The bell of the stethoscope is placed on the thoracic wall underneath the anconeus muscle. The location of the heart sounds and eventual cardiac murmurs are identified with the reference to the points of maximum intensity (**puncta maxima**). As the heart in cattle is in a nearly upright position within the thorax, the puncta maxima are located on an almost horizontal line (**Fig. 64.1**). This line is located halfway between two horizontal lines crossing the elbow and the shoulder joint, respectively. As the heart undergoes a rotary motion around its vertical axis in the course of embryogenesis, the right side of the bovine heart is aligned in a cranial direction and the left side in a caudal one. For this reason, auscultation begins at the point of maximum intensity of the left **atrioventricular valve** (mitral valve), followed by auscultation of the **aortic and pulmonary valves**. The point of maximum intensity of the left pulmonary valve is sited approximately two fingers cranially from a point of intersection formed by the caudal edge of the anconeus muscle and the horizontal line mentioned above, whereas the punctum maximum of the pulmonary valve is found by moving the bell of the stethoscope over a horizontal line beneath the shoulder as far as possible in a cranial direction. The punctum maximum of the aortic valves is located halfway between these two puncta maxima. Auscultation on the right side starts at the point of maximum intensity of the **tricuspid valve**, which is located on the base line of the heart. The stethoscope is then moved as far as possible dorsally and cranially beneath the shoulder. [21]

The most common reason for **infection and inflammation of the pericardium (pericarditis)** in cattle is **traumatic reticulopericarditis**. Foreign bodies in the lumen of the reticulum perforate the reticular and diaphragmatic walls, and finally puncture and infect the pericardium and its cavity. Infection of the pericardial cavity results in accumulation of a fibrinopurulent exudate in the pericardial cavity, which leads to a restricted filling of the heart chambers. Progressive cardiac effusion results in the congestion of blood in the peripheral circulation causing edema and vessel distension, which is most obvious in the jugular vein and the vessels of the sclera. At auscultation, the heart sounds are hardly audible or even absent. Scratching sounds are related to fibrin plaques covering the surface of the pericardial lining. If gas-forming bacteria are present in the pericardial sac, even gurgling or burbling sounds (heart bruit) can be audible at auscultation.

Bacterial infections, mainly local infections of the claws or the mammary vein can spread through the circulation and cause metastatic infections of the cardiac valves (**valvular endocarditis, Fig. 64.2**) with the tricuspid valve being most commonly affected. Due to the endocarditic changes, the closure of the valve is hindered and incomplete (valve insufficiency). As a consequence, blood leaks back to the periphery during systole causing a pulsation of the jugular vein. As the internal thoracic vein forms a shortcut between the milk vein and the right atrium, this pulse can even be palpated in the mammary vein. From time to time, bacteria containing fibrin clots can become detached from the valves, which cause embolism of the fine vessel networks of the lung or the kidney leading to infarction and metastatic pneumonia or nephritis, respectively.

Pericardiocentesis (puncture of the pericardial cavity) is performed between the 5th and 7th intercostal space of the left thoracic wall to provide drainage of the pericardial cavity in order to prevent life-threatening cardiac tamponade. In cases of chronic suppurative pericarditis, attempts can be made to drain and lavage the pericardial cavity following resection of the 5th rib and its cartilage.

ABDOMINAL WALL AND ABDOMINAL CAVITY

K. Müller, R. Berg

66 The **hair coat** of healthy cattle covers most of the body and has a smooth and glossy appearance. The length and density of the hair coat differ depending on breed and climatic conditions. In summer, the hair coat is less dense and the hairs are shorter compared to the winter months.

Healthy **skin** is smooth and soft. If lifted from the underlying tissues, healthy skin, due to its elasticity, retracts immediately into its initial position. Changes in elasticity can be related to changes in mechanical characteristics of the skin. Loss of body water reduces skin elasticity and can lead to an increased amount of time that passes until a skin fold that is lifted on the upper eyelid or the side of the neck returns back to its initial position. Emaciation is associated with extreme loss of body fat and leads to a condition where the skin becomes tightly attached to the protruding parts of the body (e.g. spinous processes of the vertebrae, spine of the scapula, ribs).

Subcutaneous injections are administered at sites where a skin fold can easily be lifted, such as the skin on the lateral aspect of the neck, the neck and on the dewlap.

The **milk vein (subcutaneous abdominal vein, Fig. 66.1)** is prominent in dairy cows. Due to the fact that this vessel forms a shortcut to the right atrium, the milk vein reflects the alterations in pressure within the right atrium of the heart. Pulsation of the milk vein is most likely related to an endocarditis accompanied by leakage of blood from the right heart to the periphery due to an insufficiency of the tricuspid valve.

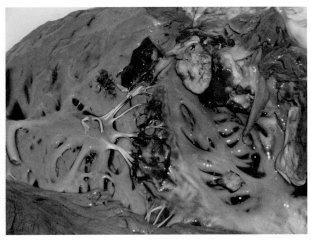

Fig. 64.2 Cauliflower-like plaques on the valves of the heart with endocarditis. (Courtesy of Ruminants and Swine Clinic, FU Berlin.)

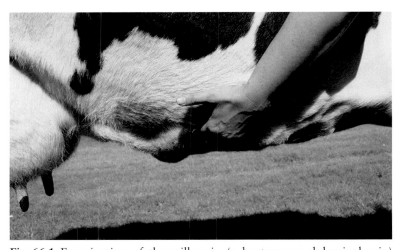

Fig 66.1 Examination of the milk vein (subcutaneous abdominal vein) checking for a pathological vein pulse. (Courtesy of Ruminants and Swine Clinic, FU Berlin.)

The **flank** is identical to the lateral abdominal region and includes those parts of the lateral body wall that do not have ribs, extending between the 13th rib, the tensor fasciae latae muscle and the tuber coxae. The flank includes the paralumbar fossa.

The **paralumbar fossa** is part of the flank and represents the most important part of the body for surgical approaches. It is located in the paralumbar abdominal region and has – from outside to inside – the following stratification (**Fig. 66.2**):

1st layer: cutis and subcutis

2nd layer: superficial layer (lamina superficialis) of the external fascia of the trunk and cutaneous trunci muscle

3rd layer: deep layer (lamina profunda) of the external fascia of the trunk

4th layer: external abdominal oblique muscle

5th layer: internal abdominal oblique muscle

6th layer: transversus abdominis muscle with iliohypogastric, ilioinguinal and genitofemoral nerves, deep ilium circumflex artery and vein.

7th layer: transversal fascia and parietal peritoneum.

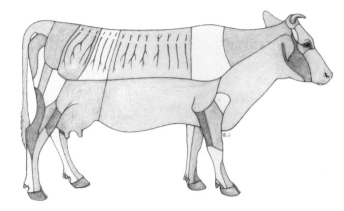

Fig. 66.3 Areas supplied by the thoracic and lumbar spinal nerves (labeled in different colors) which have to be considered for local anesthesia of the flank region.

Local anesthesia of the paralumbar fossa (flank anesthesia) is performed with the animal in a standing position. Four different approaches are commonly used (**Fig. 66.3**):

• Infiltration anesthesia (line block or inverted "L"-block anesthesia)
• Proximal paravertebral anesthesia
• Distal paravertebral anesthesia
• Segmental dorsolumbar epidural anesthesia

These procedures are suitable for abdominal surgery in the standing animal such as: rumenotomy, caecotomy, correction of conditions associated with dislocations of the abdominal organs, intestinal obstruction, volvulus, caesarian section, ovarectomy, liver biopsy, and renal biopsy.

Ad 1) Infiltration anesthesia

1a) Line Infiltration: The skin, muscle layers and parietal peritoneum are anesthetized by direct infiltration of the incision line with a local anesthetic.

1b) Inverted "L" nerve block: This technique provides anesthesia of an area located underneath and caudal to the lines of the "L"-block. The local anesthetic is injected along two lines, the first running in parallel to the edge of the last (=13th) rib and the second line running just below the transverse processes of the lumbar vertebrae extending from the last rib to the 4th lumbar vertebra (Inverted "L").

Ad 2) Proximal paravertebral anesthesia provides profound analgesia to the paralumbar fossa. It is the most suitable technique for celiotomy performed on the standing animal. The skin is punctured with a needle in a vertical direction between two spinal processus of the vertebra in a region located caudally from T13, L1 and L2 approximately 4 to 5 cm right or left of the midline of the animal. Subsequently, the needle is pushed forward along the cranial edges of the transverse processes of the lumbar vertebrae so that its end is located underneath the edge of the transverse process. By injection of a small volume of anesthetic beneath as well as just above the edge of the transverse processes, the dorsal and ventral roots of T13, L1 and L2 of the ipsilateral side are blocked. Including L3 in the anesthesia bears a risk of ataxia, which could interfere with surgery in the standing animal.

The injection sites are located on a line that runs 2.5 to 5 cm lateral to the midline. Thoracic nerve 13 is blocked just cranial to the transverse process of lumbar vertebrae 1 and 2. The first lumbar nerve is blocked just cranial to the transverse processes of L2 and the second lumbar nerve just cranial to L3. As this anesthesia induces a paralysis of the muscles of the back on one side, the back bends during surgery, which is sometimes disadvantageous for the surgeon.

Ad 3) Distal paravertebral anesthesia: This technique provides analgesia of the paralumbar fossa on the ipsilateral side. The dorsal and ventral branches of the lumbar nerves L1, L2 and L3 are blocked. The injection sites are at the lateral edges of the lumbar vertebrae L1, L2 and L4.

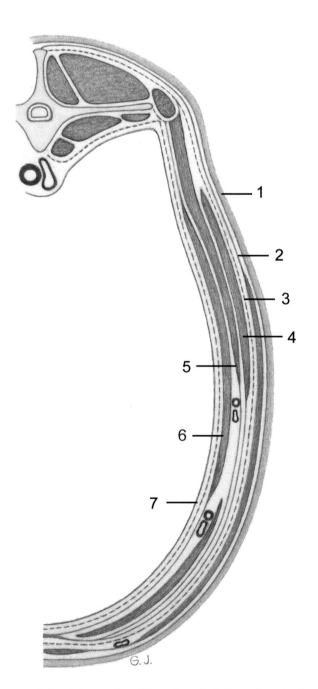

Fig 66.2 Layers of the abdominal wall (stratigraphy): (1) cutis and subcutis, (2) superficial fascia of the trunk and cutaneustrunci muscle, (3) deep fascia of the trunk, (4) external abdominal oblique muscle, (5) internal abdominal oblique muscle, (6) transversus abdominis muscle, (7) transversal fascia and parietal peritoneum.

Ad 4) Segmental dorsolumbar epidural anesthesia: This anesthesia is applied in the epidural space between L1 and L2 and results in analgesia of the flank on both sides of the midline. Depending on the dosage of the anesthetic, the 13th thoracic and the cranial lumbar nerves are blocked.

Epidural anesthesia (Fig. 66.5) is applied by inserting a needle into the epidural space either between the caudal end of the sacrum and the first vertebra of the tail or in the space between the first two vertebrae of the tail.

Cerebrospinal fluid (CSF) can be collected from the subarachnoidal space in the **lumbosacral space** with the animal either in a standing position or in sternal recumbency. The site for lumbar sampling is the depression that can be palpated between the spinous process of the last lumbar vertebra (L6) and the cranial end of the sacrum. A certain resistance can be felt when the needle passes the interarcuate ligament. As soon as the subarachnoidal space is penetrated, CSF will drain from the needle and can be aspirated into a syringe. [37]

The **stifle fold (flank fold)** is a fold formed by the skin and the superficial fascia of the trunk, which extends from the abdomen to the upper hind leg. It is suitable for subcutaneous injections. The stifle fold is located in the vicinity of the prefemoral lymph node. Grasping the fold and pulling it firmly upwards (stifle fold grip) restrains the animals and prevents it from moving and kicking.

Laparoscopy is the inspection of the organs within the abdominal and pelvic cavities using an endoscope. The endoscope is inserted transabdominally either from the right or the left paralumbar fossa with the animal in a standing position. If the animal is restrained in dorsal recumbency, the organs of the abdominal can also be inspected after insertion of the endoscope through the ventral abdominal wall.

Laparotomy is the opening of the abdominal cavity by surgical incision in the left or right paralumbar fossa or – with the animal in dorsal recumbency – in the ventral abdominal wall.

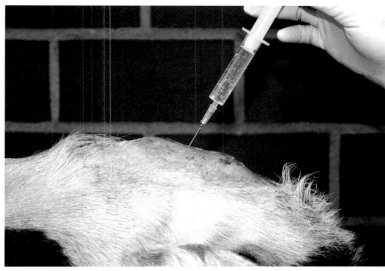

Fig. 66.5 Epidural anesthesia in the sacrococcygeal space. (Courtesy of Ruminants and Swine Clinic, FU Berlin.)

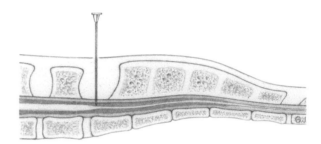

Fig. 66.6 Lumbar puncture in the lumbosacral space to collect cerebrospinal fluid (CSF).

Umbilical infections in the calf affect the umbilical cord and the umbilical vein in the region of the umbilical opening (umbilical ring). At the height of the umbilical ring, the two umbilical veins fuse to one vessel which finally enters the fetal liver. The paired umbilical arteries originate from the internal iliac arteries and run laterally along the urinary bladder to the umbilical opening and from there within the umbilical cord to the maternal placenta. The urachus which drains the fetal urine connects the bladder with the allantoic sac (**Fig. 66.4**). Infections of the umbilical structures within the abdominal cavity most often affect the umbilical vein and the urachus, less frequently the umbilical arteries. The latter phenomenon might be related to the fact that – following rupture of the umbilical cord – the umbilical arteries are retracted inside the abdomen, whereas the umbilical vein and the urachus remain in the umbilical ring where they are exposed to bacterial contamination and infection.

68 **Gastric and intestinal obstructions** as well as space-occupying masses and fluid accumulation within the abdominal cavity will cause a distended abdomen. Depending on the kind of disease, the abdomen has a characteristic outline when viewed from the back. In cases of unilateral distension of the left flank (tympany) or bilateral distension (obstructions of the small intestines) the outline resembles the shape of an apple. In cases of vagal indigestion or anterior stenosis it resembles the form of an apple in the left flank and that of a pear in the right flank (papple form). In cases of ascites, hydramnion and hydrallantois, the abdominal outline resembles a pear (**Fig. 68**).

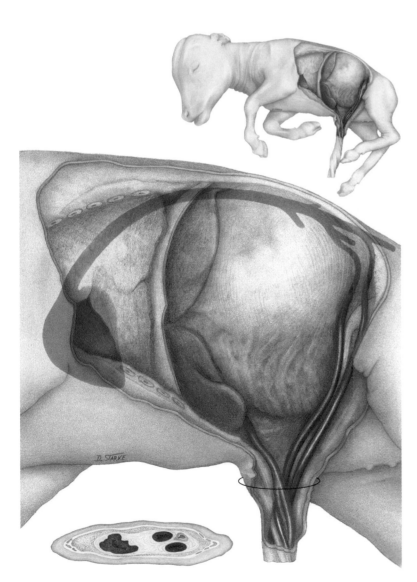

Fig. 66.4 Course of the umbilical vessels and the urachus in the fetus. The cross section of a umbilical cord close to the umbilical opening (ring) shows the structures that a visible during ultrasound examination ("smiley").

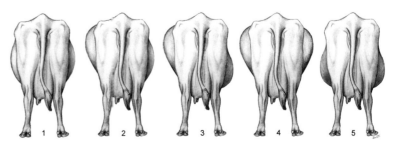

Fig. 68 Shape (outline) of the abdomen (apple or pear shape) in cases of gastrointestinal obstruction and space-occupying processes in the abdominal cavity. (1) normal, (2) left apple, (3) papple – left apple and right pear (see also Fig. 72), (4) bilateral apple, (5) bilateral pear.

Rehydration fluids and other therapeutics are injected into the abdomen (**intra-abdominal injection**) preferably by inserting a cannula through the right flank approximately 8–10 cm below the transverse processes of the lumbar vertebrae.

Abdominocentesis is performed in order to obtain peritoneal fluid for laboratory analysis or to drain excessive fluid from the abdominal cavity. The preferential site for abdominocentesis is at the lowest part of the abdominal wall right in the ventral midline.

70 A **rumenotomy** is performed following left flank laparatomy to remove foreign bodies from the reticulum of cattle suffering from traumatic reticuloperitonitis. Furthermore, toxic plants that have recently been ingested by the animal and coarse plants causing ruminal impaction can be removed by rumenotomy. **Transruminal exploration.** Following rumenotomy, the ruminal contents are removed from the proventricular compartments in order to facilitate transruminal exploration of the organs that lie in close contact to the rumen. The diaphragm, liver, spleen, omasum and abomasum can be palpated from the lumen of the reticuloruminal compartment.

If it is impossible to remove gas from the reticulorumen of a bloated animal via a nasogastric tube, the animal is at risk of dying from suffocation. In such cases the rumen is **trocarized** in the paralumbal fossa of the left flank. A permanent trocar is inserted at the same site in calves suffering from recurrent bloat.

Rumenotomy is performed on animals suffering from recurrent bloat (chronic tympany). It is also used in feeding trials when a permanent **ruminal fistula** is created. Various fistulas and fistulation techniques are available. The most feasible one is the technique in which the ruminal wall is exteriorized and sutured to the skin with part of the ruminal wall being removed. The fistula opening is covered with a plastic or rubber belt.

Traumatic reticulitis is a disease caused by sharp foreign bodies that have been ingested and have perforated the reticulum and caused an inflammation. A **reticuloperitonitis** (hardware disease) is caused by a sharp foreign body that has perforated all layers of the reticulum and subsequently infected the peritoneal cavity. This disease mainly affects adult cattle due to their different manner of feed uptake compared to young animals. Foreign bodies such as nails and pieces of wire get into the food at harvesting or during processing. They are ingested, reach the proventriuclar compartment and sink to the floor of the reticulum. The characteristic contraction pattern of the reticulum subsequently forces the foreign bodies through the reticular wall at certain predilection sites. Depending on the site of perforation, they can penetrate the liver, the diaphragm, the parietal pleura or the pericardium causing liver abscessation, peritonitis and pleuritis as well as reticulopericarditis. The resulting adhesions between the reticulum and the peritoneum are associated with disturbances in the contraction cycles of the proventricular compartment. If the disease is recognized and treated in an initial stage by the oral administration of a **rumen magnet with plastic cage**, the prognosis is fair (**Abb. 70.1**). [15]

In dairy calves and veal calves, disturbances in the gastric groove reflex give rise to the phenomenon of "ruminal drinking". If the gastric groove reflex does not function properly, the milk will enter the rumen, where it undergoes bacterial fermentation. Calves suffering from "ruminal drinking" exhibit stunted growth and recurrent bloat. The animals produce putty-like feces. "Ruminal drinking" will cause splashing sounds in the rumen while the calf is drinking from a bucket or a bottle, which are audible at auscultation of the left flank. The disorder is observed sporadically in calves suffering from severe disease and in herds in which the milk feeding does not function properly, which includes offering the calves large volumes of milk, errors in the preparation of the milk replacer (such as wrong temperature or concentrations) as well as irregular feeding intervals. [14]

Ancillary diagnostic procedures for rumen fermentation disorders include the sampling and analysis of **ruminal fluid**. Ruminal fluid is obtained using a flexible rumen sampling device made of metal that is inserted through the mouth and then pushed down the esophagus into the rumen. Alternatively, ruminal fluid can be obtained by puncture of the ventral blind sac using a hypodermic needle and a syringe. The sampling site for the ventral blind sac of the rumen is located in the left lower flank on a line drawn between the cartilaginous-bone border of the last rib and the left stifle. Sampling by puncture bears a certain risk of peritonitis. [25]

Omasal impaction, also referred to as psalter paresis, may occur sporadically in cattle. The disorder is thought to be caused by feeding chopped roughage of poor quality (primary omasal impaction). In addition, the disease may occur as a secondary complication during the course of any severe disease, mainly of the digestive tract, that is associated with vagal dysfunction (secondary omasal impaction). Animals suffering from omasal impaction are anorectic and show colic symptoms. In most cases, this disorder is diagnosed at diagnostic laparotomy. [40]

The most common disorder of the abomasum is **abomasal displacement** either to the left or the right side. This disease mainly occurs in adult dairy cows in the period around calving. Accumulation of gas in the **abomasal fundus** plays a major role in the pathogenesis of the disease. This part of the abomasum is fitted with weak muscle layers and gas accumulates in the dome-shaped part of the fundus region in cases of abomasal wall atony. This is a prerequisite for the subsequent displacement of the abomasum. Furthermore, the loose fixation of the abomasum within the abdominal cavity facilitates displacement of the stomach. During pregnancy – due to the increasing volume of the uterus – the abomasum is forced cranially

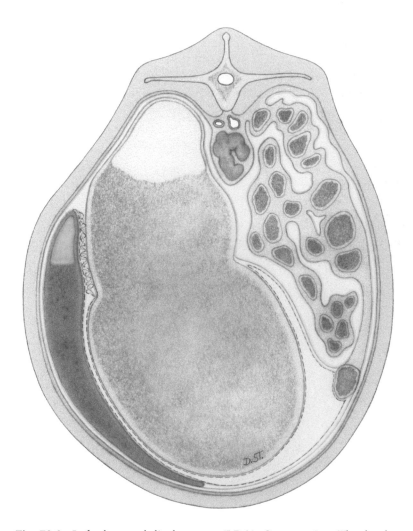

Fig, 70.2a Left abomasal displacement (LDA). Cross section. The duodenum has been pulled ventrally, the superficial sheet of the greater omentum lies ruffled up between the left longitudinal groove of the rumen and the inflated abomasum.

Fig. 70.1 Cage magnet with adherent foreign bodies. (Courtesy of Ruminants and Swine Clinic, FU Berlin.)

to a region right from the ventral midline. As the volume of the uterus decreases after calving, the abomasum shifts back into its normal position situated on the ventral body wall with its larger part lying left of the midline. The abomasum crosses the midline in an area between the end of the xyphoid and the umbilicus, and ends with the pylorus which is located near the right body wall at the height of the bone-cartilage junction of the last rib. Abomasal displacement is frequently observed in the peripartal period when dairy cows suffer from pain and diseases which interfere with feed intake and gastrointestinal motility, such as hypocalcemia, ketosis and endotoxemia.

Left-sided abomasal displacement (LDA; Fig. 70.2 a+b) is characterized by dislocation of the U-shaped abomasum, which is filled with gas and fluid, to a space underneath the ruminal atrium from where it subsequently ascends like a balloon between the left body wall and the rumen. Right-sided abomasal displacement (RDA) is characterized by a dislocation of the abomasum to the right body wall, where it lies between the right body wall and the intestines. At clinical examination, abomasal displacement can be identified by a characteristic sound in the right or left flank, which is triggered by percussion during simultaneous auscultation of the flank. As this "ping" sounds like a steel drum from Trinidad, it is also termed "steelband effect". Depending on the grade of dislocation, the sound is audible at different heights on a line that runs between the elbow and the tuber coxae. Right abomasal displacement is frequently associated with a movement of the organ around two different axes (**flexion-rotation; Fig. 70.3**). In these cases, the abomasum bends around a longitudinal axis of the animal (**flexion**), followed by a rotation around a vertical axis (**rotation**). The pyloric part shifts in a counter-clockwise fashion cranially in a way that the two sides of the U-shaped abomasum are twisted together. This causes a strangulation and obstruction of the abomasum. Such strangulations sporadically also include the omasum and the reticulum (**abomasal volvulus**). Depending on the degree of strangulation, the passage of ingesta from the abomasum to the duodenum is impaired or even totally blocked causing a reflux of abomasal contents into the rumen. The consequences of abomasal volvulus are severe disruptions of perfusion of the strangulated organs as well as severe disturbances in electrolyte and hydration status of the animal. These complications explain the fatal outcome in a large number of cases. The aim of all the approaches for the treatment of abomasal displacement is the permanent fixation of the abomasum in its normal position. The Hannover method according to Dirksen for the surgical treatment of RDA or LDA includes right flank laparotomy and omentopexy in the right flank so that the pylorus is fixated as far as possible in its normal position. The pylorus can be identified in the outer sheet of the omentum by its grey-bluish color and the typical texture.

72 Disorders associated either with impaired transport of ingesta from the **reticulorumen** to the omasum or from the **pylorus** into the duodenum, which do not originate from mechanical causes are termed **anterior functional stenosis (Hoflund Syndrome)** and **posterior functional stenosis**, respectively. Hoflund was able to reproduce the latter symptoms experimentally by transecting the vagus

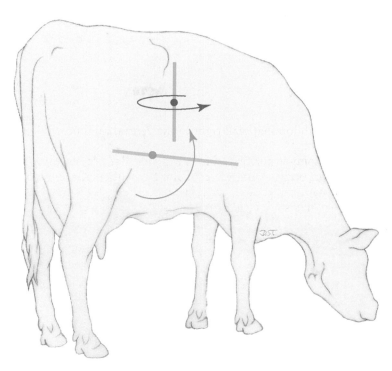

Fig. 70.3 Axes of rotation of the abomasum in right abomasal displacement (RDA) with a flexion-rotation.

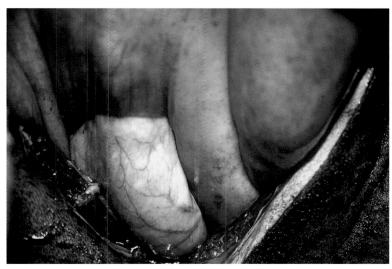

Fig. 70.4 Abomasal surgery. View in a right flank laparotomy. The pyloric region can be identified by its bluish-grey color. (Courtesy of Ruminants and Swine Clinic, FU Berlin.)

nerve at different sites. Neurectomy of the vagus at the level of the esophagus resulted in complete atony of all forestomach compartments and of the abomasum. Transection of the ventral branch of the vagal nerve at its insertion site at the reticuloomasal ostium resulted in anterior functional stenosis, whereas dissection of the ventral branch which innervates the pylorus caused a posterior functional stenosis. Impaired transport of ingesta at the reticuloomasal ostium or the pylorus results in abomasal reflux to the rumen, which subsequently becomes distended. Due to the latter alterations, the outline of the abdomen resembles an apple on the left side and a pear on the right side ("**papple**" form, Fig. 72). Only in a few cases have functional stenoses in patients been shown to originate from direct trauma to the vagal nerve. In those cases, either lesions caused by a penetrating foreign body were found at necropsy, or space-occupying masses (abscess, neoplasia) where observed in direct vicinity to the vagal nerve. The vagus contains a ratio of sensory nerve fibers to motor nerve fibers of 9 to 1. Thus, the current hypothesis concerning functional stenosis relies on the assumption that besides direct damage to the vagal nerve, disturbances in rumen function originate from afferent signals elicited in inflamed sites of the reticular wall as a consequence of foreign body disease. Interestingly, the preferential site for lesions in the reticular wall is located in an area with high receptor density. The afferent signals from the inflammatory site result in a transduction of "faulty" efferent signals from the medulla oblongata to the periphery, which subsequently cause disturbances in the fine-tuned contraction cycles of the rumen. [23] [26] [35]

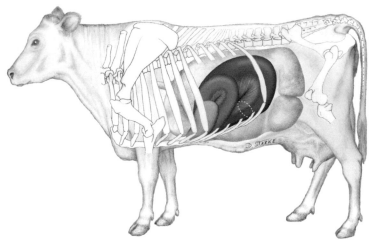

Fig. 70.2b Left abomasal displacement (LDA), lateral view. This figure shows three possible states of displacement. Dashed line = Position of the pylorus.

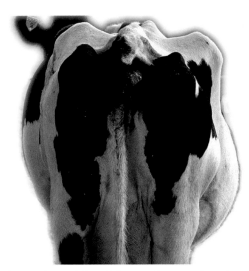

Fig. 72 "Papple" outline of the abdomen due to a functional stenosis. See also Fig. 68. (Courtesy of Ruminants and Swine Clinic, FU Berlin.)

Enlargement of the **right caudal ruminal lymph node** that is accessible to palpation on rectal examination is a highly specific and sensitive indicator for reticuloperitonitis. [46]

Abomasal ulcers occur in animals of all ages. In calves, abomasal ulcers are most often located in the pyloric region, whereas in adult cattle they are observed in the **body of the abomasum.** Perforating (grade IV) ulcers preferentially drain into the omental bursa causing a purulent infection (omental bursitis).

74 The obliterated **umbilical vein (umbilical ligament)** runs within the falciform ligament of the liver from the liver to the umbilicus. The ligament could impair attempts to replace the displaced abomasum in cases of displacement to the right. Occasionally, jejunal loops are strangulated by the ligament, leading to colic symptoms and ileus.

The greatest part of the **liver** in cattle is not accessible to clinical examination. The percussion field of the liver directly adjoins the caudal edge of the percussion field of the lung and approximately extents over two ribs and one intercostal space. **Liver biopsies** are obtained for the determination of the liver fat content in periparturient dairy cows or for the evaluation of the trace element status as well as for diagnostics in cases of suspected heavy metal intoxication. A liver biopsy is performed in the right flank in the 11th or 12th intercostal space, a hand width ventral to the longissimus dorsi muscle. The appropriate site for the biopsy can be identified by percussing the area of dullness caused by the liver beneath the body wall. The skin above the 11th intercostal space is shaven approximately 8–10 cm underneath the transverse vertebral processes. Following local anesthesia and a stab incision, a biopsy needle is inserted aimed at the contralateral elbow and the biopsy specimen is obtained. Liver percussion will help in detecting the optimal site for sampling (**Fig. 76**). [47]

76 Occasionally, a functional stenosis is observed at the sigmoid curve of the duodenum at diagnostic laparotomy in cattle with colic symptoms. In such cases, the **proximal part of the duodenum** is dilated and overloaded whereas the remainder of the duodenum is empty and shows normal motility. The impaired transport function of the proximal duodenum causes distension of the abomasum and abomasal reflux. [49]

Intussusception is a displacement of the intestines, which is characterized by invagination of one part of the intestine (intussuscipiens) into its adjacent segment (intussuscept), giving the intestine a telescope-like appearance. In cattle, most intussusceptions are observed in the jejunum; a predisposition site is the transition between the jejunum and ileum. Only sporadically does the cecum invaginate into either the colon or the jejunum. The prerequisites for intussusceptions are local disturbances of intestinal motility (e.g. parasitic infections or local inflammatory processes). If the intussusception is within the reach of the arm at rectal examination, a firm mass formed like a "snails shell" can be palpated. [14]

Intestinal **volvulus** is an abnormal twisting of the intestine causing obstruction. Besides affecting the abomasum and the cecum, this condition particularly affects the intestinal loops which are mobile due to their long mesentery. This is especially true for the jejunum in cattle.

Remnants of the umbilical vessels and a patent urachus or newly formed bridges of connective tissue on opposing organs in the course of chronic peritonitis bear a risk of causing strangulation of intestinal loops. Furthermore, rents or preformed openings of the abdominal wall, the mesentery or the **broad ligament of the uterus** can lead to herniation of abdominal organs. There have been individual reports of obstructions of the small intestines by phyto- or trichobezoars and foreign bodies in cattle.

Cecal dilatation and volvulus are mainly observed in adult cattle. The disease evolves from an accumulation of intestinal contents in the cecum and the curved proximal part of the colon due to intestinal atony in the course of gastrointestinal disorders. The distension of the cecum is diagnosed by rectal palpation of the gas-filled cecum in the pelvic cavity, which can be recognized by its characteristic blind end (**cecal apex**). In cecal volvulus, the cecum and the ansa proximalis of the colon are extremely extended and make a clockwise or counterclockwise movement resembling a corkscrew. In the latter disorder, the passage of feces is impaired or absent. [18]

A dramatic strangulating disease of the gastrointestinal tract in the bovine is the **torsion of the mesenteric root.** The complete intestinal convolute is twisted around the mesenteric root with the **cranial mesenteric artery** in its centre. The associated impairment of the venous and lymphatic drainage results in severe edema of the mesenteric root. At rectal palpation, the abdominal cavity is filled with distended intestinal loops of small and large calibers. [42]

At an early stage of **Johne's disease (paratuberculosis)** the causal agent *Mycobacterium paratuberculosis* colonizes the **colonic lymph nodes.** The clinical disease, however, is not observed until the animals have reached an age of at least three to four years.

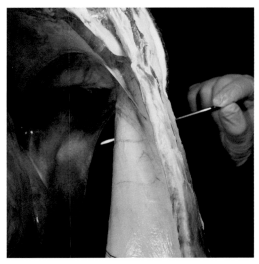

Fig. 74 Liver biopsy: Position of the biopsy needle in the 11th intercostal space on the right side (anatomical specimen). (Courtesy of Ruminants and Swine Clinic, FU Berlin.)

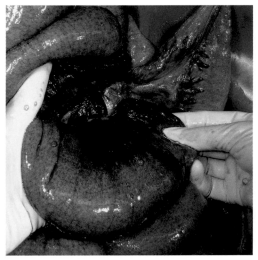

Fig. 76.1 Invagination of the jejunum. The index finger of the right hand is positioned within the invaginated fold of the intestine lying between the intussuscepted and intussuscepting segment of the intestine. (Courtesy of Ruminants and Swine Clinic, FU Berlin.)

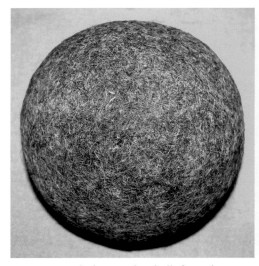

Fig. 76.2 Trichobezoar (hairball) from the stomach of a calf. (Courtesy of Ruminants and Swine Clinic, FU Berlin.)

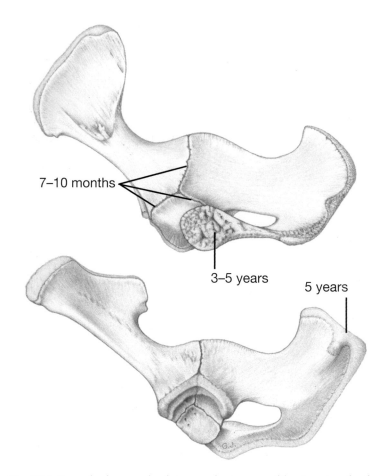

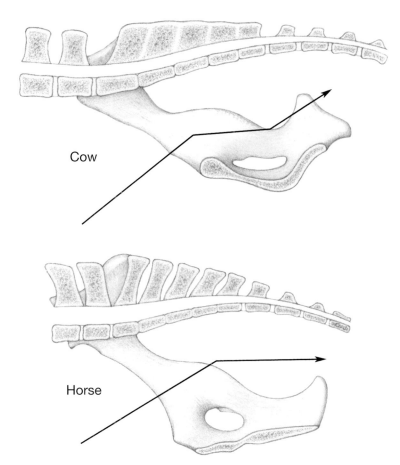

Cow

Horse

Fig. 78.1 Growth plates and pelvic symphysis as predilection sites for fractures (the ages refer to the time of closure of the growth plates).

7–10 months

3–5 years

5 years

Fig. 78.2 Guiding line for delivery of the fetus through the pelvic cavity. The birth canal has 2–3 bends in direction in the cow (complex), whereas it forms a continuous curve in the horse (optimal).

PELVIC CAVITY AND PUDENDUM

P. S. GLATZEL

78 **Fractures of the pelvis** normally occur along the **growth plates** of the affected bones (**Fig. 78.1**). With evulsion fractures of the bony protuberances recognizable under the skin (i.e. the **tuber coxae or ischial tuber**), an obvious asymmetry of the two sides of the animal can be seen. Pelvic fractures or **pubic symphysis separation** occurring as a consequence of incorrect obstetrical assistance, especially in heifers (use of so-called mechanical calving aids) are associated with typical **changes in gait and often downer cow syndrome**. The tentative diagnosis of such conditions can be confirmed by transrectal examination.

The **floor of the pelvis** has a concave structure, which provides a great deal of problems for the **birth canal** and therefore for parturi-

tion. This concavity results in the **axis of the pelvis** being divided into three separate sections (**Fig. 78.2**), resulting in a particularly long calving process in cattle, which can last up to 12 hours.

The caudal edge of the **sacrosciatic ligament** can be used for clinical recognition of estrogen dominance. Phytoestrogen-containing feed (such as young clover, etc.) or contaminated bedding and cystic ovaries (**Fig. 78.3**) can induce an obvious relaxation of this ligament, which can then lead to the development of an **elevated tailhead** (**Fig. 78.4**). During **estrus**, the relaxation of the ligaments in cattle under breeding conditions is indistinct and can only be recognized as sign of estrus by experienced milkers.

Physiologically, the **approaching birth** in the last trimester of pregnancy is characterized by increasing estrogen production. This is expressed in the development of edema of the connective tissue and ligaments (**Fig. 78.5**). The cow is conspicuous due to its uncertain gait, difficulties in getting up, as well as edema and changes in the udder. In addition, there is **relaxation of the pelvic ligaments**. In

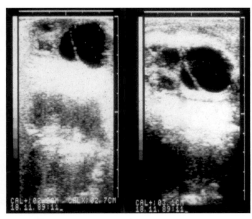

Fig. 78.3 Sonograms showing cystic ovaries. (Courtesy of Prof. P. Glatzel.)

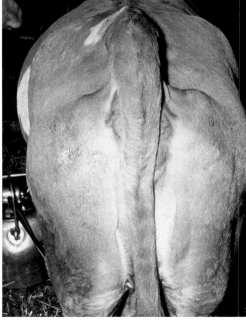

Fig. 78.4 Elevation of the tail due to the effect of extreme estrogen levels. (Courtesy of Prof. P. Glatzel.)

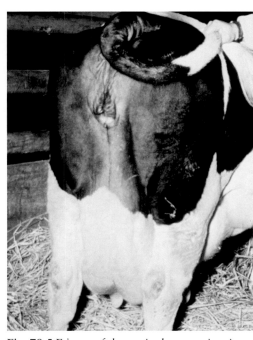

Fig. 78.5 Edema of the vaginal connective tissue due to increasing estrogen secretion. (Courtesy of Prof. P. Glatzel.)

149

practice, the resulting bending over of the tail tuft with the end of the tail being held vertically is a sign of impending birth. Due to this relaxation, improper obstetrical assistance can easily lead to crushing, overextension and tearing of the affected joints or ligaments and so to permanent damage.

80 In bulls, the **processus vaginalis peritonei** (Nuck's diverticulum) is developed during the descent of the testes. This double outgrowth of the peritoneum can lead to the escape of peritoneal contents (usually intestinal loops) and the development of an **inguinal hernia** when the opening of the diverticulum and the **inguinal canal** are too large. Other diseases can arise due to the loss of fluid into the diverticulum from the abdomen, which is known as a **hydrocele** with watery contents and a **hematocele** with bloody ones. Both sides of the scrotum are affected in these conditions. The scrotum is obviously swollen but without any signs of inflammation. Immediate clarity concerning the genesis of such swelling can be achieved by the careful palpation of the inguinal region with displacement of the individual testes, the **rectal examination of the abdominal inguinal ring** and finally, the **ultrasonography** of the scrotum including its contents.

Care must be taken when doing **bloodless castration** using a Burdizzo forceps in bull calves for **bullock rearing** that all the structures within the diverticulum, especially the spermatic cord with its supply vessels, are crushed so that both **sperm production and transportation** are permanently prevented.

Sterilization to prevent just the transport of sperm while retaining the animal's sexual function is used for **fattening bulls** or for the preparation of a **teaser bull**. The diverticulum is opened and the spermatic cord is closed using two ligatures close to the body of the epididymis. The section between the ligatures is either removed or left in place. A more simple method is the **resection of the tail of the epididymis**. After opening Nuck's diverticulum in the distal scrotum, the prominently offset tails of the epididymis are constricted using two clips turned in opposite directions to each other.

The **cremaster muscle** is partially responsible for testicular movement in bulls (raise, lower) and so for the **thermoregulation of testicular temperature**. This is absolutely essential for undisturbed **spermatogenesis**, which can only be achieved at a temperature 2–3 °C below the core body temperature. With high ambient temperatures, the muscle relaxes and the testes are dropped low into the scrotum so that air can circulate around the sack and cool its contents. If it is cold or if the temperature is above the animal's body temperature (tropics), then the cremaster muscles contract and the testicles are drawn towards the body wall.

The **external spermatic fascia** is also involved in testicular thermoregulation together with the scrotal skin. The external spermatic fascia is fused with the **modified subcutis (Tunica dartos)** on the inner side of the scrotal wall, which in turn is firmly attached to the dermis. To aid in thermoregulation, contraction of the smooth muscles of the dartos fascia raises the testes towards the body wall or they are lowered when the muscle fibers relax. During opening of the scrotum (e.g. during castration), the fused fasciocutaneous layers of the skin should be cut with scissors.

The **caudal preputial muscle** develops from the **external spermatic fascia**. This muscle aids in the shortening of the **preputial sheath** during **erection of the penis** or **micturition**. The branches of this muscle must be protected as much as possible during **surgical displacement of the penis**. This complex operation is preferentially used in ruminants for the preparation of **teaser bulls or rams**. The advantages of this operation mainly outweigh the disadvantages as the animal's sexual function is maintained with full libido, while complete **coitus** (vaginal introitus) is prevented; this means that in contrast to vasectomy the transmission of genital disease is prevented.

URINARY TRACT

K. Müller, R. Berg

82 **Cysto-uretro-pyelonephritis** in cattle is characterized by a usually unilateral inflammation of the pelvis of the kidney (**renal calices** in cattle) and the urine conducting system. The condition is referred to as inflammation of the pelvis of the kidney even though the kidney in cattle has individual calices and not a fused pelvis. Parts of the kidney and the **renal calices** ("pelvis") in particular become necrotic (melt down) and have a fluctuating consistency under transrectal palpation.

In cases of amyloid nephrosis, pathologically altered protein compounds are deposited in the kidney. These deposits stain blue with iodine solution (**amyloidosis**). The kidneys are enlarged, and one can hardly differentiate the individual lobules.

Puncture of the urinary bladder: A urinary bladder which contains only very little urine can be punctured through the rectum. If the bladder is moderately filled, puncture can be performed through the ventral abdominal wall.

Reposition of a prolapsed urinary bladder: The urinary bladder may prolapse through the urethra in cases of a prolapse of the rectum, vagina or uterus. Under epidural anesthesia, one attempts to stretch and widen the urethra with an index finger. The prolapsed wall of the bladder is repositioned by pushing it through the urethra starting in the region of the external urethral opening.

Collection of urine (urine sampling) in cattle is difficult because of the suburethral diverticulum as the catheter easily slides into the blind ending diverticulum first of all when introduced into the vaginal vestibule.

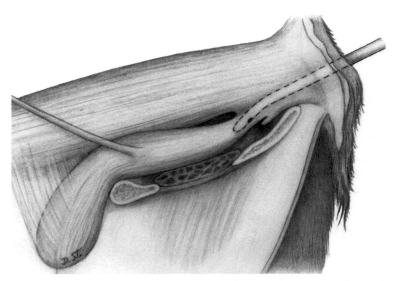

Fig. 82 Collection of urine with a catheter showing the position of the suburethral diverticulum.

FEMALE REPRODUCTIVE TRACT

P. S. Glatzel

86 **Endocrine control of reproduction by the CNS**
The **central nervous system (CNS)** is a crucial center for the **endocrine control** of metabolic processes. Through stimulation of the sensory system, psychological experiences or internal processes within the body, specific reactions are induced in the brain. With respect to the reproductive processes, information is sent neurally either directly or indirectly from the cortex – via the limbic system – to the structures of the diencephalon and from there to the endocrine centers of the **hypothalamus**. In these centers, specific releasing hormones (oligopeptides) are formed, which are transferred to the hypophysis with the blood flowing in the hypophyseal portal circulation. In the **adenohypophysis** (anterior pituitary), these hormones stimulate the production and release of proteohormones (glycoproteins such as ACTH, FSH, LH, STH, and TSH). These hormones reach their target **endocrine organs** via the blood (e.g. adrenals, ovaries, testes, and thyroid). This type of hormonal information achieves its effects by stimulating the peripheral glands via specific receptors. In their target glands, such proteohormones stimulate the production and release of specific hormones mainly **steroid hormones** (estrogen, testosterone, progesterone, cortisone,

etc.). These steroid hormones when released in the blood induce specific effects in their **target organs** (e.g. muscles, bones, vagina, uterus, ovarian or testicular parenchyma); for example, mucous secretion or retention, production of germ cells (eggs, sperm) or muscle development as well as the synthesis and release of tissue hormones such as prostaglandins or serotonin. In addition to this, the steroid hormones have a **feedback** effect on the CNS and subsequently initiate specific behavioral patterns, such as heat or rutting behavior, or the facilitation or inhibition of the release of the releasing hormones. This effect, therefore, closes the **hormonal autoregulation feedback control system** (Fig. 86.1A).

A special role is played in this system by the **pineal gland**, known also as the **epiphysis** or "third eye". This gland reacts specifically to light stimuli coming from the **retina**, with the release of catecholamines, in particular **melatonin**. The gland is, therefore, directly involved in the animal's biorhythms: its circadian and diurnal vital functions such as seasonality of sexual function or day-night rhythms of the metabolism or sleep-wake behavior (**Fig. 86.1B**).

The **neurohypophysis** or caudal lobe of the hypophysis is another important endocrine structure. In this lobe, the formation of **oxytocin**, an octapeptide, is stimulated by **direct neural information** and released in the blood. Oxytocin is important for the stimulation of milk let-down and the uterine contractions during birth.

The **adrenals** are also vitally important endocrine glands. Their hormones have a fundamental significance for the metabolism, **sexual** function and the sympathetic nervous system. They are subdivided into hormones of the adrenal cortex (mineralocorticoids, glucocorticoids and androcorticoids) and the adrenal medulla (adrenaline and noradrenaline). For further information see biochemistry textbooks.

The **uterine artery,** lying lateral to the body of the uterus in the broad uterine ligament, is easily palpable from the 8th–10th week after conception during a transrectal examination (*see page 158*). In particular, the so-called **uterine thrill**, which is triggered by a light compression of the well-filled artery, can be considered an indirect indication of pregnancy. This blood vessel is inconspicuous in the non-pregnant uterus.

A clinical examination of the **female reproductive tract** is divided into the **inspection** and **palpation** of the external genitalia (pudendum and surroundings). This is followed by an inspection of the vagina up to the external cervix with the aid of a speculum. The examination is finished with the **transrectal palpation** of the uterus and ovaries, including the mesentery. All the results should be recorded with the aid of a specific abridged code (comparison to the size of different fruits, nuts, and bird eggs, hand measurements such as thumb width or general instruments and colors). For further elucidation and documentation, **ultrasonographic examinations** and **quick hormonal analyses** can be done in the stall.

The ovaries are palpated to check more exactly the state of the **estrous cycle**. During the **transrectal palpation**, the ovaries can be felt as bean- to walnut-sized (during disease they can reach fist-sized) structures on the left or right outer edge of the non-pregnant uterus which is collected in the hand and pushed gently into the pelvic cavity. To palpate the ovaries, the investigator's hand should

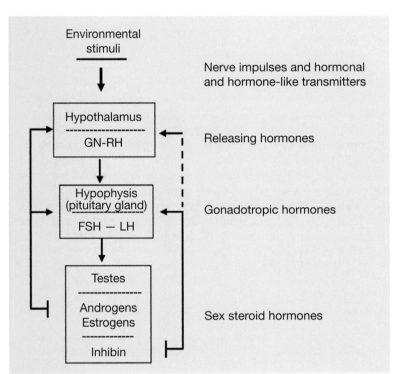

Fig. 86.1A Feedback regulation of hormones (bull).

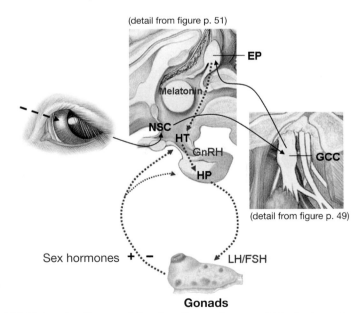

Fig. 86.1B Light stimuli control the circadian and seasonal biorhythms via the epiphysis (pineal gland). NSC Suprachiasmatic nucleus, GCC Cranial cervical ganglion, EP Epiphysis, HT Hypothalamus, HP Hypophysis. Black, continuous arrows = neuronal pathways; red, dashed arrows = hormonal influence.

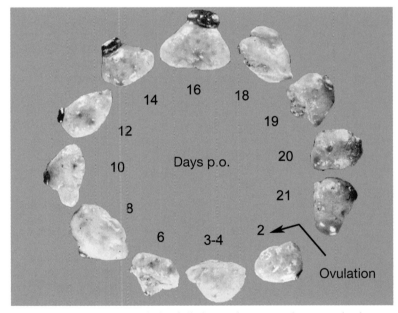

Fig. 86.2 Development of the follicles and corpora lutea in the bovine ovary during the estrous cycle. (Courtesy of Prof. P. Glatzel.)

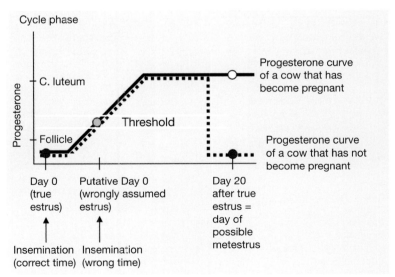

Fig. 86.3 Diagram showing a schematic progesterone profile in the milk during the estrous cycle (produced with a practicable quick test used in the stall; visual assessment can be done within 15–20 minutes; see Fig. 86.4). The threshold value (continuous line) between the progesterone phase (active C. luteum) and the follicle phase lies at 2–3 ng progesterone/ml milk (Homonost Easy Test, Biolab GmbH Munich, Germany).

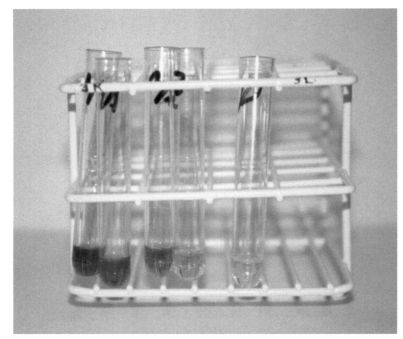

Fig. 86.4 Semi-quantitative quick test (Homonost Easy Test, Biolab GmbH Munich, Germany; see Fig. 86.3): dark blue = no progesterone; medium blue = threshold value, C. luteum either developing or regressing; colorless or only faintly blue = fully developed C. luteum. (Courtesy of Prof. P. Glatzel.)

glide over the greater curvature of the uterus and move either left or right to the tip of the rolled-up uterine horn, where the ovaries can be readily felt. Depending on the stage of the cycle, the uterus can be easily felt as a sensitive (exhibiting spontaneous contractions), firm, finger- to thumb-thick structure during estrus (estrogen influence) and a less definite, slack and less sensitive structure in the interestrus phase (progesterone influence).

The state of **ovarian function** is recognizable by the presence of either mature ova in the cyclically formed **follicles** or the **corpora lutea** which are formed from the follicle wall after ovulation. The estrous cycle is the time between two successive ovulations and lasts for ca. 21 ± 2 days. This cycle is divided according to the external physical appearance of the cow into estrus (heat), metestrus, diestrus (no sexual behavior), proestrus and then again estrus. The follicles or corpora lutea can be palpated transrectally or seen on ultrasonography and these structures are used to classify the stage

of the cycle according to this classification. The largest follicles occurring during proestrus are ca. 0.5 cm in diameter (pea-sized). During estrus, mature vesicular (Graafian) follicles are present (ca. 1–2 cm, cherry-sized). There are no palpable structures present during metestrus, while corpora lutea (diameter 0.5 to ca. 1.5 cm) develop in the diestrus (**Fig. 86.2**).

In addition, the **sex hormones** produced by each of these structures are dominant and measurable during the various phases of the cycle: estrogen [its precursor (androgen) is produced by the ovarian theca interna cells and this is then aromatized by the epithelial cells in the follicle] and **progesterone** (formed by the corpus luteum; **Fig. 86.3**). This knowledge is of great importance for clinical **diagnosis** and **therapy**, as well as the **strategic intervention in the estrous cycle**. The clearly interpretable **progesterone profile** can be used as it dominates almost 3/4 of the cycle. With **quick tests** for this steroid hormone in the milk, clinical results or causes of the patient's problems can be **quickly** and **objectively** interpreted. Additionally, the **time for insemination** or the **absence of pregnancy** can be determined; e.g. by using enzyme immunoassay (EIA). One such test, the Hormonost easy Test (Biolab GmbH, Munich, Germany) gives the progesterone values in various shades of blue (**Fig. 86.4**). The threshold value of 3–5 ng progesterone/ml milk indicates the presence of the transitional period between the estrogen-dominated follicular phase to the progesterone-dominated luteal phase. Such tests have become even more valuable since it has been known that **prostaglandin F2-alpha** can initiate **luteolysis** at any time, thereby allowing control of the cycle. This makes a **calendrically planned** and **genetically selective mating** in association with artificial insemination possible. This knowledge is also important for other biotechnical methods such as **embryo transfer (ET)**.

Another prerequisite for such methods and **in-vitro fertilization** (including **cloning**) is knowledge about the above-mentioned cyclic processes in the ovaries as well as the associated **follicular dynamics**, which run as an integrated **biocybernetic regulation system**. This includes the phases during which the **follicles are formed** and the **eggs mature** and the associated hormones show their effects. Generally in cattle, there are **two waves of follicle formation** during a single cycle. At the start of the first wave is the so-called **recruitment phase** (activation of inactive primordial follicles). This is followed by the **growth phase** of the secondary follicles and the **selection phase of the dominant follicles**, then the **dominance and plateau phase** and finally, the **regression or atretic phase**. The **second wave** of follicular development that starts during the selection phase of the first wave begins around the 5th–7th day of the cycle. It does not end with follicular atresia but with an **ovulation phase**. In

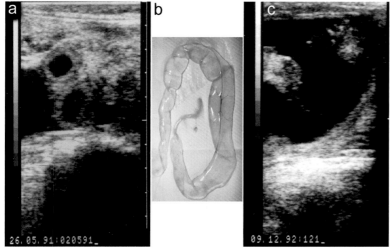

Fig. 86.5a–c
a Sonogram of an early pregnancy in a cow (26 days after conception). The lumina uterine horns are visible as anechogenic (dark) round areas in the transverse section. They contrast with the echo-rich (white) wall of the uterine horn that surrounds them. The ovaries are recognizable lying on right, above the somewhat oval pregnant uterine horn.
b Fetus in a cow ca. 26–27 days after insemination. The development of the placental anchorage system (cotyledons) has not started. The chorionic sac has expanded unevenly into the two uterine horns, so that the embryo has settled in the apical third of the pregnant uterine horn.
c Sonogram of a ca. 4-week-old fetus in its amniotic vesicle. Parts of the fetus (head, vertebral column and abdomen) can be seen as whitish structures lying in the dark amniotic fluid (amniotic cavity). (Courtesy of Prof. P. Glatzel.)

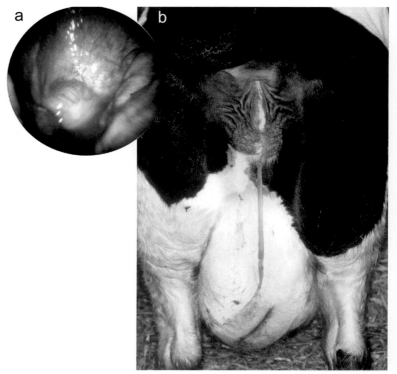

Fig. 86.6 a+b
a The external os of the uterus is closed until ca. 6 days *ante partum* with a thick, whitey-grey, sticky mucous plug (endoscopic view).
b Loss of the cervical mucus plug ca. 3–5 days *ante partum*. (Courtesy of Prof. P. Glatzel.)

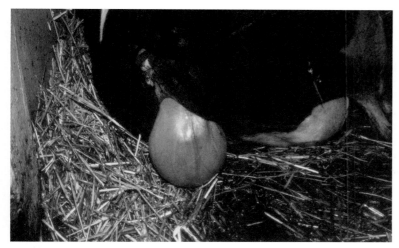

Fig. 86.7 Fetus during the expulsion phase, the forelegs covered by remnants of the amniotic sac are protruding from the vulva. (Courtesy of Prof. P. Glatzel.)

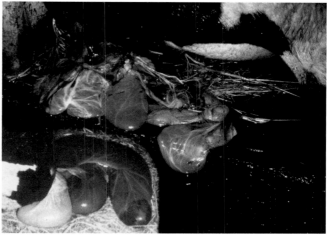

Fig. 86.8 Complete, normal afterbirth (insert: intact amniotic sac). The amniotic sac appears whitey-pink, the allantoic sac dark bluish and the tough chorionic sac with its cotyledons ruddy-yellow. (Courtesy of Prof. P. Glatzel.)

this phase, the egg is released for fertilization. This occurs at the end of the cycle around day 21. These clinically definable processes can be differentiated with the aid of **hormone measurements** (e.g. progesterone quick tests; **Figs. 86.3, 86.4**) or ultrasonography. The biotechnically interesting phase is when the two waves overlap, around the 5th–7th day of the cycle, as during this period **numerous small follicles** (up to 20) can be stimulated by the application of **FSH** or its analog **eCG**. These small follicles can be induced to ovulate without going through the dominance phase by using **LH** or its analog **hCG** (**superovulation**). After insemination, a number of viable embryos can be collected from these animals, e.g. for embryo transfer.

The **bicornate uterus** of cattle has a **bifurcation** in the intercornual ligaments that run deep into the body of the uterus. This structure ensures that a **single-fetus pregnancy** occurs only within a **single uterine horn**. Sometimes this septum can extend into the cervix so that the animal has a double external cervical orifice, in other words a **cervix duplex**.

The **cervix** is an important orientation aid for **artificial insemination (AI)**. It can be fixed **transrectally** by the hand and stretched cranially so that the **insemination pipette** can be inserted. The cervix with its 3 to 4 **annular rings or folds** forms a hermetic closure of the uterine lumen. This and the **external os of the uterus** that projects into the vaginal fornix both form a barrier to the introduction of the AI apparatus, the achievement of which determines the success or lack of success of the insemination.

During the whole **pregnancy**, the cow is under the influence of **progesterone**, which is mainly produced by the **corpus luteum graviditatis** formed on the ovary. The earliest direct proof of an implanted embryo can be gained by the experienced investigator with a **transrectal ultrasonographic examination** on the 26th day after insemination. The tube-like amniotic sac that extends through the uterine horn can be seen on the sonogram as a round anechogenic, i.e. dark area (**Fig. 86.5a**). This dark area with a diameter of ca. 1 cm is surrounded by the contrasting echo-rich (white) wall of the uterus. In the sonogram in **Fig. 86.5a**, both uterine horns are visible. The **fetus** can be seen on the right, lying above the somewhat oval pregnant horn. The amniotic sac is characterized by the two (lower and upper) lines of sonic reflections as well as the already very thin and so less clearly visible wall of the uterus. In **Fig. 86.5b**, a similar embryo is shown macroscopically *in situ*. It is clear that the placental anchorage, the development of the **chorion** (with the cotyledons), has not started. In addition, it is obvious that **the amniotic sac has expanded into both uterine horns**. The two ends of the amniotic sac are of unequal lengths because the embryo has settled in the apical third of the pregnant uterine horn. A definite confirmation of pregnancy by transrectal palpation is possible 4–6 weeks after insemination. At this time, one talks about an "**amniotic vesicle**". The approx. goose-egg-sized amniotic vesicle can be felt through the thin wall of the pregnant uterine horn. In a **sonogram** (**Fig. 86.5c**), parts of the **fetus** (head, vertebral column, abdomen) can be recognized as whitish structures in the dark-appearing amniotic fluid. During the ultrasound examination, **fetal cardiac activity** can be used to prove the presence of a viable fetus.

In the **last trimester**, the synthesis of **estrogen and formation of relaxin** increases, particularly in the **placenta**. All of the body's ligaments become softer, which can be readily observed in the **sacrosciatic ligament**. At this stage, the **cervix** starts to become upright and softer. The erection of the cervix occurs because the caudal part of the uterine neck is pulled down into the abdomen towards the end of the second trimester due to the weight of the fetus and due to the descending fetus being pushed into the pelvic area. The reappearance of the outer os of the uterus can be seen towards the end of the last trimester. This observation is important for the prediction of the birth in ca. 5–6 days. The relaxation of the cervix starts at the internal os of the uterus. The external os of the uterus is closed by a thick, whitey-grey sticky mucous plug until roughly 6 days *ante partum* (**Fig. 86.6a**). Under the influence of estrogen, this plug liquefies and flows out of the vagina as a thick slimy thread approx. 3–5 days before birth (**Fig. 86.6b**). This sign is another criterion for the impending birth.

Individual irregular uterine contractions can already be observed about 2 weeks before the birth. These so-called **premonitory signs of labor** are initially caused by the **expansion of the uterine muscles**. At the same time, the skin between the thighs (between the base of the udder and the lower vaginal commissure) becomes taut, so that **sebum**, which is produced under the influence of high **estrogen levels**, is pressed out of the hair follicles. This area, as a result, becomes smooth and shiny. This change in the skin consistency is considered to be a clear sign that the birth will occur in ca. 3–5 days. The sebum serves in the **olfactory imprinting** of the **neonate calf** on its dam and its dam's udder. This is achieved via the **pheromones** dissolved within the fatty sebum, which the calf takes up as its first olfactory signal as it slithers over this area during birth. The frequency and regularity of the **premonitory contractions** increase up to the 4th–3rd day *ante partum*. This is associated with the – at this time increasing – production of the **prostaglandin PgF2-alpha** and so the **degeneration of the corpus luteum graviditatis**. The contractions of the uterus cause the fetus to move from its position in the lateral part of the uterus to a position in front of the internal os of the uterus, the birth position. At the same time, the **myogenic progesterone block** desists. The uterine contractions become more frequent and the fetus is pushed towards the pelvic inlet. The calf stretches itself out so that it lies in front of the internal os of the uterus, thereby inducing an increasing amount of pressure on this structure. This stimulates the nerve endings at this site, which communicate with the hypothalamus and **neurohypophysis** via the nervous system. The resulting release of **oxytocin** in the blood circulation causes an increase in the strength of the uterine contractions (neurohormonal feedback system: the Ferguson reflex).

In "**Stage 1**" of normal calving, the cervix is dilated by the effects of the **labor contractions** that occur rhythmically in a cranial to caudal direction about every 5–10 minutes. The **chorionic sac** tears open. This is the outer layer of the three membranes surrounding the fetus (the middle one is the allantoic sac, the internal one the amniotic sac). The fetus within its **membranes** is pushed into the dilating cervical canal, widening it even further. "**Stage 2**" of calving starts with the beginning of the **expulsive contractions** and abdominal pressing. The **allantoic sac** breaks releasing its fluid contents to lubricate the vagina. The fetus is pushed into the vagina and the **amniotic sac** tears and its slimy contents lubricate the birth canal. In exceptional cases, such as premature births, both the

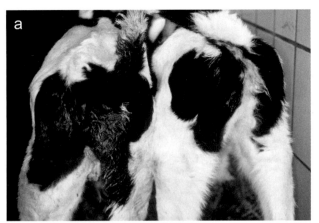

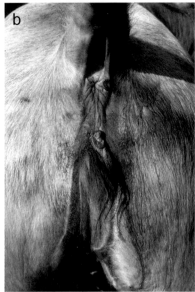

Fig. 86.9 a+b
a Freemartin calf produced as a result of dizygotic twins of two different sexes. The outer female genitalia are conspicuous due to their increased hairiness. The male twin is normal.
b Hermaphroditism, genetic defect. The genitals show a mixture of both, male and female anlages.

time after Europe was Christianized and is associated with the Festival of Saint Martin, the protector of the poor and serfs. At this festival, the lord of the manor gave the cows that had proven to be infertile in the previous calving period to his peasants for slaughter as provisions for the winter. For the term **hermaphrodite**, it is clear that a divine influence was involved. The hermaphrodite was the child of Hermes and Aphrodite. A hermaphrodite is a creature that is like both **Hermes** (male) and **Aphrodite** (female).

The structure, size and organization of the **vagina** should be considered with respect to its function as birth canal and mating organ. Its form is fitted to the bull's penis. The time taken for the **mating reflexes** with successful ejaculation occurs very quickly (2–3 minutes). The thrusting action of the bull with its long extended penis lying deep in the female genitalia causes the vagina to be maximally stretched so that the sperm can be deposited deep in the cranial section of the **cervical canal**. This also prevents the **vaginal fornix** from being used as a storage space for the sperm.

Lacerations can occur in the **external vagina** as a result of a difficult birth, which can lead to the formation of a **cloaca**. Smaller lacerations that only affect the **vestibule** or the **lips** can be treated conservatively. Deeper injuries, perineal lacerations or **rectovaginal fistulas** must be treated surgically.

Inspecting the external vagina and the **perineum** will provide information about any changes in the **vestibule, vagina** or even **uterus**. Every extensive inflammation of the mucous membranes will cause the production of secretions that flow out of the vagina and so can be seen externally. Especially catarrhal secretions caused by specific infectious agents [such as IBR (infectious bovine rhinotracheitis), IPV (infectious pustular bulbovaginitis), BVD (bovine viral diarrhea), etc.] collected from the **clitoral fossa** can be used for the laboratory diagnosis of these diseases. This information can then be used to determine treatment where necessary. Even slight inflammations should also be treated as they, as a rule, negatively affect the animal's fertility.

allantoic sac and amniotic sac may remain intact during the birth, which should be considered as an alarm signal as the life of the fetus is endangered (suffocation). The forelegs of the calf then become visible between the labia of the vagina (**Fig. 86.7**) and then after ca. 15–20 minutes the calf's nose can be seen. The intermittent compression of the umbilical blood vessels against the pubic bone leads to **fetal hypoxia** and therefore the calf must pass through the last two narrow places within the birth canal, the **vestibule and pubis**, very quickly. With completion of the birth, the calf starts to breathe, the umbilical blood vessels tear, and the arteries retract immediately into the calf's abdomen.

The Ferguson reflex is once again set into action during the ejection of the placenta and leads to a facilitation of the milk let-down, and so to **lactation**. First of all, **colostrum** is produced which provides the newborn calf with the necessary **antibody protection**, nutrients and buffer compounds immediately after birth (within ca. 2 hours). In "Stage 3" of calving, the maturation of the afterbirth is finished under the influence of various hormonal, hemodynamic and immune changes as well as mechanical forces. The connections between the cotyledons and the caruncles in the **placentomes** are relaxed so that the placenta can be completely ejected at the end of the birthing process either in the expulsion phase or directly afterwards, at the latest after 12 hours. If the third stage of parturition is not completed properly, then one talks about a **retained placenta**.

The **maternal caruncles** of the placentome have a mushroom-like form. During twin pregnancies, the settlement of the caruncles by the **cotyledons** of the placentome is subjected to a certain degree of competition, so that a number of caruncles are settled by cotyledons from both calves. Due to this situation, there can be an exchange of **immune, hormonal and cellular components**. In dizygotic **twins of different sexes**, this exchange can result in the inhibition of the normal development of the female genital tract and a **masculinization** of the female twin resulting in a freemartin (**Fig. 86.9a**). This (intrauterine-)**acquired malformation** must be differentiated from **genetic abnormalities** such as **hermaphroditism** (**Fig. 86.9b**).

The origin of terms such as freemartin and hermaphrodite is interesting as it indicates that malformations associated with infertility were known in early times. The term **freemartin** comes from the

UDDER

D. Döpfer

[88] To prevent irreversible damage to the **udder and its functions** as well as to alleviate the clinical consequences of udder inflammation, it is very important to be able to recognize and treat any deviations in udder health in the individual animal as quickly as possible. With this in mind, the clinical investigation of the udder utilizing the functional anatomy of the organ is an integral part of modern udder health management. Before undertaking a systematic clinical investigation of the individual cow, the overall appearance of the animal should be considered as well as the udder health status of the whole herd.

Diseases of the udder can be associated with a whole gamut of conditions ranging from just local changes affecting the **gland, teats** or **surrounding tissues** (including the associated **lymph nodes**) but with no effects on the cow's general health to serious changes in the cow's general health including inappetence, fever and even downer cow syndrome.

The assessment of the udder and its surrounding tissues starts at the door of the cow's stall; for example, an abnormal smell can be the first sign of disease arising from an **eczema affecting the inner thighs** or with some forms of **gangrenous udder inflammation**. The animal's general appearance is then assessed, including its reactions to its environment and its general medical condition.

The **normal form of the lactating udder** is described as being bowl-like, with the gland lying firmly against the abdominal wall, allowing it to be milked **easily**. [37] The udder form is also dependent on the animal's breed, whether it is being used for milking or as a foster cow, its **lactation number** and **lactation stage**.

The physical inspection of the udder and its surrounding tissues enables changes in form to be recognized, such as asymmetry due to **swelling, damage to the support apparatus** or separation of the skin from the deeper lying structures. Swelling can be due to the **physiological swelling** that occurs before **parturition**, udder inflammation (**intramammary infection, so-called mastitis**) or even hemorrhages caused by trauma to the organ. Abnormal asymmetry can also be the consequence of a tearing of the udder's suspensory ligaments. If the **lateral laminae** of the suspensory apparatus have been

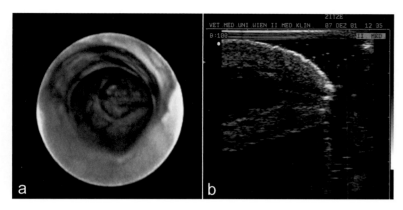

Fig. 88.1 a Teat cistern as seen via the streak canal (endoscopic image). b Streak canal (sonogram). (Courtesy of Dr. S. Franz, Second Medical Clinic, Vetmeduni Vienna.)

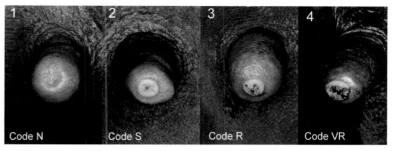

Fig. 88.2 Four-point system for the assessment of teat canal cornification: (1) normal, (2) smooth ring at the end of the teat, (3) rough ring at the end of the teat, (4) severe fraying of the end of the teat. (Courtesy of Dr. ir. F. Neijenhuis, Animal Sciences Group of Wageningen University, and Research Centre, Lelystad.)

partially or completely torn, then any parts of the udder lying outside of their elasticated support will appear to be enlarged asymmetrically and are abnormally mobile. In comparison, rupture of the **medial laminae** or of the rectus abdominis muscle can cause the whole of the udder to "drop down" to below the level of the tarsal joint.

A superficial investigation of the **skin of the udder and teats** with respect to reddening, blue discoloration or the presence of well-circumscribed hemorrhages is essential. Tumor-like changes to the skin of either the udder or teats (e.g. **papillomas**) are undesirable as they can lead to milking problems or due to tears in their surfaces can lead to blood contaminating the milk. As the teat skin has neither sweat glands nor sebaceous glands, the mechanical effects of milking can lead to the skin becoming friable and sore. This can be prevented by the application of **milking grease** or **skin care products in the form of teat sprays**.

Excretions produced by the skin covering the udder and teats, which can be transparent, cloudy or bloody, can also be seen during the clinical inspection and can complete the clinical picture in certain conditions; for example, damage to the skin at the level of the gland and teats.

The extent of severe hemorrhages, for example with a teat injury, can indicate whether or not the **venous plexus** lying at the base of the teat and in the teat wall is involved. This plexus usually serves to hold the milk back following physiological stimuli. The tendency of the udder's parenchyma to severe hemorrhaging (which can even lead to death) means that great care must be taken in the arresting of bleeding (haemostasis), especially during the collection of udder biopsies or during udder operations involving incision of the parenchyma.

The individual **teats** are also inspected superficially, whereby the direction of the tips of the teats should be checked to see if they deviate from the vertical (dependent on the degree of filling of the udder) as this can lead to the air being sucked into the teat when the teat cups are placed on the cow. This intake of air can result in a reduction in milkability and a predisposition to udder inflammation. Deviation from the normal cylindrical **teat form** that widens slightly towards the base of the teat can be seen as conical or step-like teats which are partially or completely narrowed.

The normal **teat canal** opens on the half-moon-shaped teat apex as a smoothly demarcated aperture (**Fig. 88.1**). Irregular or extreme keratinization of the **teat canal opening** prolongs the closing of the canal, prevents the restoration of the keratin plug within the teat canal after milking and is associated with an increased risk of bacterial invasion which can lead to udder inflammation. Such dyskeratosis is evaluated according to its degree of severity (**Fig. 88.2**) and the evaluation can be used in conjunction with the form and appearance of the teats after being milked (i.e. after being affected by the milking machine and its vacuum) as part of an udder health management scheme to assess the functionality of the milking machine. [32] Particularly the presence of flat teats, petechiae on the tip of teats and ring-like swellings affecting the skin at the base of the teat following the removal of the teat cups indicate a faulty interaction between the milking machine and the teats, which can lead to permanent damage to the **tip of the teat** and the **teat mucosa**. The occurrence of milk leaking from the tip of the teat long after milking has ceased (i.e. longer than 30 minutes) or occurring between milking sessions is a sign that there is a defect in the closure of the teat, indicating possible damage to the **sphincter muscles** or

Furstenberg's rosette. Normally, the teat canal closes after milking through muscle contraction and there is a shortening of the teat with respect to the teat canal, which is stretched out lengthwise, and so closes the canal's lumen.

Certain abnormalities should be taken into consideration while **palpating the udder skin, parenchyma, teats and the regional lymph nodes**. The skin of the udder can be overly warm due to the presence of inflammation, but it may feel cold if there are necrotic changes present. Normally, the skin of the udder can be easily displaced over the underlying glandular tissue. It can, however, be under a great deal of tension when there is an acute swelling of the udder and the investigator will not be able to pick up a skin fold between his or her fingers. Such swelling may be due to the normal physiological swelling of the udder that occurs just before parturition (udder edema). In contrast, the normal skin over the teats is tightly attached to the subcutis, therefore, the teat should be **gently rolled** between investigator's fingers as this allows the investigator to gain an impression of the thickness of the mucosa in the teat canal's lumen and feel the presence of any narrowing of the canal caused by freely movable clots or tumor-like processes. This is important in judging the milkability of the udder.

The udder cistern flows into the teat cistern at the transition from the udder parenchyma to the base of the teat, and can be pressed inwards with a finger, in the direction of the abdomen. This enables the investigator to palpate any narrowing or enlargement of the cistern with respect to the milk flow. During the **palpation of the udder parenchyma**, each of the four quarters should be tested individually by gently lifting and releasing the udder to see if it has a soft elastic consistency or whether there are any irregularities in the parenchyma (e.g. lumps due to abscessation, sequestration or chronic udder inflammation) (**Fig. 88.3**). Starting from the proximal part, each quarter should then be palpated with one hand on the medial side and one on the lateral side. The deeper tissues can be palpated by pressing the fingers towards each other. The investigator then gradually works his or her hands towards bottom of each quarter. Pain reactions may occur in the cow as a consequence of the local or general pressure being applied to the udder. If an indentation from a finger does not disappear, this indicates the presence of edema. Crackling sounds in the subcutis are an indication of the presence of gas caused by gas-producing infections; however, gas in the subcutis can also arise due to a physical connection between the deeper layers of the dermis with the outer world.

90 The **palpation of the udder lymph nodes (superficial inguinal lymph nodes)** requires a simultaneous lifting of the respective side of the udder and a palpation of the lymph nodes using a pincer-like movement in the depths of the tissue between the inner side of the knee and the outer wall of the udder (**Figs. 88.3 and 90**). Attention should be paid to the **size, consistency** and the **surface structure of each lymph node**. In cases of acute udder inflammation, the associated lymph nodes may be tense and enlarged, whereas chronic inflammation may lead to induration of the lymph nodes. Palpation of the **subiliac lymph nodes** (lying in the flank fold) and a rectal investigation of the **medial iliac lymph nodes** can provide more information about the cause of udder dermatitis and inflammation.

An **investigation of the milk** (e.g. during foremilk stripping) is an integral part of an udder investigation and a number of **quick tests** can be used to aid in the assessment of the **cell content**, the presence of bacteria and the **determination of the milk's pH**. The changes in

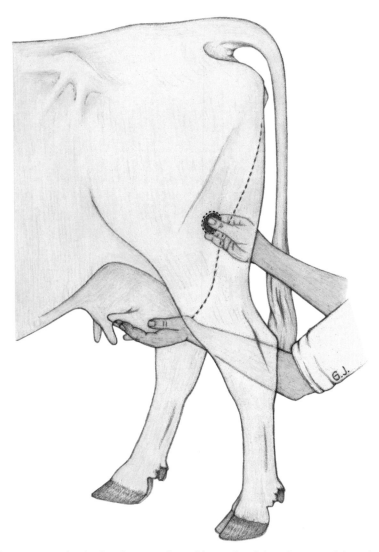

Fig. 88.3 Method of palpating the udder's glandular tissue and lymph nodes while simultaneously lifting the udder.

milk pH during udder inflammation has consequences for the permeability of the so-called "blood-udder barrier". The physiological blood-udder barrier is the barrier between the blood system and the udder parenchyma. This is a transition from the hydrophilic medium of the **blood** with a **pH value of ca. 7.4** to the lipophilic medium of the **milk** with a **pH of ca. 6.4**. This is important for the choice of systemically applied therapeutic agents as they have to pass this

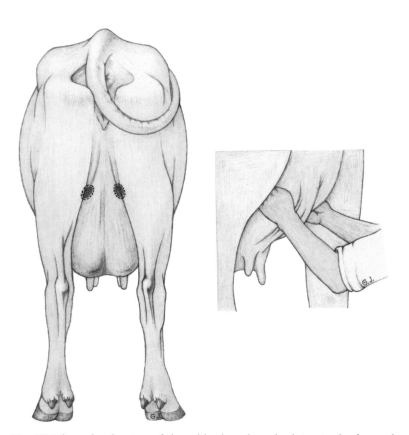

Fig. 90 Bilateral palpation of the udder lymph nodes lying in the femoral canal.

barrier and penetrate into the milk to be effective. As soon as the pH of the milk increases (e.g. due to udder inflammation), dissociation of the antibiotic's ions may occur so that their penetrability of the blood-udder barrier, and therefore therapeutic effectivity, may be increased or reduced. Knowledge about the pharmacotherapeutic characteristics of the agents being used with respect to the blood-udder barrier is essential (e.g. when choosing medications for the treatment of udder inflammation).

Modern developments, such as **automated milking with milk robots,** are a challenge for the functional anatomy of the udder and have consequences for the selection of cows suitable for this type of milking parlor. The selection may, on the one hand, be dictated by the form of the udders and teats which can be recognized and handled by the robots or on the other hand, by the increase in udder parenchyma caused by frequent milking. In-line sensors for assessing the health of the udder are at the moment at an advanced stage of development and are oriented at **udder investigation** and **udder physiology.** Knowledge of the functional anatomy of the udder remains essential for the assessment of udder health especially in such highly technological situations.

MALE REPRODUCTIVE TRACT

P. S. GLATZEL

92 The inspection and **palpation of the scrotum including its contents** are irreplaceable parts of an **andrological examination.** The results are recorded with the help of a suitable key as done in gynecology. First of all, the development of the freely hanging, bottle-shaped, symmetrical scrotal contents with their typical contours should be assessed visually with respect to the age and breed of the bull. Then palpation is undertaken, whereby attention is paid to **free displacement, signs of inflammation** and **pain.** Any bilateral changes indicate either a congenital abnormality (such as **bilateral cryptorchidism** or **microorchidia**) or a systemic infection (e.g. brucellosis or tuberculosis). Unilateral abnormalities can be an indication of a **congenital inhibition malformation** such as **unilateral cryptorchidism (Fig. 92.1)** or trauma. The results of these two examinations should be reinforced by ultrasonography **(Fig. 92.2a–c).**

So that the **testes** can fulfill their function of producing **sperm,** they must have an internal temperature that is ca. 3°C below the animal's body temperature; otherwise **sperm production** is incomplete and the sperms are not fertile. An important structure for the necessary thermoregulation is the **pampiniform plexus,** in which an intensive temperature exchange between the incoming warmth-providing **arterioles** (their pulsation can be clearly seen during ultrasonography) and the outgoing colder **venules** occurs. In a transcutaneous sonogram **(Fig. 92.2a),** the plexus is easily recognized by its sieve-like structure. As a consequence of swelling (e.g. in a post-traumatic hematoma), the structures within the plexus can be consolidated and their function destroyed.

The **testes** should be firm, elastic, ovoid structures with a smooth surface that can be easily moved around in their capsules. Their **internal texture** has a homogenous "salt and pepper" structure on a sonogram **(Fig. 92.2b–c).** Changes caused by trauma or infection can be easily recognized by the presence of densities (white patches) and collections of fluid (black = clear serous fluid or cloudy grey = purulent or bloody secretions) within the testicular capsule. Deposition of minerals such as calcium can also occur. The undisturbed functioning of the testes is expressed in the production of perfect sperm. This is assessed in breeding bulls by the **collection of semen** using an **artificial vagina (Fig. 92.3)** and subsequent microscopic analysis of the sperm.

The biological function of the **epididymis** consists of the **transfer, storage, maturation** and **selection of the sperm,** whereby the latter is achieved by selective phagocytosis. Indications that these functions are normal can be revealed by palpation, starting from the distal end of the testes. The delimitation of the **tail of the epididymis** from the knitting-needle-thick **body of the epididymis** that runs medially over the testis and the cap-like **head of the epididymis** situated at the proximal end of the testis is useful. Thickening of these structures can indicate a reduction or occlusion of the epididymis with the formation of cyctoceles and stasis, which can negatively influence sperm quality or completely prevent semen flow (azoospermia).

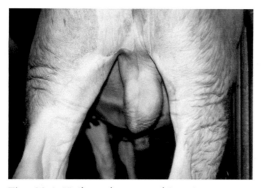

Fig. 92.1 Unilateral cryptorchism in a young bull. (Courtesy of Prof. P. Glatzel.)

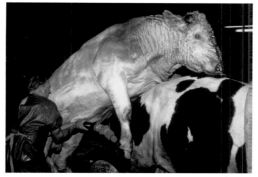

Fig. 92.3 Sperm collection in a bull. (Courtesy of Prof. P. Glatzel.)

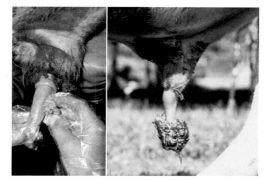

Fig. 92.4 Penile papillomas in two bulls. (Courtesy of Prof. P. Glatzel.)

On palpation, a harder, more movable and obviously rounded structure running parallel to the body of the epididymis is apparent, the **spermatic cord.** The flow of semen is prevented by surgery on this organ during sterilization.

The **function of the accessory sex glands** involves the provision of the ejaculate with nutrients and protectants (sugars, starch, mucous, prostaglandins, etc.). These glands also induce changes in the pH value of the semen leading to the removal of the **inhibition of the sperm's motility (anabiosis)**; sperm are unable to move until this influx of the accessory sex glands' secretions. Abnormalities such as malformation, inflammation or neoplasia directly affect the **characteristics of the ejaculate** and so the fertility of the sire.

The **bulbourethral glands,** which also belong to the accessory sex glands, are paired structures lying at the level of the **sciatic arch,** dorsal to the urethra. They are totally covered by the **urethral muscle** and partially by the **bulbospongiosus muscle.** They can only be palpated or recognized clinically when they are diseased. Their secretions flow after the initiation of the sexual reflex (excitation) as an **initially crystal-clear, slightly viscous fluid** for the preparation of the ejaculation and cleaning of the urethra.

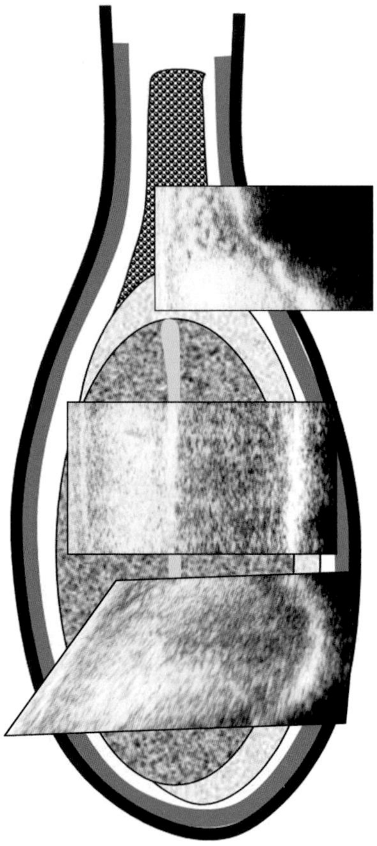

The **instigation and the course of the sexual reflex (foreplay:** emission and erection of the penis; **coitus:** mounting, embracing, touching, intromission, friction, ejaculation in the vagina, propulsion with or without ejaculation; **postcoital phase:** calming, dismounting, relaxation and retraction of the penis) can be clearly assessed by watching the bull's penile movements. **Sensory and tactile stimuli** with their respective receptors are responsible for the initiation of the individual parts of the reflex chain. **Nerve endings** are present on the glans and shaft of the penis (free nerve endings, Ruffini corpuscles, small lamellar corpuscles and Vater-Pacini corpuscles), which register temperature stimuli, slippage and pressure and are transmitted as a **mating impulse,** which in turn initiate the bull's thrusting actions and ejaculation .

The **penis** can be affected by **congenital, genetic** and **acquired defects.** The congenital defects include **hypospadia, hypoplasia, distortions, dysfunction of the retractor penis muscle** and **diphallia.** The acquired defects include traumatic non-infectious injuries and inflammations as well as infectious **swellings, diseases of the mucous membranes and abscesses** (Fig. 92.4).

Prolapse of the preputial mucous membrane, **preputial prolapse,** is of clinical importance. It occurs habitually in tropical cattle breeds of the *Bos indicus* **type (Fig. 92.5).** In these breeds this phenomenon is physiological and aids in the thermoregulation of the whole body. In contrast, preputial prolapse is not acceptable in **taurine cattle breeds** as it is due to a connective tissue weakness. The prepuce is also associated with congenital or inflammatory **phimosis, preputial adhesions** (possibly with formation of a persistent frenulum) as well as being the site of abscesses, inflammation (posthitis), neoplasia (e.g. papilloma), granulomas (e.g. actinomycoma) or ulceration. The preputial sheath is also the **reservoir** for **sexually transmitted diseases** such as *Tritrichomas fetus, Campylobacter fetus,* infectious pustular vaginitis (IPV), infectious vaginal catarrhal complex and genital tuberculosis. This is the reason why all breeding bulls should be regularly checked for these infectious agents using preputial washing samples.

Fig. 92.2a–c Sonograms of a normal bull scrotum, transcutaneous images.
a Neck of the scrotum, perpendicular section: junction between the pampiniform plexus shown as a light/dark "sieve-like" structure and the head of the epididymis seen as a light, compact transverse stripe.
b Testis, perpendicular section: the internal texture of the testis has a homogenous "salt and pepper" texture. The rete testis can be seen in the center as a white axial column. The tissue under the coupling site of the ultrasonic probe is artificially dense due to being compressed by the probe
c Testis, horizontal section: the internal region of the testis has a homogenous "salt and pepper" texture. The rete testis can be seen as a white dot in the center.

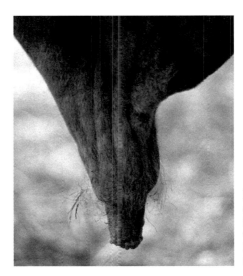

Fig. 92.5 Habitual prolapse of the preputial mucosa for thermoregulation (of the whole body) in a *Bos indicus* bull. (Courtesy of Prof. P. Glatzel.)

TRANSRECTAL EXAMINATION

P. S. GLATZEL, K.-D. BUDRAS

The **structures of the pelvis** (especially the **body of the ilium, pectineal line of the pubis** and the **sacrum**) act as important landmarks to the abdominal organs during **transrectal examination**. Before starting a transrectal exploration, the **anal and perineal region** should be inspected for the presence of fecal staining, bloody mucous or blood (rectal injury due to previous examinations!), swelling, tumors, or parasites. In order to be prepared for any possible forensic conflicts, documenting the situation with photographs is recommended. In addition, the degree of resistance to moving the animal's tail to one side should be registered (more elastic under the effects of estrogen).

The animal should then be professionally **restrained** by an assistant. Before introducing the gloved and richly lubricated hand and arm into the animal's rectum, the **fingers should be put together to form a cone.** The hand is then pushed through the **anal sphincter muscle** with a slight screwing movement. Subsequently, the hand is slowly and carefully pushed forwards cranially, parallel to the spine. After manual clearing out of the **rectal ampulla**, the hand is then pushed even further forwards, whereby force should be avoided at all costs. Any feces present should be removed. The **peristaltic movements of the intestines** should be allowed to run over the hand and arm. If **spasms** of the intestines occur, then these are released using vibrating massaging movements of the fingers and hand. Whilst in the **rectum**, the degree of filling, the consistency of its contents, the spatial relationships of the different structures, the rectal temperature, and the consistency of the rectal wall should be assessed.

The pelvic organs are then investigated; i.e. the **vagina**, which can be found lying on the floor of the pelvis underneath the investiga-

tor's hand, roughly a hand's length inside the pelvis. Using pendulum-like movements of the bent hand, the vagina can be felt with the finger tips as a flabby inconspicuous tube, with the width of roughly a child's arm. Cranially, the vagina joins the **cervix** (thickness = approx. a thumb; length = a small finger). The consistency of the cervix varies according to the stage of the estrus cycle: from hard (under progesterone) to soft-elastic (under estrogen). The neck of the uterus lies over **the pectineal line** of the pubis in the cranial pelvic aperture.

Further into the abdomen — though depending on its degree of filling — a round bottle-shaped, thin-walled, firm structure can be felt: the **urinary bladder**. If one lets the bladder glide under ones hand, then the paired, **broad lateral uterine ligaments** will fall into the slightly curved fingers at the level of the cervix. In the middle of these ligaments (starting from the short body of the uterus) lie the freely movable and cranioventrally rolled **uterine horns** (these do not have any special ligamentous supports as, for example, in the horse). In the non-gravid or early gravid cow, once these structures have been collected under the hand, the whole of the uterus is displaced into the pelvic cavity to enable better palpation. This occurs either by the dorsal flexion and retraction of the filled hand or by holding the (double) intercornual ligament with the middle or index finger. This leads to a dorsocaudal displacement of both uterine horns. The consistency of the uterine horns varies according to stage of the estrous cycle. In proestrus and estrus, the horns are firm, sensitive (contractile) and easy to discern. During diestrus and interestrus, they are flabby, less sensitive and difficult to differentiate.

The ovaries are attached to the tips of the uterine horns and can be found by palpating along the coiled uterine horns, reminiscent of a ram's horn or a snail's shell. The ovaries lie within the inner coil of the uterine horn tip. Palpation of the oviduct is only possible if it has pathological changes.

The terminal branches of the aorta lie in the dorsocranial area of the pelvic cavity. They can be easily palpated due to their typical firmness and pulsation. Lying lateral to these pulsating structures are the iliosacral joints, which can be palpated without any difficulty and particularly after trauma.

A good orientation guide in the transrectal investigation of the accessory glands in the bull (**Fig. 92.6**) is provided by the contractile reaction to palpation of the urethral muscle lying on the floor of the pelvis. Lying at the cranial end of this ca. 2- to 3-cm-wide, rounded strongly contractile annular muscle (length = roughly one hand) is a smooth, ca. 4- to 5-mm-wide, signet-ring-like structure: the prostate. Right and left of the prostate lie the seminal vesicles (thumb-

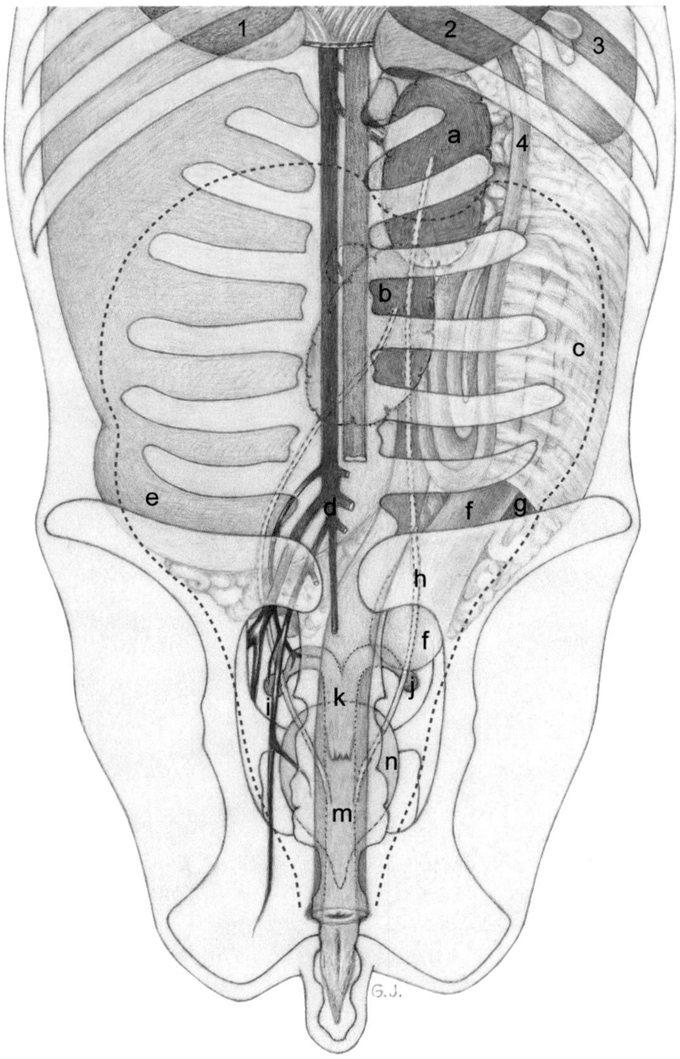

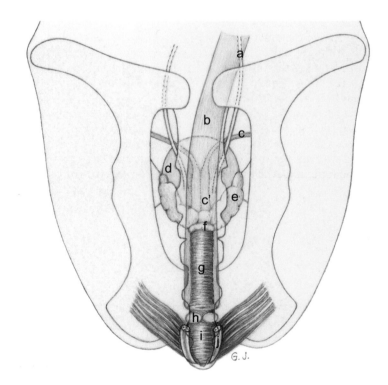

Figs. 86.9 + 92.6 Organs of the abdomen and pelvic cavity, dorsal view. Extent of the conic area of examination during a transrectal examination (dotted line). **86.9 Female pelvic organs.** (a) right kidney, (b) left kidney, (c) colon (lying covered by greater omentum in the supraomental recess), (d) branches of the aorta, (e) dorsal rumen sack, (f) cecum, (g) jejunum and ilium, (h) right ureter, (i) uterine artery, (j) ovary, (k) uterus, (m) vagina, (n) bladder; (1) spleen, (2) liver, (3) abomasum, (4) descending duodenum.

Fig. 92.6 Male pelvic organs. (a) ureter, (b) rectum, (c) vas deferens, (c') ampulla of the vas deferens, (d) bladder, (e) seminal vesicle, (f) prostate, (g) bulbourethral muscle, (h) bulbourethral gland, (i) bulbospongiosus muscle, (j) retractor penis muscle.

thick with the length of a middle finger), which extend along the body of the ilium. The knitting-needle-thick deferent ducts run out of the inguinal canal on each side of the bladder. They can be felt with the finger tips — whilst the hand rests on top of the bladder — running alongside the narrow bladder neck. The deferent ducts can be palpated best where it runs into the pencil-wide and 2-cm-long vas deferens ampulla. The final section of the deferent ducts run underneath the prostate together with the seminal vesicles into the ejaculatory duct on the seminal hillock.

In the standard transrectal palpation of the abdominal organs, it should be remembered that the field of investigation resembles a cone opened cranially (Fig. 86.9). The craniodorsal limit lies at the level of the 1st to 2nd lumbar vertebra, where the furrowed right kidney can be found (assuming an investigator with an average arm's length and a medium-sized cow). Laterally, the cone is limited by the rumen on the left. If there is a left-handed displacement of the abomasum with bloat, then this organ can extend to the level of half the left costal arch and can be easily palpated. The right-hand lateral limit of the cone is formed by the intestines within the greater omentum. In a right-handed displacement of the abomasum, the organ pushes itself underneath the intestines on the right and can be palpated as a gas-filled "balloon".

For the palpation of the abdominal organs, the hand is pushed forwards into the distal section of the ascending colon. This is possible when the arm is inserted up to the middle of the upper arm. Once there, investigators should orientate themselves on the left kidney, which is displaced by the rumen into the region of the 4th to 5th lumbar vertebra.

Left in the entrance to the pelvic cavity is the dorsal sack of the rumen, while the ventral sack lies over the (left) pectineal line of the pubis. The dorsal sack can be circumscribed by the hand, while the ventral sack can only be partially differentiated cranioventrally, depending on its amount of filling. The middle area of both sacks, which can be palpated by running the hand around the dorsal section, enables an assessment to be made about the degree of rumen filling and stratification as well as determining the presence of pain in association with adhesions. The individual sections of the intestinal loops lying to the right of the rumen can only be palpated when excessively filled, distended with gas, or when there is a hardening of the walls. Under these conditions, for the diagnosis of colic, the cecum lying in front of the pelvic inlet can be palpated, including its tip which may even extend into the pelvic cavity itself. In addition, the section of the colon lying in the right upper flank region or the jejunum and ileum lying underneath it (and under the cecum) can be palpated, too.

The pelvic lymph nodes (sacral, medial iliac, and lateral iliac lymph nodes) and the caudal mesenteric lymph nodes can only be felt when they are pathologically swollen.

The lining of the abdomen, the peritoneum, should be smooth and insensitive. Its examination should be undertaken in connection with the rumen diagnostics.

In bulls, the internal inguinal ring with its surroundings a hand-length in front of the pubis should be investigated a hand's width next to the medial plane, especially if there is suspicion of colic (inguinal hernia) (Fig. 92.6).

The liver can only be palpated in cases of severe enlargement lying cranial to the right paralumbar fossa. The organs which cannot be palpated rectally at all under any circumstances are the spleen (adhered together with the dorsal rumen sack to the dorsal body wall), the reticulum, the omasum, and the cranial two-thirds of the rumen.

APPLIED ANATOMY OF THE CARCASS

K.-D. Budras, R. Fries, R. Berg

(Numbers in parentheses: Roman numerals refer to the figures in Table 1 on page 34; Arabic numerals refer to the respective page number in the bovine anatomy atlas 2002/anatomical description). The midline split carcass is further cut transversely between the 12th and 13th rib (North America) at a right angle to the vertebral column. With this cut, the carcass is divided into a front and hind quarter.

Processing of the front quarter:

Further processing of the front quarter continues with a vertical cut between the 5th and 6th ribs, separating the ribs (IV) and flank (V) from the chuck (I) and brisket/shank (II and III). The ribs are separated from the hind quarter by cutting between the 12th and 13th ribs. The ventral flank (V) is separated from the ribs (IV) by a longitudinal cut through the lower third of the ribs.

The ribs are divided into:
1. rib (longissimus dorsi, spinalis and semispinalis thoracis, complexus, multifidi, internal and external intercostal muscles and bones from the 6th to 12th rib [7 bones])
2. rib eye (longissimus dorsi, spinalis and semispinalis thoracis muscles)
3. back ribs (including the musculature between the transverse and spinous processes of the thoracic vertebrae)

A longitudinal cut through the middle of the radius creates the chuck (I) and the brisket/shank (II and III).

The chuck is divided into:
1. chuck roll (longissimus dorsi, spinalis and semispinalis thoracis, subscapularis, rhomboideus, complexus, serratus ventralis, serratus dorsalis, and the internal intercostal muscles.)
2. top blade – chuck tender (supraspinatus muscle)
3. top blade – flat iron (infraspinatus muscle)
4. shoulder clod (deltoideus, teres major, triceps brachii [long, medial, lateral heads] and infraspinatus muscles.)
5. clod tender (teres major muscle)
6. chuck tail flat (chuck short ribs) (serratus ventralis, pectoralis superficialis, scalenus dorsalis, and intercostal muscles.)

The brisket (II; deep pectoral, serratus ventralis, cutaneus trunci and intercostal muscles) is separated from the shank (III). The latter is divided into:
1. hind shank (flexor muscles of the foreleg)
2. fore shank (extensor muscles of the foreleg)

Processing of the hind quarter:

The hind quarter is divided into three major parts:
1. sirloin/loin (VI and VII)
2. flank/plate (VIII)
3. round (IX and X)

The loin is composed of the strip loin and tenderloin, which lie respectively over and beneath the transverse processes of the lumbar vertebrae. The sirloin is cut into:
1. top sirloin (gluteus medius, longissimus dorsi, biceps femoris, gluteus accessorius, gluteus profundus, and tensor fasciae latae muscles)
2. bottom sirloin (rectus femoris, vastus lateralis, vastus medialis muscles).

Each of these cuts can be further subdivided to meet the demands of the market.

The tenderloin (XI) consists of the psoas major, psoas minor and iliacus muscles.

The flank is cut into:
1. flank steak (rectus abdominis muscle)
2. beef short ribs (serratus ventralis muscle)
3. skirt steaks (inside: transversus abdominis muscle; Outside: costal part of the diaphragm).

The remainder of the carcass is referred to as the round (IX). After the hind shank (X) is removed the round is divided into five pieces:
1. knuckle – sirloin tip (vastus intermedius, vastus lateralis, vastus medialis, rectus femoris, tensor fasciae latae muscles)
2. eye of round, semitendinosus muscle)
3. outside round (semitendinosus, biceps femoris, gastrocnemius, superficial digital flexor muscles; may contain the gluteus medius, gluteus accessorius and gluteus profundus muscles)
4. outside flat (biceps femoris muscle; may contain the gluteus medius, gluteus accessorius and gluteus profundus muscles)
5. inside round (semimembranosus, gracilis, adductor femoris, pectineus, sartorius, obturator externus/internus muscles; may contain the iliopsoas muscle).

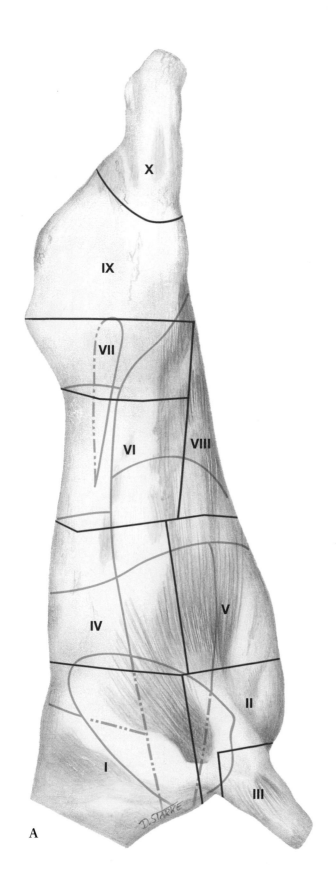 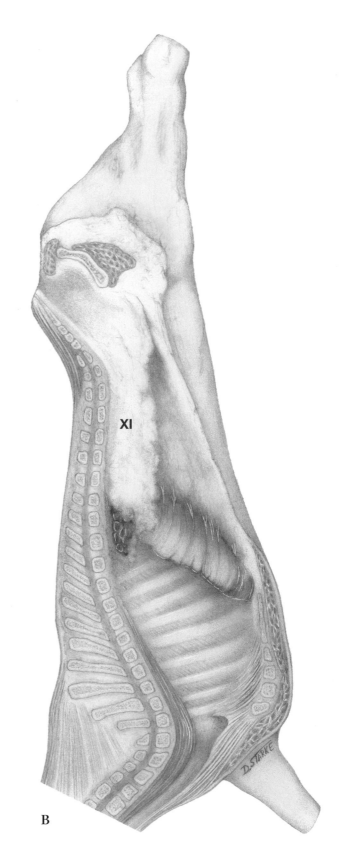

Table 1. Anatomy of the carcass/beef cuts.
(A) lateral view with German cuts as grey lines and North American/Canadian cuts as red lines, (B) medial view.

I	chuck
II	brisket
III	shank
IV	ribs
V	flank/plate
VI	sirloin/loin
VII	sirloin/loin
VIII	flank/plate
IX	round
X	hind shank
XI	tenderloin

REFERENCES

Monographs, textbooks, reference books

Ashdown, R.R. and S. Done, 1984: Color Atlas of Veterinary Anatomy. The Ruminants. Univ. Park Press, Baltimore

Barone, R., 1976-1996: Anatomie comparée des mammifères domestiques. T. 1–5, Laboratoire d'Anatomie, Ecole Nationale Vétérinaire, Lyon; Vigot Frères, Paris

Baum, H., 1912: Das Lymphgefäßsystem des Rindes. A. Hirschwald, Berlin

Benzie, D. and A.J. Phillipson, 1957: The alimentary tract of the ruminant. Oliver and Boyd, Edinburgh

Berg, R., 1995: Angewandte und topographische Anatomie der Haustiere. Gustav Fischer, Jena, Stuttgart

Budras, K.-D., McCarthy, P., W. Fricke and R. Richter, 2002: Anatomy of the Dog. 4th ed., Schlütersche, Hannover

Budras, K.-D., W.O. Sack and S. Röck, 2001: Anatomy of the Horse, 4th ed., Schlütersche, Hannover

De Lahunta, A. and R.E. Habel, 1986: Applied Veterinary Anatomy. W.B. Saunders Co., Philadelphia

Dyce, K.M. and C.J.G. Wensing, 1983: Anatomie van het Rund. Bohn, Scholtema and Holkema, Utrecht

Dyce, K.M., W.O. Sack and C.J.G. Wensing, 1987: Textbook of veterinary anatomy. W.B. Saunders, Philadelphia

Dyce, K.M., W.O. Sack and C.J.G. Wensing, 1991: Anatomie der Haustiere. Lehrbuch für Studium und Praxis. Ferdinand Enke Verlag, Stuttgart

Ellenberger, W. und H. Baum, 1943: Handbuch der vergleichenden Anatomie der Haustiere. 18. Aufl., J. Springer, Berlin

Ensminger, M.E., 1977: Animal Science, 7. ed., Danville, Illinois. Interstate Printers and Publishers

Frewein, J., R.E. Habel and W.O. Sack, editors, 1994: Nomina Anatomica Veterinaria. 4th ed., Internat. Com. Vet. Gross Anat. Nomenclatur, Zürich and Ithaca, New York

Fürstenberg, M.H.F., 1868: Die Milchdrüsen der Kuh, ihre Anatomie, Physiologie und Pathologie. Leipzig

Getty, R., 1975: Sisson and Grossman's The Anatomy of the Domestic Animals. 5th ed., W.B. Saunders Co., Philadelphia

Ghoshal, N.G., T. Koch, and P. Popesko, 1981: The venous drainage of the domestic animals. W.B. Saunders Co. Philadelphia

Habel, R.E., 1992: Guide to the Dissection of Domestic Ruminants. 4th ed., Published by author, Ithaca, New York

Hofmann, R.R., 1969: Zur Topographie und Morphologie des Wiederkäuermagens im Hinblick auf seine Funktion. Nach vergleichenden Untersuchungen an Material ostafrikanischer Wildarten. Parey, Berlin, Hamburg

Hofmann, R.R. und B. Schnorr, 1982: Die funktionelle Morphologie des Wiederkäuer-Magens. Schleimhaut und Versorgungsbahnen. Enke, Stuttgart

King, A.S., 1999: The Cardiorespiratory System. Blackwell Science Ltd., Oxford

Koch, T. und R. Berg, 1992: Lehrbuch der Veterinär-Anatomie. Bd. 1-3. 5. Aufl., Fischer, Jena, Stuttgart

König, H.E. und H.-G. Liebich, 1999: Anatomie der Haussäugetiere. Lehrbuch und Farbatlas für Studium und Praxis. Bd. 1 u. 2, Schattauer, Stuttgart, New York

Martin, P. und W. Schauder, 1938: Lehrbuch der Anatomie der Haustiere. Bd. 3: Anatomie der Hauswiederkäuer. 3. Aufl., Schickhardt u. Ebner, Stuttgart

Montané, L. et E. Bourdelle, 1917: Anatomie régionale des animaux domestiques. 2e vol.: Ruminants. J.-B. Baillère et Fils, Paris.

Nickel, R., A. Schummer und E. Seiferle, 1992-2001: Lehrbuch der Anatomie der Haustiere. Bd. 1-4, Parey, Berlin

Pavaux, Cl., 1982: Farbatlas der Anatomie des Rindes. Splanchnologie. Schober, Hengersberg

Popesko, P., 1998: Atlas der topographischen Anatomie der Haustiere. Enke, Stuttgart

Prince, H., C.D. Diesem, J. Eglitis and al. 1960: Anatomy and Histology of the Eye and Orbit in Domestic Animals. Charles C. Thomas, Springfield, Ill.

Salomon, F.-V., H. Geyer und U. Gille, 2008: Anatomie für die Tiermedizin, Enke, Stuttgart.

Schaller, O., 1992: Illustrated Veterinary Anatomical Nomenclature. Enke, Stuttgart

Schmaltz, R., 1895: Topographische Anatomie der Körperhöhlen des Rindes. Schoetz, Berlin

Ziegler, H. und W. Mosimann, 1960: Anatomie und Physiologie der Rindermilchdrüse. Paul Parey, Berlin und Hamburg

Chapter 1. Thoracic limb

Badawi, H. und H. Wilkens, 1961: Zur Topographie der Arterien an der Schultergliedmaße des Rindes, unter besonderer Berücksichtigung der Versorgung des Vorderfußes. Zbl. Vet. Med. A 8: 533-550

Baum, H., 1911: Die Lymphgefäße der Gelenke der Schultergliedmaße des Rindes. Anat. Hefte 44: 439-456

Baum, H., 1911: Die Lymphgefäße der Muskeln und Sehnen der Schultergliedmaße des Rindes. Anat. Hefte 44: 623-656

Bruchmann, W., 1965: Untersuchungen über die Punktionsmöglichkeiten am Schulter-, Ellenbogen- und Hüftgelenk des Rindes. Diss. med. vet. Hannover

Cuq, P., 1962: Les articulations du carpe ou genou chez le boeuf. Rec. Méd. Vét. 138: 849-868

Desrochers, A., G. St.-Jean, W.C. Cash, et al. 1997: Anatomic communications among the antebrachiocarpal, middle carpal, and carpometacarpal joints in cattle. Am. J. Vet. Res. 58: 7-10

De Vos, N., 1964: Description topographique des artères du pied chez le boeuf. Econ. Méd. anim. 5: 367-401

De Vos, N., 1964: Vergelijkende studie van de arteries van het voorste lidmaat bij de huisdieren. Mededel. Veeartsenijschool Rijksuniv. Gent 8: 1-176

Fölger, A.F., 1906: Über die unteren Sehnenscheiden des Rindes. Mh. prakt. Tierheilkd. 17: 445-452

Frewein, J., 1963: Die Vv. communicantes an den Schultergliedmaßen einiger Säugetiere (Rind, Pferd, Schwein, Hund und Katze). Verh. Anat. Ges., Jena 59: 304-309

Frewein, J., 1967: Die Faszien an den Schultergliedmaßen von Schwein, Rind und Pferd. Anordnung, Struktur und Bedeutung für den Einbau der Leitungsbahnen. Acta anat., Suppl. 53: 1-100

Frewein, J. und M.-B. Morcos, 1962: De arteries van de voorvoet bij het rund. Vlaams diergeneesk. Tijdschr. 31: 161-170

Funk, Kl., 1966: Röntgenanatomische Untersuchungen am Karpalskelett des Rindes. Diss. med. vet. Hannover

Ghoshal, N.G. and R. Getty, 1967: Innervation of the forearm and foot in the ox, sheep and goat. Iowa State Univ. Vet. 29: 19-29

Ghoshal, N.G. and R. Getty, 1970: Comparative morphological study of the major arterial supply to the thoracic limb of the domestic animals (Bos taurus, Ovis aries, Capra hircus, sus scrofa domestica, Equus caballus). Anat. Anz. 127: 422-443

Habel, R.E., 1950: The nerves and arteries of the bovine foot. Proc. Amer. Vet. Med. Assoc., 78. meet., Miami Beach, 323-327

Habermehl, K.H., 1961: Dorsale Corpora sesamoidea an den Zehen einiger Wiederkäuer. Festschr. für Schreiber, Wien. Tierärztl. Monatschr.: 213-224

Hartung, O., 1923: Das Verbindungsgewebe zwischen Radius und Ulna bei den Haustieren mit besonderer Berücksichtigung von Schwein und Rind. Diss. med. vet. Berlin

Horowitz, A., 1964: The veins of the thoracic limb of the ox. Speculum, Ohio State Univ. 17(2): 21-30

Langer, P., R. Nickel, 1953: Nervenversorgung des Vorderfußes beim Rind. Dtsch. Tierärztl. Wschr. 60: 307-309

Lauwers, H., en N.R. De Vos, 1967: Systematische en topografische beschrijving van de venen van de voor – en achtervoet bij het rund. Vlaams diergeneesk. Tijdschr. 36: 81-90

Münster, W. und R. Schwarz, 1968: Venen der Schultergliedmaße des Rindes. Zbl. Vet. Med. A 15: 677-717

Nickel, R. und P. Langer, 1953: Zehengelenke des Rindes. Berl. Münch. Tierärztl. Wschr. 66: 237-246

Nickel, R. und H. Wissdorf, 1964: Vergleichende Betrachtung der Arterien an der Schultergliedmaße der Haussäugetiere (Katze, Hund, Schwein, Rind, Schaf, Ziege, Pferd). Zbl. Vet. Med. A 11: 265-292

Peters, E., 1965: Zur Anatomie der gemeinsamen digitalen Sehnenscheide am Vorder- und Hinterfuß des Rindes. Diss. med. vet. Hannover

Richter, H., 1927: Querschnittformen vom Metacarpus und Metatarsus bei einigen unguligraden und digitigraden Haustieren und Wild. (equus, bos, canis, tarandus rangifer (Rentier) und alces alces (Elch) mit Erklärung in physiologischer und biologischer Hinsicht. Anat. Anz. (Erg. H) 63: 220-228

Richter, B. und Riessner, 1973: Morphologische Untersuchungen an den Venen der Vorder- und Hintergliedmaße des Rindes im Hinblick auf den Blutrückfluß. Diss. med. vet. Berlin

Schmidtchen, P., 1906: Die Sehnenscheiden und Schleimbeutel des Rindes. Mschr. prakt. Tierheilk. 18: 1-60

Schraml, O., 1931: Untersuchung am Carpalgelenk des Rindes. Diss. med. vet. München

Schreiber, J., 1956: Die anatomischen Grundlagen der Leitungsanaesthesie des Rindes. III. Teil: Die Leitungsanaesthesie der Nerven der Vorderextremität. Wien. Tierärztl. Mschr. 43: 273-287

Shively, M.J. and J.E. Smallwood, 1979: Normal radiographic and xerographic anatomy of the bovine manus. Bovine Pract. 14: 74-83

Simoens, P., N.R. De Vos, H. Lauwers et al., 1980: Illustrated anatomical nomenclature of the arteries of the thoracic limb in the domestic mammals. Mededel. Fac. Diergeneesk., Rijksuniv. Gent 22: 1-50

Sussdorf, M. von, 1889: Die Verteilung der Arterien und Nerven an Hand und Fuß der Haussäugetiere. Festschr. 25j. Regierungsjubiläum S.M. König Karl von Württemberg. Verlag W. Kohlhammer, Stuttgart

Taylor, J.A., 1960: The applied anatomy of the bovine foot. Vet. Rec. 72: 1212-1215

Vollmerhaus, B., 1965: Topographisch-anatomische Darstellungen mit Hinweisen zu Injektionstechnik an Gelenken, Sehnenscheiden und Schleimbeuteln bei Pferd, Rind und Hund. Farbwerke Hoechst AG, Marburg

Wilkens, H., 1955: Arterien des Unterarms in vergleichender Betrachtung beim Menschen und bei unseren Haussäugetieren. Zbl. Vet. Med. A2: 193-198

Zniniewicz, V., 1908: Beiträge zur Anatomie und Mechanik des Schultergelenks beim Pferd und Rind. Diss. med. vet. Bern

Chapter 2. Pelvic limb

Barone, R. et M. Lombard, 1968: Le jarret du boeuf et son fonctionnement. Rev. Méd. Vét. 31: 1141-1166

Baum, H., 1896: Besteht beim Rinde eine Verbindung zwischen der Kniescheibenkapsel und der Kapsel des Femoro-Tibialgelenkes, bzw. zwischen den beiden Säcken der letzteren? Arch. wiss. prakt. Thierheilk. 22: 333-337

Bragulla, H. und Ch. Mülling, 1997: Veränderungen der Architektur der Hornzellen und des Hornzellverbandes bei Klauenerkrankungen. Anat. Histol. Embryol. 26: 51-52

Bragulla, H., Reese, S., Mülling, Ch. et al., 1997: Die hinfällige Klauenkapsel des Rindes. Anat. Histol. Embryol. 26: 62

Bruchmann, W., 1965: Untersuchungen über die Punktionsmöglichkeiten am Schulter-, Ellenbogen- und Hüftgelenk des Rindes. Diss. med. vet. Hannover

Budras, K.-D. und Ch. Mülling, 1997: Die Hornbildungsrate im Wandsegment der Rinderklaue. Anat. Histol. Embryol. 26: 52

Cerveny, C., 1965: Die Gelenkbänder am Sprunggelenk des Rindes. (Dtsch. Zus.fassg.) Vet. Med. 10 (38): 111-118

Desrochers, A., G.St. Jean, W.C. Cash, et al. 1996: Anatomic communications between the femoropatellar joint and lateral and medial femorotibial joints in cattle. Am. J. Vet. Res. 57: 798-802

Dirks, Cl., 1985: Makroskopische, Licht- und elektronenmikroskopische Untersuchungen über den Rückenteil der Rinderklaue. Diss. med. vet. Freie Universität Berlin

Dottrens, E., 1946: Les phalanges osseuses de Bos taurus domesticus. Rev. Suisse Zool. 53: 739

Engel, E., 1919: Vergleichend-anatomische Untersuchungen über die Zehenknochen von Pferd, Rind, Ziege und Schaf. Diss. med. vet. Leipzig

Fürst, A., 1992: Makroskopische und mikroskopische Anatomie der Rinderklaue. Diss. med. vet. Zürich

Fürst, C.M., 1914: Über die Entwicklung und Reduktion der Fibula beim Rinde. Z. Morph. Anthrop. 18: 93-110

Hagenbuch, K., 1938: Das Sprunggelenk des Rindes. Bau und Bewegungsart. Diss. med. vet. München

Heinze, W. und H. Kantor, 1972: Morphologisch-funktionelle Untersuchungen über das Blutgefäßsystem der Rinderklaue. Morph. Jb. 117: 472-482, 118: 139-159

Hirschberg, R., 1999: Die Feinstruktur der Blutgefäße an der gesunden und erkrankten Rinderklaue. Diss. med. vet. Freie Universität Berlin

Hirschberg, R.M., Ch. Mülling and H. Bragulla, 1999: Microvasculature of the bovine claw demonstrated by improved micro-corrosions casting technique. Microsc. Res. Techn. 45: 184-197

Hochstetter, T., 1998: Die Hornqualität der Rinderklaue unter Einfluß einer Biotinsupplementierung. Diss. med. vet. Freie Universität Berlin

Howlett, C.R., 1971: Anatomy of the arterial supply to the hip joint of the ox. J. Anat. 110: 343-348

Ippensen, E., 1969: Venen der Beckengliedmaße des Rindes. Diss. med. vet. Hannover

Kolesnikow, W.W., 1932: Zur vergleichenden Anatomie des M. glutaeobiceps der Säugetiere. Z. Anat. Entw.gesch. 99: 538-570

Lauwers, H., en N.R. De Vos, 1967: Systematische en topografische beschrijving van de venen van de voor – en achtervoet bij het rund. Vlaams diergeneesk. Tijdschr.36: 81-90

Müller-Calgan, H., 1954: Interosseus-Apparat bei Wiederkäuern. Diss. med. vet. Gießen

Mülling, Ch., 1993: Struktur, Verhornung und Hornqualität in Ballen, Sohle und Weißer Linie der Rinderklaue und ihre Bedeutung für Klauenerkrankungen. Diss. med. vet. Freie Universität Berlin

Mülling, Ch., Bragulla, H., Budras, K.-D. et al., 1997: Der Aufbau der Weißen Linie in Abhängigkeit von der Papillarkörperform. Anat. Histol. Embryol. 26: 71

Mülling, Ch. und K.-D. Budras, 1998: Der Interzellularkitt (Membrane Coating Material MCM) in der Epidermis der Rinderklaue. Wien. Tierärztl. Mschr. 85: 216-223

Nickel, R. und P. Langer, 1953: Zehengelenke des Rindes. Berl. Münch. Tierärztl. Wschr. 66: 237-246

Pavaux, C., H. Chahrasbi et J.Y. Sautet et al., 1981: Les rameaux musculaires distaux du nerf tibial chez le boeuf (Bos taurus). Anat. Histol. Embryol. 10: 15-25

Pavaux, C., Y. Lignereux, and J.Y. Sautet, 1983: Anatomie comparative et chirugical du Tendon calcanéen commun des mammifères domestiques. Anat. Histol. Embryol. 12: 60-69

Peters, E., 1965: Zur Anatomie der gemeinsamen digitalen Sehnenscheide am Vorder- und Hinterfuß des Rindes. Diss. med. vet. Hannover

Petersen, G., 1921: Untersuchungen über das Fußskelett des Rindes. Morph. Jb. 51: 291-337

Pötschke, H.-P., 1969: Der Plexus lumbosacralis des Rindes und die Blockstellen für die Paravertebralanästhesie sowie für die Anästhesie der Nerven der Dammgegend. Diss. med. vet. Freie Universität Berlin

Prentice, D.E., 1973: Growth and wear rates of hoof horn in Ayrshire cattle. Res. Vet. Sci. 14: 285-290

Reimers, H., 1913: Plexus lumbalis und sacralis von Rind und Schwein. Diss. med. vet. Leipzig

Reinsfeld, R., 1932: Die Mechanik des Kniegelenkes vom Rinde. Diss. med. vet. München u. Z. Anat. Entw.gesch. 97: 487-508

Richter, H., 1927: Querschnittformen vom Metacarpus und Metatarsus bei einigen unguligraden und digitigraden Haustieren und Wild (equus, bos, canis, tarandus rangifer (Rentier) und alces alces (Elch) mit Erklärung in physiologischer und biologischer Hinsicht. Anat. Anz. (Erg. H) 63: 220-228

Richter, B. und Riessner, 1973: Morphologische Untersuchungen an den Venen der Vorder- und Hintergliedmaße des Rindes im Hinblick auf den Blutrückfluß. Diss. med. vet. Berlin

Schmidtchen, P., 1906: Die Sehnenscheiden und Schleimbeutel des Rindes. Mschr. prakt. Tierheilk. 18: 1-60

Schreiber, J., 1956: Die anatomischen Grundlagen der Leitungsanaesthesie des Rindes. IV. Teil: Die Leitungsanaesthesie der Nerven der Hinterextremität. Wien. Tierärztl. Mschr. 43: 673-705

Smallwood, J.E. and M.J. Shively, 1981: Radiographic and xeroradiographic anatomy of the bovine tarsus. Bovine Pract. 2: 28-46

Smith, R.N., 1956: The proximal metatarsal sesamoid of the domestic ruminants. Is it vestige of a second metatarsal? Anat. Anz. 103: 241-245

Stuhlenmiller, M., 1922: Untersuchungen am Hüftgelenk des Rindes. Diss. med. vet. München

Sussdorf, M. von, 1889: Die Verteilung der Arterien und Nerven an Hand und Fuß der Haussäugetiere. Festschr. 25j. Regierungsjubiläum S.M. König Karl von Württemberg, Verlag W. Kohlhammer, Stuttgart

Szenes, J., 1923: Zur Anatomie des Sprunggelenks des Rindes mit Beziehung auf die Wirkung seiner Bänder und Muskeln. (Dtsch. Zus.fassg.) Diss. med. vet. Budapest

Taylor, J.A., 1960: The applied anatomy of the bovine foot. Vet. Rec. 72: 1212-1215

Vollmerhaus, B., 1965: Topographisch-anatomische Darstellungen mit Hinweisen zur Injektionstechnik an Gelenken, Sehnenscheiden und Schleimbeuteln bei Pferd, Rind und Hund. Farbwerke Hoechst AG, Marburg

Wackwitz, B., 1967: Beiträge zur topographischen Anatomie der Extremitas pelvina des Rindes. Diss. med. vet. Berlin (Humboldt-Univ.)

Westerfeld, I., 2003: Struktur und Funktion des bovinen Klauenbeinträgers. Diss. med. vet. Berlin

Wilkens, H., 1964: Zur makroskopischen und mikroskopischen Morphologie der Rinderklaue mit einem Vergleich der Architektur von Klauen- und Hufröhrchen. Zbl. Vet. Med. A 11: 163-234

Wilkens, H. und H. Badawi, 1962: Beitrag zur arteriellen Blutgefäßversorgung vom Fuß der Beckengliedmaße des Rindes. Berl. Münch. Tierärztl. Wschr. 75: 471-476

Wünsche, A., 1966: Die Nerven des Hinterfußes vom Rind und ihre topographische Darstellung. Zbl. Vet. Med. A 13: 429-443

Chapter 3. Head

Baldwin, B.A., 1964: The anatomy of the arterial supply to the cranial regions of the sheep and ox. Amer. J. Anat. 115: 101-118

Barzt, W., 1910: Über die Epithelkörperchen, die Thyreoidea und die Nebenschilddrüsen beim Rind, Schaf, Schwein und Hund. Diss. med. vet. Bern

Baum, H., 1898: Die Nasenhöhle und deren Nebenhöhlen beim Rinde. Arch wiss. prakt. Thierheilk. 24: 337-374

Baum, H., 1928: Die Lymphgefäße des Kehlkopfes der Haustiere (Pferd, Rind, Schwein und Hund). Festschr. E. Fröhner, Stuttgart, Enke Verlag

Brandt, K., 1928-29: Die Entwicklung des Hornes beim Rinde bis zum Beginn der Pneumatisation des Hornzapfens. Gegenb. Morph. Jb. 60: 428-468

Butler, W.F., 1967: Innervation of the horn region in domestic ruminants. Vet. Rec. 80: 490-492

Cummings, J.F. and R.E. Habel, 1965: The blood supply of the bovine hypophysis. Amer. J. Anat. 116: 91-114

Dahmen, E., 1970: Die embryonale Entwicklung des Waldeyer'schen Rachenringes beim Rind. Diss. med. vet. München

Davies, R., M. Kare, R. Cagan, 1979: Distribution of taste buds in fungiform and circumvallate papillae of bovine tongue. Anat. Rec. 195: 443-446

Dougherty, R.W., K.J. Hill, F.L. Campeti, R.C. Mc Clure and R.E. Habel, 1962: Studies of pharyngeal and laryngeal activity during eructation in ruminants. Amer. J. Vet. Res. 23: 213-219

Egehöj, J., 1934: Das Lymphsystem des Kopfes beim Rinde. Dtsch. Tierärztl. Wschr. 42: 333-336

Forster, A., 1934: L'articulation temporomaxillaire chez les ruminants (mouton, chèvre, bovins) et les solipèdes (cheval). Étude d'anatomie comparée. Arch. d'Anat. 18: 327-371

Godinho, H.P. and R. Getty, 1971: The branches of the ophthalmic and maxillary nerves to the orbit of goat, sheep and ox. Arquivos da Escola de Veterinaria (Brazil) 23: 229-241

Hauser, H., 1937: Über Bau und Funktion der Wiederkäuerparotis. Zschr. mikrosk.-anat. Forsch. 41: 177-228

Heinze, W., 1963: Die Morphologie der Kaumuskulatur des Rindes, der Ziege und des Schafes sowie Erörterungen einiger myologischer Fragen. Anat. Anz. 112: 101-128

Helm, F.Chr., 1957: Die Gefäßverzweigung in der Schilddrüse des Rindes. Zbl. Vet. med. A4: 71-79

Himmelreich, H.A., 1964: Der M. tensor veli palatini der Säugetiere unter Berücksichtigung seines Aufbaus, seiner Funktion und seiner Entstehungsgeschichte. Anat. Anz. 115: 1-26

Iwanoff, St., 1940/41: Das Relief des harten Gaumens beim Rind unter Berücksichtigung der Variabilität der Gaumenstaffeln. (Dtsch. Zus.fassg.) Jb. Univ. Sofia, Vet. med. Fak. 17: 555-572

Lassoie, L., 1952: Les sinus osseux de la tête, chez la béte bovine. Ann. Méd. Vét. 96: 300-322

Lauwers, H. and N.R. De Vos, 1966: Innervatie van de hoorn bij het rund in verband met het verloop van de N. ophthalmicus. Vlaams Diergenesk Tijd. 35: 451-464

Lechner, W., 1941: Die A. alveolaris mandibulae beim Wiederkäuer. Anat. Anz. 91: 273-320

Le Roux, J.M.W., 1959: Die Venen am Kopf des Rindes. Diss. med. vet. Hannover

Le Roux, J.M.W. und H. Wilkens, 1972: Zur Angiographie der Kopfarterien des Rindes. Dtsch. tierärztl. Wschr. 79: 342-346

Mc Cormack, J.E., 1974: Variations of the ocular fundus of the bovine species. Scope 18: 21-28

Modes, E., 1936: Das Blutgefäßbild des Augenhintergrundes bei den Haussäugetieren. Arch. wiss. prakt. Tierheilk. 70: 449-472

Mosimann, W., 1954: Die sensiblen Nerven von Horn und Ohrmuschel beim Rind und die Möglichkeit ihrer Anaesthesie. Schweiz. Arch. Tierheilk. 96: 463-469

Müller, A., 1969: Das Bild des normalen Augenhintergrundes beim Rind. Berl. Münch. Tierärztl. Wschr. 82: 181-182

Nickel, R. und R. Schwarz, 1963: Vergleichende Betrachtung der Kopfarterien der Haussäugetiere (Katze, Hund, Schwein, Rind, Schaf, Ziege, Pferd). Zbl. Vet. Med. A10: 89-120

Paulli, S., 1923: Ein Os rostri bei Bos taurus. Anat. Anz. 56: 249-252

Peters, J., 1904: Untersuchungen über die Kopfspeicheldrüsen bei Pferd, Rind und Schwein. Diss. med. vet. Gießen

Pichler, Fr., 1941: Über die Gaumenkeilbeinhöhle des Rindes. Wien. Tierärztl. Mschr. 28: 413-414

Prodinger, F., 1940: Die Artmerkmale des Kehlkopfes der Haussäugetiere (Pferd, Rind, kleine Wiederkäuer, Schwein, Hund, Katze, Kaninchen). Z. Anat. Entwickl.gesch. 110: 726-739

Salomon, S., 1930: Untersuchungen über das Nasolabiogramm des Rindes. Diss. med. vet. Hannover

Schachtschabel, A., 1908: N. facialis und trigeminus des Rindes. Diss. med. vet. Leipzig

Schmidt, K., 1910: Die arteriellen Blutgefäße des Rindes. Diss. med. vet. Zürich

Schmidt, W.J. und H. Sprankel, 1954: Bildet sich im Stratum corneum des Rinderhornes Röhrchenstruktur aus? Z. Morph. u. Ökol. der Tiere 42: 449-470

Schmuck, U., 1986: Die Zunge der Wiederkäuer. Vergleichend-anatomische und histologische Untersuchungen an 42 Haus- und Wildwiederkäuerarten (Ruminantia scopdi 1777). Diss. med. vet. Gießen

Schreiber, J., 1955: Die Leitungsanästhesie der Kopfnerven beim Rind. Wien. Tierärztl. Mschr. 42: 129-153

Schreiber, J., 1959: Das Ganglion cervicale superius von Bos taurus. Morph. Jb. 99: 821-837

Somers, M., 1957: Saliva secretion and its function in ruminants. Australian Vet. J. 33: 297-301

Steven, D.H., 1964: The distribution of external and internal ophthalmic arteries in the ox. J. Anat. 98: 429-435

Vollmerhaus, B., 1957: Über tonsilläre Bildungen in der Kehlkopfschleimhaut des Rindes. Berl. Münch. Tierärztl. Wschr. 70: 288-290

Wilhelm, J., 1924: Zur Entwicklungsgeschichte der Hinterhauptsschuppe des Rindes. Anat. Anz. 59: 1-11

Wilkens, H., 1958: Zur Topographie der Nasenhöhle und der Nasennebenhöhlen beim Rind. Dtsch. Tierärztl. Wschr. 65: 580-585, 632-637

Zhedenov, V.N., 1937: On the question of the obliteration of the internal carotid artery in cattle. (russ.) Arkh. Anat. Histol. Embryol. 16: 490-508

Ziegler, H., 1927: Beiträge zum Bau der Unterkieferdrüse der Haussäugetiere: Rind, Ziege und Schaf. Zschr. Anat. 82: 73-121

Zietzschmann, O., 1906: Traubenkörner der Haussäugetiere. Arch. mikrosk. Anat. 65: 611-622

Zietzschmann, O., 1942: Horn und Geweih. Dtsch. Tierärztl. Wschr. 50: 55-57

Chapter 4. Central nervous system

Dellmann, H.D., 1960: Zur makroskopischen Anatomie der subkortikalen Kerne des Telencephalon und des Pallidum beim Rind. Zbl. Vet. med. 7: 761-768

Frewein, J., 1962: Die Partes abdominalis, pelvina und coccygea systematis autonomici und deren periphere Geflechte bei Bos taurus L. Morph. Jb. 103: 361-408

Goller, H., 1958: Vergleichende Rückenmarkstopographie unserer Haustiere. Tierärztl. Umschau 4: 107-110

Goller, H., 1962: Segmentquerschnitte des Rinderrückenmarkes. Zbl. Vet. 9: 943-950

Goller, H., 1965: Zytoarchitektonik der Medulla oblongata des Rindes. Paul Parey, Berlin

Hopkins, G.S., 1935: The correlation of anatomy and epidural anesthesia in domestic animals. Ann. Report NYS Vet. College 1934-35: 46-51

Kaufmann, J., 1959: Untersuchungen über die Frühentwicklung des Kleinhirns des Rindes. Diss. med. vet. Bern

Lang, K., 1959: Anatomische und histologische Untersuchungen der Epiphysis cerebri von Rind und Schaf. Diss. med. vet. München

Seiferle, E., 1939: Zur Rückenmarkstopographie von Pferd und Rind. Z. Anat. u. Entwicklgesch. 110: 371-384

Weber, W., 1942: Anatomisch-klinische Untersuchungen über die Punktions- und Anästhesiestellen des Rückenmarkes und die Lage des Gehirns beim Rind. Schweizer Arch. Tierheilk. 84: 161-173

Chapter 5. Skeleton of the trunk and neck

Bölck, G., 1961: Ein Beitrag zur Topographie des Rinderhalses. Diss. med. vet. Berlin

Donat, K., 1972: Der M. cucullaris und seine Abkömmlinge (M. trapezius und M. sternocleidomastoideus) bei den Haussäugetieren. Anat. Anz. 131: 286-297

Frewein, J., 1970: Die Haemapophysen an den Schwanzwirbeln von Katze, Hund und Rind. Zbl. Vet. Med. A17: 565-572

Hagström, M., 1921: Die Entwicklung des Thymus beim Rind. Anat. Anz. 53: 545-566

Luckhaus, G., 1966: Die Pars cranialis thymi beim fetalen Rind. Morphologie, Topographie, äußere Blutgefäßversorgung und entwicklungsgeschichtliche Betrachtungen. Zbl. Vet. Med. A13: 414-427

Mietzner, C., 1920: Die Dornfortsätze des Rindes. Diss. med. vet. Leipzig

Smuts, M.M.S., 1974: The foramina of the cervical vertebrae of the ox. Part I: Atlas and Axis. Zbl. Vet. Med. C3: 289-295

Smuts, M.M.S., 1975: The foramina of the cervical vertebrae of the ox. Part II: Cervical vertebrae 3-7. Zbl. Vet. Med. C4: 24-37

Smuts, M.M.S., 1976: Mm. intertransversarii cervicis of the ox (Bos taurus L.). Zbl. Vet. Med. C5, 135-146

Smuts, M.M.S. and J.M.W. le Roux, 1975: Mm. scaleni of the ox (Bos taurus L.). Zbl. Vet. Med. C4: 256-267

Smuts, M.M.S. and J.M.W. le Roux, 1976: Areas of muscular attachment and their correlation with foraminous area of the cervical vertebrae of the ox (Bos taurus L.). Zbl. Vet. Med. C5: 253-266

Stuckrad, U. v., 1954: Zur Statik der Wirbelsäule des Rindes. (Speziell über den Richtungswechsel des Dornfortsatzes des 7. Halswirbels). Diss. med. vet. Freie Universität Berlin

Chapter 6. Thoracic cavity

Agduhr, E., 1927/28: Morphologische Beweise für das Vorhandensein intra-vitaler Kommunikationen zwischen den Kavitäten der Pleurasäcke bei einer Reihe von Säugetieren. Anat. Anz. 64: 276-298

Barone, R., 1956: Bronches et vaisseaux pulmonaires chez le boeuf (Bos taurus). C.R. Assoc. Anat. Lisbonne

Barone, R. et A. Collin, 1951: Les artères du coeur chez les ruminants domestiques. Rev. Méd. Vét. 102: 172-181

Baum, H., 1911: Die Lymphgefäße der Pleura costalis des Rindes. Z. f. Infektionskrankh. d. Haust. 9: 375-381

Bühling, H., 1943: Die Venae pulmonales des Rindes. Diss. med. vet. Hannover

Bürgi, J., 1953: Das grobe Bindegewebsgerüst in der Lunge einiger Haussäuger (Rind, Schwein, Pferd, Ziege, Schaf, Hund und Katze) mit besonderer Berücksichtigung der Begrenzung des Lungenläppchens. Diss. med. vet. Zürich

Calka, W., 1967: Bronchial arteries with extrapulmonary course in domestic cattle. Folia Morph. Warszawa 26: 359-367

Calka, W., 1969: Präkapilläre Anatomosen zwischen der A. bronchalis und der A. pulmonalis in den Lungen von Hausrindern. Folia morphol. Warszawa 28: 65-74

Calka, W., 1969: The blood supply of the lungs through direct branches of the aorta in domestic cattle. Folia Morphol. Warszawa 28: 442-450

Fize, M., 1965: Anatomie der Lungen und des Bronchialgefäßbaumes bei Wiederkäuern. Thèse doct. vét. Lyon

Grau, H., 1933: Beiträge zur vergleichenden Anatomie der Azygosvenen bei unseren Haustieren (Pferd, Hund, Rind, Schwein) und zur Entwicklung der Azygosvenen des Rindes. Z. Anat. Entwicklgesch. 100: 119-148, 256-276, 295-329

Hausotter, E., 1924: Das Herzskelett der Haussäuger Pferd, Rind, Schaf, Schwein, Hund u. Katze. Wien. Tierärztl. Mschr. 11: 311

Hegazi, A. el H., 1958: Die Blutgefäßversorgung des Herzens von Rind, Schaf und Ziege. Zbl. Vet. Med. 5: 776-819

Koch, T. und R. Berg, 1961: Die mediastinalen Pleuraumschlagslinien am Sternum und das Lig. sterno- bzw. phrenicopericardiacum bei einigen Haustieren. Anat. Anz. 110: 116-126

Palmgren, A., 1928: Herzgewicht und Weite der Ostia atrioventricularia des Rindes. Anat. Anz. 65: 333-342

Schorno, E., 1955: Die Lappen und Segmente der Rinderlunge und deren Vaskularisation. Diss. med. vet. Zürich

Schmack, K.-H., 1975: Die Ventilebene des Herzens bei Pferd, Rind und Hund. Diss. med. vet. Gießen

Seiferle, E., 1956: Grundsätzliches zu Bau und Benennung der Haussäuger-Lunge. Okajima's Folia Anat. Jap. 28: 71-81

Simoens, P., N.R. De Vos and H. Lauwers, 1978/79: Illustrated anatomical nomenclature of the heart and the arteries of head and neck in the domestic mammals. Mededel. Fac. Diergeneesk. Rijksuniv. Gent, 21: 1-100

Stamp, J.T., 1948: The distribution of the bronchial tree in the bovine lung. J. Comp. Path. 58: 1-8

Stroh, G., 1923: Untersuchungen an Rinderherzen über das Offenbleiben des Foramen ovale. Münch. Tierärztl. Wschr. 74: 293-297

Strubelt, H., 1925: Anatomische Untersuchungen über den Verschluß und die Rückbildung des Ductus Botalli bei Kälbern und Rindern. Diss. med. vet. Berlin

Vaerst, G., 1888: Vorkommen, anatomische und histologische Entwicklung der Herzknochen bei Wiederkäuern. Dtsch. Z. Thiermed. vergl. Path. 13: 46-71

Ziegler, H. und H. Hauser, 1939: Anatomie für die Praxis. II. Zur Lage der Speiseröhre und intrathorakalen Bauchorgane beim Rind. Schweiz. Arch. Tierheilk. 81: 366-390

Zsebök, Z., A. Székely und E. Nagy, 1955: Beiträge zur Anatomie des Bronchialsystems und der Lungenangioarchitektur des Rindes. Acta vet. acad. sci. Hung. 5: 307-332

Chapter 7. Abdominal wall and abdominal cavity

Arnold, J.P. and R.L. Kitchel, 1957: Experimental studies of the innervation of the abdominal wall of cattle. Amer. J. Vet. Res. 18: 229-240

Baum, H., 1911: Die Lymphgefäße der Milz des Rindes. Z. f. Infektionskh. d. Haust. 10: 397-407

Christ, H., 1930: Nervus vagus und die Nervengeflechte der Vormägen der Wiederkäuer. Z. Zellforsch. 11: 342-374

Dietz, O. et al., 1970: Untersuchungen zur Vagusfunktion, zur Vagusbeeinflussung und zu Vagusausfällen am Verdauungsapparat des erwachsenen Rindes. Arch. Exp. Veterinärmed. 24: 1385-1439

Eichel, J., 1925: Maße, Formen und Gewichte der Lebern von Rindern und Schafen. Diss. med. vet. Berlin

Florentin, P., 1953: Anatomie topographique des viscères abdominaux du boeuf et du veau. Rev. Méd. Vét. 104: 464-493

Geyer, H., G. Aberger und H. Wissdorf, 1971: Beitrag zur Anatomie der Leber beim neugeborenen Kalb. Topographische Untersuchungen mit Darstellung der Gallenwege und der intrahepatischen Venen. Schweiz. Arch. Tierheilk. 113: 577-586

Ghoshal, N.G. and R. Getty, 1968: The arterial blood supply to the appendages of the ox (Bos taurus). Iowa State J. Sci. 43: 41-70

Grau, H., 1955: Zur Funktion der Vormägen, besonders des Netzmagens der Wiederkäuer. Berl. Münch. Tierärztl. Wschr. 15: 271-278

Grau, H. und P. Walter, 1957: Über die feinere Innervation der Vormägen der Wiederkäuer. Acta anat. 31: 21-35

Grossman, J.D., 1949: Form, development and topography of the stomach of the ox. J. Amer. Vet. Med. Assoc. 114: 416-418

Habel, R.E., 1956: A Study of the innervation of the Ruminant Stomach. The Cornell Vet. 46 (4): 555-633

Harms, D., 1966: Über den Bau und Verschluß des Ductus arteriosus Botalli der Rinder. Z. Zellforsch. 72: 344-363

Hofmann, R.R., 1976: Zur adaptiven Differenzierung der Wiederkäuer; Untersuchungsergebnisse auf der Basis der vergleichenden funktionellen Anatomie des Verdauungstraktes. Prakt. Tierarzt 57: 351-358

Hummel, R. und B. Schnorr, 1982: Das Blutgefäßsystem des Dünndarms vom Wiederkäuer. Anat. Anz. 151: 260-280

Jones, R.S., 1962: The position of bovine abomasum. An abattoir survey. Vet. Rec. 74: 159-163

Koch, T., 1954: Die Innervation der Bauchdecke des Rindes. Mhefte Vet.-Med. 9: 541-544

Lagerlöf, N., 1929: Investigations of the topography of the abdominal organs in cattle and some clinical observations and remarks in connection with the subject. Skand. Veterinärtidskr. 19: 253-265

Lambert, P.S., 1948: The development of stomach in the ruminant. Vet. J. 104: 302-310

Lauwers, H., N.R. De Vos et H. Teuchy, 1975: La vascularisation du feuillet du boeuf. Zbl. Vet. Med. C 4: 289-306

Maala, C.P. and W.O. Sack, 1981: The arterial supply to the ileum, cecum and proximal loop of the ascending colon in the ox. Zbl. Vet. Med. C Anat. Histol. Embryol. 10: 130-146

Maala, C.P. and W.O. Sack, 1983: The venous supply of the cecum, ileum and the proximal loop of the ascending colon in the ox. Zbl. Vet. Med. C Anat. Histol. Embryol. 12: 154-166

Martin, P., 1890: Zur Entwicklung der Bursa omentalis und der Mägen beim Rinde. Österr. Mschr. Tierheilk. 14: 49-61

Martin, P., 1890/91: Die Entwicklung des Wiederkäuermagens und -Darmes. Festschr. f. K.W. Naegeli u. A. v. Kölliker, Albert Müllers Verlag, Zürich

Martin, P., 1895: Zur Entwicklung des Netzbeutels der Wiederkäuer. Österr. Mschr. Tierheilk. 19: 145-154

Martin, P., 1896: Die Entwicklung des Wiederkäuermagens. Österr. Mschr. Tierheilk. 21: 385-400, 433-444

Moritz, A., 1957: Verlauf und Verbreitung der Nervi vagi am Rindermagen. Diss. med. vet. Wien

Morrison, A.R. and R.E. Habel, 1964: A quantitative study of the distribution of vagal nerve endings in the myenteric plexus of the ruminant stomach. J .Comp. Neurol. 122: 297-309

Nickel, R. u. H. Wilkens, 1955: Zur Topographie des Rindermagens. Berl. Münch. Tierärztl. Wschr. 68: 264-271

Pernkopf, E., 1931: Die Entwicklung des Vorderdarmes, insbesondere des Magens der Wiederkäuer. Z. Anat. Entwickl.gesch. 94: 490-622

Pospieszny, N., 1979: Die Versorgung des Magens und einiger Lymphknoten durch den Nervus vagus beim Schaf in der praenatalen Periode. Anat. Anz. 146: 47-59

Sack, W.O., 1971: Das Blutgefäßsystem des Labmagens von Rind und Ziege. Diss. med. vet. München, Zbl. Vet. Med. C1: 27-54 (1972)

Schaller, O., 1956: Die periphere sensible Innervation der Haut am Rumpfe des Rindes. Wien. Tierärztl. Mschr. 43: 346-368, 534-561

Schnorr, B. u. B. Vollmerhaus, 1967: Das Oberflächenrelief der Pansenschleimhaut bei Rind und Ziege. I. Mitteilung zur funktionellen Morphologie der Vormägen der Hauswiederkäuer. Zbl. Vet. Med. A14: 93-104

Schnorr, B. und B. Vollmerhaus, 1968: Das Blutgefäßsystem des Pansens von Rind und Ziege. IV. Mitt. zur funktionellen Morphologie der Vormägen der Hauswiederkäuer. Zbl. Vet. Med. A 15: 799-828

Schreiber, J., 1953: Topographisch-anatomischer Beitrag zur klinischen Untersuchung der Rumpfeingeweide des Rindes. Wien. Tierärztl. Mschr. 40: 131-144

Schreiber, J., 1955: Die anatomischen Grundlagen der Leitungsanaesthesie des Rindes. II. Teil: Die Leitungsanaesthesie der Rumpfnerven. Wien. Tierärztl. Mschr. 42: 471-491

Schummer, A., 1932: Zur Formbildung und Lageveränderung des embryonalen Wiederkäuermagens. Diss. med. vet. Gießen Z. Anat. Entwickl.gesch. 99: 265-303

Schwarz, E., 1910: Zur Anatomie und Histologie des Psalters der Wiederkäuer. Diss. med. vet. Bern

Seidler, D., 1966: Arterien und Venen der Körperwand des Rindes. Diss. med. vet. Hannover

Smith, D. F., 1984: Bovine intestinal surgery, Part I, Mod. Vet. Pract., 65: 705-710

Smith, R.N. and G.W. Meadows, 1956: The arrangement of the ansa spiralis of the ox colon. J. Anat. 90: 523-526

Spörri, H., 1951: Physiologie der Wiederkäuer-Vormägen. Schweiz. Arch. Tierheilk. 93: 1-28

Walter, P., 1959: Die Innervation der Flankengegend des Rindes. Tierärztl. Umschau 14: 302-304

Warner, E.D., 1958: The organogenesis and early histogenesis of the bovine stomach. Am. J. Anat. 102: 33-63

Warner, R.G. and W.P. Flatt, 1965: Anatomical development of the ruminant stomach. In: Physiology of digestion in the ruminant. Butterworth Inc., Washington, D.C.

Wass, W.M., 1965: The duct systems of the bovine and porcine pancreas. Am. J. Vet. Res. 26: 267-272

Wensing, C.J.G., 1968: Die Innervation des Wiederkäuermagens. Tijdschr. Diergeneesk. 93: 1352-1360

Wester, J., 1930: Der Schlundrinnenreflex beim Rind. Berl. Tierärztl. Wschr. 46: 397-402

Williamson, M.E., 1967: The venous and biliary systems of the bovine liver. M.S. Thesis, Cornell Univ. Ithaca

Ziegler, H., 1934: Anatomie für die Praxis. I. Von den Vormägen des Rindes. Schweiz. Arch. Tierheilk. 76: 449-461

Chapter 8. Pelvic cavity, inguinal region, and urogenital organs

Amselgruber, W. und F.-H. Feder, 1986: Licht- und elektronenmikroskopische Untersuchungen der Samenblasendrüse (Glandula vesicularis) des Bullen. Anat. Histol. Embryol. 15: 361-379

Ashdown, R.R., 1958: The arteries and veins of the sheath of the bovine penis. Anat. Anz. 105: 222-230

Ashdown, R.R., 1971: Angioarchitecture of the sigmoid flexure of the bovine corpus cavernosum penis and its significance in erection. J. Anat. 106: 403-404

Ashdown, R.R. and M.A. Coombs, 1968: Experimental studies on spiral deviation of the bovine penis. Vet. Rec. 82: 126-129

Ashdown, R.R. and H. Gilanpour, 1974: Venous drainage of the corpus cavernosum penis in impotent and normal bulls. J. Anat. 117: 159-170

Ashdown, R.R. and H. Pearson, 1973: Studies on "corkscrew" penis in the bull. Vet. Rec. 93: 30-35

Ashdown, R.R.; S.W. Ricketts and R.C. Wardley, 1968: The fibrous architecture of the integumentary covering of the bovine penis. J. Anat. 103: 567-572

Ashdown, R.R. and J.A. Smith, 1969: The anatomy of the corpus cavernosum penis of the bull and its relationship to spiral deviation of the penis. J. Anat. 104: 153-160

Barone, R., 1957: La vascularisation utérine chez quelques mammifères. Assoc. Anat. C.R. 44: 124-131

Barone, R. und B. Blavignac, 1964: Les vaisseaux sauguins des reins chez le boeuf. Bull. Soc. Sci. Vét., Lyon 66: 114-130

Becker, R.B. and P.T. Dix Arnold, 1942: Circulatory system of the cow's udder. Fla. Agric. Exp. Sta. Bull. 379: 1-18

Bjoerkman, N. and G. Bloom, 1957: On the fine structure of the fetal-maternal junction in the bovine placentome. Z. Zellforsch. 45: 649-659

Blavignac, B., 1964: Recherche sur la vascularisation et l'innervation des reins chez le boeuf. Thèse doct. vét. Lyon

Böhm, A., 1969: Zur Innervation der Glans penis beim Rind. Diss. med. vet. München

Bressou, C. et J. le Gall, 1936: Contribution à l'étude de la vascularisation de l'utérus des ruminants. Recueil Méd. vét. 112: 5-9

Brown, R.E. and R.E. Carrow, 1963: Vascular anatomy of the bovine tail. J. Amer. vet. med. Ass. 156: 1026-1029

Budras, K.-D., F. Preuss, W. Traeder et al., 1972: Der Leistenspalt und die Leistenringe unserer Haussäugetiere in neuer Sicht. Berl. Münch. Tierärztl. Wschr. 22: 427-431

Comuri, N., 1972: Untersuchungen über zyklusabhängige Strukturveränderungen am distalen Gangsystem der Milchdrüse des Rindes. Diss. med. vet. Gießen

Daigo, M., Y. Sato, M. Otsuka et al., 1973: Stereoroentgenographical studies on the peripheral arteries of the udder of the cow. Bull. Nippon vet. zootech. Coll. 22: 31-39

Desjardins, C. and H.D. Hafs, 1969: Maturation of bovine female genitalia from birth through puberty. J. Anim. Sci. 28: 502-507

Dohm, H., 1936: Anatomische Unterschiede an den Geschlechtsorganen von Kalb und Kuh. Diss. med vet., Leipzig

Drothler, G., 1977: Makroskopisch-morphologische Grundlagen des Descensus testiculorum beim Rind (Fotografischer Atlas des bovinen Hodenabstiegs). Diss. med. vet. Gießen

Edwards, M.J., 1965: Observations on the anatomy of the reproductive organs of cows. With special reference to those features sought during examination per rectum. New Zealand Vet. J. 13: 25-37

Egli, A., 1956: Zur funktionellen Anatomie der Bläschendrüse (Glandula vesiculosa) des Rindes. Acta anat. 28: 359-381

El Hagri, M.A.A.M., 1945: Study of the arterial and lymphatic system in the udder of the cow. Vet. J. 101: 27-33, 51-63, 75-88

Erasha, A.M.M., 1987: Topographisch-anatomische Untersuchung zur Homologisierung der Arterien des Perineums beim Rind. Diss. Med. vet. Hannover

Erickson, B.H., 1966: Development and senescence of the postnatal bovine ovary. J. Anim. Sci. 25: 800-805

Fabisch, H., 1968: Die operative Entfernung von Harnleitersteinen bei Kühen. Wien. Tierärztl. Mschr. 55: 409-411

Fehér, G. und A. Haraszti, 1964: Beiträge zur Morphologie und zu den altersbedingten Veränderungen der akzessorischen Geschlechtsdrüsen von Stieren. Acta vet., Budapest 14: 141-145

Fricke, E., 1968: Topographische Anatomie der Beckenorgane bei Haussäugetieren (Pferd, Rind, Schaf, Ziege, Schwein, Hund, Katze). Diss. med. vet. Berlin

Garcia, O.S.; M. de Almeida and J. Biondini, 1965: Anatomical study of the terminal parts of the excretory ducts of the vesicula seminalis and the ductus deferens in cattle. Arqu. Esc. Vet. 17: 76-82

Geiger, G., 1954: Die anatomischen Grundlagen des "Hymenalringes" beim Rinde. Tierärztl. Umschau 9: 398-403

Ghoshal, N.G., and R. Getty, 1967: Applied anatomy of the sacrococcygeal region of the ox as related to tail-bleeding. Vet. Med.-SAC 62: 255-264

Glättli, H., 1924: Anatomie des Venensystems des Kuheuters. Diss. med. vet. Zürich

Godina, G., 1939: Le fosse ischio-rettale dei bovini. Nuovo Ercolani 44: 353-363

Goyal, H.O., 1985: Morphology of the bovine epididymis. Amer. J. Anat. 172: 155-172

Habel, R.E., 1956: A source of error in the bovine pudendal nerve block. J. Amer. Vet. Med. Assoc. 128: 16-17

Habel, R.E., 1966: The topographic anatomy of the muscles, nerves and arteries of the bovine female perineum. Am. J. Anat. 119: 79-96

Habel, R.E. and K.-D. Budras, 1992: Anatomy of the praepubic tendon in the horse, cow, sheep, goat and dog. Am. J. Vet. Res. 53: 2183-2195

Hampl, A., 1965: Lymphonodi intramammarii der Rindermilchdrüse. I. Makroskopisch-anatomische Verhältnisse. Anat. Anz. 116: 281-298

Hampl, A., 1967: Die Lymphknoten der Rindermilchdrüse. Anat. Anz. 121: 38-54

Harris, G.W., 1958: The central nervous system, neurohypophysis and milk ejection. Proc. Roy. Soc. B 149: 336-353

Heinemann, K., 1937: Einige Muskeln des männlichen Geschlechtsapparates der Haussäugetiere (M. bulbocavernosus, M. ischiocavernosus, M. retractor penis). Diss. vet. med. Hannover

Heinze, W. und W. Lange, 1965: Beitrag zum artifiziellen Penisprolaps unter besonderer Berücksichtigung der anatomischen Verhältnisse beim Bullen. Mh. Vet. Med. 20: 402-412

Heinze, W. und W. Ptak, 1976: Vergleichende morphologische Untersuchungen am Blutgefäßsystem des Hodens von Rind, Schwein, Pferd und Hund unter funktionellen Aspekten. Arch. exp. Vet. Med. 30: 669-685

Henneberg, B., 1905: Abortivzitzen des Rindes. Anat. Hefte 1: 25

Hilliger, H.-G., 1957: Zur Uterus-Karunkel des Rindes und ihrer Vaskularisation unter Berücksichtigung der zuführenden Uterusgefäße. Diss. med. vet. Berlin u. Zbl. Vet. Med. A5: 51-82 (1958)

Höfliger, H., 1943: Die Ovarialgefäße des Rindes und ihre Beziehungen zum Ovarialzyklus. Berl. Münch. Tierärztl. Wschr. 1943: 179

Höfliger, H., 1948: Das Ovar des Rindes in den verschiedenen Lebensperioden unter besonderer Berücksichtigung seiner funktionellen Feinstruktur. Acta anat., Suppl. 5: 1-196

Höfliger, H., 1952: Drüsenaplasie und –hypoplasie in Eutervierteln des Rindes – eine erblich bedingte Entwicklungsanomalie. Schweiz. Arch. Tierheilkd. 94: 824-833

Hofmann, R.R., 1960: Die Gefäßarchitektur des Bullenhodens, zugleich ein Versuch ihrer funktionellen Deutung. Zbl. Vet. Med. A7: 59-93

Kainer, R.A.; L.C. Faulkner and R.M. Abdel-Raouf, 1969: Glands associated with the urethra of the bull. Am. J. Vet. Res. 30: 963-974

Koch, T., 1956: Die Milchdrüse (Glandula lactifera, Mamma) des Rindes. Mhefte Vet.-Med. 11: 527-532

Küng, W.B., 1956: Weiterer Beitrag zur Kenntnis einer erblich bedingten Drüsenaplasie – und –hypoplasie in Eutervierteln des Rindes. Diss. med. vet. Zürich

Lamond, D.R. and M. Drost, 1974: Blood supply to the bovine ovary. J. Anim. Sci. 38: 106-112

Larson, L.L., 1953: The internal pudendal nerve block for anesthesia of the penis and relaxation of the retractor penis muscle. J. Amer. Vet. Med. Ass. 123, 18-27

Larson, L.L. and R.L. Kitchel, 1958: Neural mechanisms in sexual behavior. II. Gross neuroanatomical and correlative neurophysiological studies of the external genitalia of the bull and ram. Am. J. Vet. Res. 19: 853-865

Lewis, J.E.; D.F. Walker; S.D. Beckett and R.I. Vachon, 1968: Blood pressure within the corpus cavernosum penis of the bull. J. Reprod. Fertil. 17: 155-156

Le Roux, J.M.W. and Wilkens, 1959: Beitrag zur Blutgefäßversorgung des Euters der Kuh. Dtsch. tierärztl. Wschr. 66: 429-435

Linzell, J.L., 1960: Valvular incompetence in the venous drainage of the udder. J. Physiol. 153: 481-491

Long, S.E., and P.G. Hignett, 1970: Preputial eversion in the bull – a comparative study. Vet. Rec. 86: 161-164

Mac Millan, K.L. and H.D. Hafs, 1969: Reproductive tract of Holstein bulls from birth through puberty. J. Anim. Sci. 28: 233-239

Meissner, R., 1964: Beiträge über den anatomischen Bau des elastisch-muskulösen Systems der Rinderzitze. Diss. med. vet. Berlin

Merkt, H., 1948: Die Bursa ovarica der Katze. Mit einer vergleichenden Betrachtung der Bursa ovarica des Hundes, Schweines, Rindes und Pferdes sowie des Menschen. Diss. med. vet. Hannover

Mosimann, W., 1949: Zur Anatomie der Rindermilchdrüse und über die Morphologie ihrer sezernierenden Teile. Diss. med. vet. Bern, Acta anat. 8: 347-378

Mosimann, W., 1969: Zur Involution der bovinen Milchdrüse. Schweiz. Arch. Tierheilkd. 111: 431-439

Neuhaus, U., 1956: Die Bedeutung des Oxytocins für die Milchsekretion. Dtsch. Tierärztl. Wschr. 63: 467-496

Nickel, R., 1954: Zur Topographie der akzessorischen Geschlechtsdrüsen bei Schwein, Rind und Pferd. Tierärztl. Umschau 9: 386-388

Nitschke, Th. und F. Preuss, 1971: Die Hauptäste der A. iliaca interna bei Mensch und Haussäugetieren in vergleichend-anatomisch häufiger Reihenfolge. Anat. Anz. 128: 439-453

Oelrich, T.M., 1980: The urethral sphincter muscle in the male. Am. J. Anat. 158: 229-246

Oelrich, T.M., 1983: The striated urogenital sphincter muscle in the female. Anat. Rec. 205: 223-232

Otto, A., 1930: Beiträge zur Anatomie der Cervix uteri des trächtigen Rindes. Diss. med. vet. Hannover

Pastea, E., 1973: Contribution à l'étude macroscopique de l'innervation et de la vascularisation des glandes surrénales chez le boeuf. Anat. Anz. 134: 120-126

Perk, K., 1957: Über den Bau und das Sekret der Glandula bulbourethralis (Cowperi) von Rind und Katze. Diss. med. vet. Bern

Popesko, P., 1965: Vaskularisation des Hodens des Bullen: A. spermatica interna. (slowak.) Folia vet. 9: 137-146

Porthan, L., 1928: Morphologische Untersuchungen über die Cervix uteri des Rindes mit besonderer Berücksichtigung der Querfaltenbildung und des Kanalverlaufs. Diss. med. vet. Leipzig

Preuss, F., 1953: Beschreibung und Einteilung des Rinderuterus nach funktionellen Gesichtspunkten. Anat. Anz. 100: 46-64

Preuss, F., 1954: Die Tunica albuginea penis und ihre Trabekel bei Pferd und Rind. Anat. Anz. 101: 64-83

Preuss, F., 1959: Die A. vaginalis der Haussäugetiere. Berl. Münch. Tierärztl. Wschr. 72: 403-406

Reuber, H.W. and M.A. Emerson, 1959: Arteriography of the internal genitalia of the cow. J. Am. Vet. Med. Assoc. 134: 101-109

Röder, O., 1898: Über die Gartnerschen Gänge beim Rind. Arch. wiss. prakt. Tierhkeilk. 24: 135-141

Rubeli, O., 1913: Besonderheiten im Ausführungsgangsystem der Milchdrüsen des Rindes. Mitt. nat. forsch. Ges. Bern

Rubeli, O., 1914: Bau des Kuheuters. Verl. Art. Inst. Orell Füssli, Zürich

Ruoss, G., 1965: Beitrag zur Kenntnis der Euterarterien des Rindes mit besonderer Berücksichtigung der Beziehung zwischen Feinbau und Funktion. Diss. med. vet. Zürich

Schenker, J., 1950: Zur funktionellen Anatomie der Prostata des Rindes. Acta anat. 9: 69-102

Schlumperger, O.-R.V., 1954: Der Nebenhoden und seine Lage zum Hoden bei Rind, Schaf und Ziege. Diss. med. vet. Hannover

Schummer, A. und B. Vollmerhaus, 1960: Die Venen des trächtigen und nichtträchtigen Rinderuterus als Blutstrom regulierendes funktionelles System. Wien. Tierärztl. Mschr. 47: 114-138

Seidel, G.E., and R.H. Foote, 1967: Motion picture analysis of bovine ejaculation. J. Dairy Sci. 50: 970-971

Seiferle, E., 1933: Über Art- und Altersmerkmale der weiblichen Geschlechtsorgane unserer Haussäugetiere: Pferd, Rind, Kalb, Schaf, Ziege, Kaninchen, Meerschweinchen, Schwein, Hund und Katze. Z. ges. Anat. 101: 1-80

Seiferle, E., 1949: Neuere Erkenntnisse über Bau und Funktion der Milchdrüse der Kuh. Schriften d. Schweiz. Vereinigung f. Tierzucht, Euter u. Milchleistung. Banteli AG, Bern-Bümpliz

Skjervold, H., 1961: Überzählige Zitzen bei Rindern. Hereditas, Lund 46: 1960, Landw. Zbl.: 1156

Smollich, A., 1958: Gestalt, Topographie, Masse und Gewichtsverhältnisse der Nebennieren des Rindes. Anat. Anz. 105: 205-221

St. Clair, L.E., 1942: The nerve supply to the bovine mammary gland. Amer. J. Vet. Med. Assoc. 129: 405-409

Tgetgel, B., 1926: Untersuchungen über den Sekretionsdruck und über das Einschießen der Milch in das Euter des Rindes. Diss. med. vet. Zürich

Thon, H., 1954: Zur Struktur der Hodensackwand des Rindes. Diss. med. vet. München

Traeder, W., 1968: Zur Anatomie der Leistengegend des Rindes. Diss. med. vet. Freie Universität Berlin

Überschär, S., 1961: Zur makroskopischen und mikroskopischen Altersbestimmung am Corpus luteum des Rindes. Diss. med. vet. Hannover

Vau, E., 1960: Die Blutabflußwege des Kuheuters. Wien. Tierärztl. Mschr., Festschr. Prof. Schreiber: 312-319

Vierling, R., 1956: Das Zwischenhirn-Hypophysensystem und die Laktation. Z. Tierzüchtg., Zücht. – Biol. 66: 317-322

Vollmerhaus, B., 1963: Die Arteria und Vena ovarica des Hausrindes als Beispiel einer funktionellen Koppelung viszeraler Gefäße. Anat. Anz. 112: Erg. H. 258-264

Vollmerhaus, B., 1964: Gefäßarchitektonische Untersuchungen am Geschlechtsapparat des weiblichen Hausrindes (Bos primigenius f. taurus, L. 1758.) Teil I u. Teil II Zbl. Vet. Med. A 11: 538-596, 597-646

Weber, A.F., 1955: The identity and characterization of the smallest lobule unit in the udder of the dairy cow. Am. J. Vet. Res. 16: 255-263

Wille, K.-H., 1966: Das Blugefäßsystem der Niere des Hausrindes. (Bos primigenius f. taurus, L., 1758) Diss. med. vet. Gießen

Wille, K.-H., 1968: Gefäßarchitektonische Untersuchungen an der Nierenkapsel des Rindes. (Bos primigenius f. taurus, L.). Zbl. Vet. Med. A15: 372-381

Yamauchi, S. and F. Sasaki, 1970: Studies on the vascular supply of the uterus of a cow. Jap. J. Vet. Sci. 32: 59-67

Ziegler, H., 1954: Zur Hyperthelie und Hypermastie (überzählige Zitzen und Milchdrüsen) beim Rind. Schweiz. Arch. Tierheilkd. 96: 344-350

Ziegler, H., 1959: Das Lymphgefäßsystem der Rindermilchdrüse und dessen Bedeutung für die Milchsekretion. Bull. Schweiz. Akad. med. Wiss. 15: 105-120

Zietzschmann, O., 1910: Bau und Funktion der Milchdrüse. In: Grimmer, W. (Ed.): Chemie und Physiologie der Milch. Paul Parey Berlin

Zietzschmann, O., 1917: Die Zirkulationsverhältnisse des Euters einer Kuh. Dtsch. Tierärztl. Wschr. 25: 361-365

Zingel, S., 1959: Untersuchungen über die renkulare Zusammensetzung der Rinderniere. Zool. Anz. 162: 83-99

Zwart, S.G., 1911: Beiträge zur Anatomie und Physiologie der Milchdrüse des Rindes. Diss. med. vet. Bern

Anatomical aspects of bovine spongiform encephalopathy

Borchers, K., 2002: TSE, Alte Krankheiten mit neuer Brisanz. Berl. Münch. Tierärztl. Wschr.; 115: 81-90

Editorial, Jour. Am. Vet. Med. Assoc. 2002; 221: 1670

Eggers, T., S. Buda, K.-D. Budras, R. Fries, G. Hildebrandt und K. Rauscher, 2001: Ganglien als Risikomaterial in der Fleischgewinnung. Proc. 42. Arbeitstagung des Arbeitsgebietes Lebensmittelhygiene der Deutschen Veterinärmedizinischen Gesellschaft, Garmisch-Partenkirchen, 25.–28.09.2001

Hörnlimann, B., D. Riesner, H. Kretzschmar (Hrsg.), 2001: Prionen und Prionkrankheiten. DeGruyter

Mabbott, N.A., and M.E. Bruce, 2001: The immunbiology of TSE diseases. Journal of General Virology, 82: 2307 – 2318

McBride, P.A., W.J. Schulz-Schaeffer, M. Donaldson, M. Bruce, H. Diringer, H.A. Kretzschmar, M. Beekes, 2001: Early spread of scrapie from the gastrointestinal tract to the central nervous system involves autonomic fibers of the splanchnic and vagus nerves. J Virol. Oct; 75 (19): 9320-7

Sigurdson, C.J., T.R. Spraker, M.W. Miller, 2001: PrP^{CWD} in the myenteric plexus, vagosympathetic trunk, and endocrine glands of deer with chronic wasting disease. Jour. General Virology 82: 2327-2334

U.S. Dept. of Agriculture, Animal and Plant Health Inspection Service, 2001: Washington, D.C. 20250

Venturini, M., P. Simoens, C. de Jaeger, 2000: Obductie van Runderhersenen voor het BSE-Onderzoek. Vlaams diergeneesk. Tijdschr. 69: 377-381

Contributions to Clinical-Functional Anatomy

[1] Berg. R., 1995: Angewandte topographische Anatomie der Haustiere. 4. Aufl., Gustav Fischer Jena Stuttgart

[2] Braun, U., F. Salis, C. Gerspach, K. Feige and T. Sydler, 2004: Pharyngeal perforation in three cows caused by administration of a calcium bolus. Vet. Rec. 154:240-242

[3] Breukink, H.J., K. Kroneman, 1963: The "steelband effect" a new diagnostic aid in inspection of the cow concerning the presence of abomasal dilatation and/or dislocation in the cow. Tijdschr. Diergeneesk. 88:8-12

[4] Breukink, H.J., Th. Wensing, and A. van Weeren-Keverling Buisman, 1988: Consequences of the failure of the reticular groove reflex in veal calves fed milk replacer. Vet. Quarterly 10:126-135

[5] Bruchmann, W., 1965: Untersuchungen über die Punktionsmöglichkeiten am Schulter-, Ellbogen- und Hüftgelenk des Rindes. Vet. med. Diss. Hannover.

[6] De Lahunta, A. und Habel, R.E., 1986: Applied Veterinary Anatomy. Saunders Co. Philadelphia

[7] Dietz, O., 1957: Zur Grenzstrangblockade beim Tier. Arch. exper. Vet. med. 11:310-330

[8] Dietz, O., Koch, T., Nagel, E. und Berg, R., 1961: Die Topographie des Perikards und chirurgische Eingriffsmöglichkeiten am Herzbeutel des Rindes. Dtsch. tierärztl. Wschr. 68:317-321

[9] Dietz, O., Schaetz, F., Schleiter, H., Teuscher, R., 1988: Anästhesie und Operationen bei Gross- und Kleintieren. 4. Aufl., VEB Fischer Jena

[10] Dirksen, G., 1962: Die Erweiterung, Verlagerung und Drehung des Labmagens beim Rind. Hannover, Tierärztl. Hochsch., Habilschr., Verlag Parey, Berlin und Hamburg

[11] Dirksen, G., H.-D. Gründer und M. Stöber, 2002: Innere Medizin und Chirurgie des Rindes. 4. Aufl., Blackwell Verlag GmbH, Wien und Berlin

[12] Dirksen, G., K. Doll, 2002: Dünndarmverschlingung. In: Dirksen et al. Innere Medizin und Chirurgie des Rindes. 4. Aufl., Parey Buchverlag im Blackwell Verlag GmbH Berlin, Wien, 525-527

[13] Dirksen, G., K. Doll, 2002: Einklemmung, Abschnürung, Kompression des Darmes. In: Dirksen et al. Innere Medizin und Chirurgie des Rindes. 4. Aufl., Parey Buchverlag im Blackwell Verlag GmbH Berlin, Wien 530-531.

[14] Dirksen, G., K. Doll, 2002: Darminvagination. In: Dirksen et al. Innere Medizin und Chirurgie des Rindes. 4. Aufl., Parey Buchverlag im Blackwell Verlag GmbH Berlin, Wien, 517-525

[15] Dorresteijn, J., 1973: Further studies on acute indigestion and traumatic reticuloperitonitis in cattle. Tijdsch. Diergeneesk. 98:831– 839

[16] Dyce, K.M. and Wensing, C.J.G., 1971: Essentials of bovine anomty. Lea & Febiger, Philadelphia

[17] Fischer, W., 1978: Zu Diagnose- und Behandlungsmöglichkeiten von Kehlkopferkrankungen beim Kalb. Dtsch. Tierärztl. Wschr. 85:168-170

[18] Geishauser Th., C. Pfänder, Untersuchungen zur Topographie von Blinddarm und Anfangsschleife des Grimmdarmes bei Blinddarmerweiterung des Rindes. Dtsch. Tierärztl. Wschr. 103: 205-209

[19] Getty, R., 1975: In: Sisson and Grossman's The Anatomy of the Domestic Animals. Vol. 1, 5th edition, W.B. Saunders Co. Philadelphia

[20] Habel, R., 1982: Guide to the dissection of domestic ruminants. Self published Ithaca, U.S.A.

[21] Hajer R., J. Hendrikse, L.J.E. Rutgers, M.M. Sloet van Oldruitenborgh-Oosterbaan, B. Van der Weyden, 1993: Het klinisch onderzoek bij grote huisdieren. Wetenschappelijke Uitgeverij Bunge, Utrecht, Niederlande

[22] Haven, M.K., 1990: Bovine Esophageal Surgery. The Vet. Clin North Am. 6:359-369

[23] Hoflund, S., 1940: Untersuchungen über Störungen in den Funktionen der Wiederkäuermägen durch Schädigung des Nervus vagus verursacht. Svensk. Vet. Tidskr. 45, Suppl.

[24] Hollack, K., 2003: Auskultation und Perkussion, Inspektion und Palpation. 13. Auflage, Georg Thieme Verlag Stuttgart

[25] Kleen, J. L., G.A. Hooijer, J. Rehage, and J.P. Noordhuizen, 2004: Rumenocentesis (rumen puncture): a viable instrument in herd health diagnosis. Dtsch. Tierärztl. Wschr., 111: 458-462

[26] Kuiper, R., and H.J. Breukink, 1987: Das Hoflundsche Syndrom nach 47 Jahren. Dtsch. Tierärztl. Wschr. 94:271–273

[27] Kuiper, R., 1980: Reflux van lebmaaginhoud bij het rund. Proefschrift, Utrecht

[28] Lehmann, B. (1986): Untersuchungen zur praxisnahen Dauertropfinfusion beim Rind (Behälter, Lösungen, Infusionstechnik). Hannover, Tierärztl. Hochsch., Diss.

[29] Merkal, R.S., D.L. Whipple, J.M. Sacks, G.R. Snyder, 1987: Prevalence of Mycobacterium paratuberculosis in ileocecal lymph nodes of cattle culled in the United States. J. Am. Vet. Med. Assoc., 190:676-680

[30] Müller, M., S. Platz, J. Ehrlein, T. Ewringmann, G. Molle, A. Weber, 2005: Bakteriell bedingte Thromboembolie bei Milchkühen – eine retrospektive Auswertung von 31 Fällen unter besonderer Berücksichtigung des Ursachenkomplexes. Berl. Münch. Tierärztl. Wschr., 118:121-127

[31] Muir, W.W., Hubbell, J.A.E., 2000: Veterinary Anesthesia. 3rd edition. Mosby, St. Louis

[32] Neijenhuis, F., H.W. Barkema, H. Hogeveen und J.P.T.M. Noordhuizen, 2000: Classification and longitudinal examination of callused teat ends in dairy cows. J. Dairy Science 83, 12:2795-804

[33] Pearce, S.G., C.L. Kerr, L.P. Bcure, K. Thompson and H. Dobson, 2003: Comparison of the retrobulbar and PETERSON'S nerve block technique via magnetic resonance imaging in bovine cadavers. JAVMA 223:852-855

[34] Pusterla, N., and U. Braun, 1996: Prophylaxis of intravenous catheter-related thrombophlebitis in cattle. Vet. Rec. 139:287– 289

[35] Rehage, J., M. Kaske, N. Stockhofe-Zurwieden, and E. Yalcin, 1995: Evaluation of the pathogenesis of vagus indigestion in cows with traumatic reticuloperitonitis. J. Amer. Vet. Med. Ass. 207:1607–1611

[36] Reinhold, P., 2001: Untersuchungen zur Bestimmung pulmonaler Funktionen beim Kalb. Habilitationsschrift. Fachbereich Veterinärmedizin der Freien Universität Berlin, 25-28

[37] Rosenberger, G., 1990: Die klinische Untersuchung des Rindes. 3. Aufl., Verlag Paul Parey, Berlin und Hamburg

[38] Schreiber, J., 1949: Die Beziehungen zwischen Topik und Trauma des Plexus brachialis beim Pferd. Wien. tierärztl. Mschr. 36:569-582

[39] Schreiber, J., 1956: Die anatomischen Grundlagen der Leitungsanästhesie beim Rind. III. Teil. Die Leitungsanästhesie der Nerven der Vorderextremität. Wien. tierärztl. Mschr. 43, 273-287

[40] Simkins, K.M., and M.J. Nagele 1997: Omasal and abomasal impaction in beef suckler cows. Vet. Rec. 141:466–468

[41] Smallwood, J. E., 1999: A guided tour of veterinary anatomy. Domestic ungulates. 2nd edition. Laser Image Corporate Publishing, Durham, NC

[42] Smith, D.F., 1990: Surgery of the bovine small intestine. Vet. Clin North Am. Food Anim. Pract., 449-460

[43] Stöber, M., 1990: Intravenöse Injektion und Infusion in: Rosenberger, G. Die klinische Untersuchung des Rindes, 3. Aufl. Verlag Paul Parey, Berlin, Hamburg, 689– 695

[44] Sugimoto, M., H. Furuoka and Y. Sugimoto, 2003: Deletion of one the duplicated HSP 70 genes cause hereditary myopathy of diaphragmatic muscles in Holstein-Friesian cattle. Anim. Genet. 34:191-197

[45] Tadic, M., S. Murgaski, B. Misic und Jeremic, 1975: Serijska biopsija rebarna kosti u goveda za procenjivanje stanja mineralnich re zervi skeletal (Serienmässige Biopsie der Rippen beim Rind zwecks Beurteilung der Mineralstoffreserven des Skeletts). Veter. Glasnik 29, 15-18

[46] Taffe, B., 1993: Untersuchung der Brauchbarkeit des Käfigmagneten CAP, Super II zur Vorbeuge und Behandlung der Fremdkörpererkrankung des Rindes. Diss. Vet. med. Hannover

[47] Van den Top, A.M., Th. Wensing, M.J.H.Geelen, G.H. Wentink, A.Th. van`t Klooster und A.C. Beynen, 1995: Time trends o plasma lipids and hepatic triacylglycerol synthesizing enzymes during post partum fatty liver development in dairy cows with unlimited access to feed during the dry period. J. Dairy Sci. 78:2208-20

[48] Van der Velden, M.A., 1981: De lebmaagdislocatie naar rechts bij het rund: topografische en therapeutische aspecten. Proefschrift, Utrecht, Niederlande

[49] Van der Velden, M.A., 1983: Functional stenosis of the sigmoid curve of the duodenum in cattle. Vet. Rec. 112:452-453

[50] Vollmerhaus, B., 1965: Topographisch-anatomische Darstellungen für die Injektionstechnik an Gelenken, Sehnenscheiden und Schleimbeuteln. Behringwerke Marburg/Lahn

INDEX

Klaus-Dieter Budras · Patrick H. McCarthy ·
Wolfgang Fricke · Renate Richter

Anatomy of the Dog

with Aaron Horowitz and Rolf Berg

Fifth, revised edition

2007. 224 pp., 71 largesized color plates including
several illustrations, radiographs, drawings and
photographs, 9 3/4 x 13 1/2", hardcover
ISBN 978-3-89993-018-4

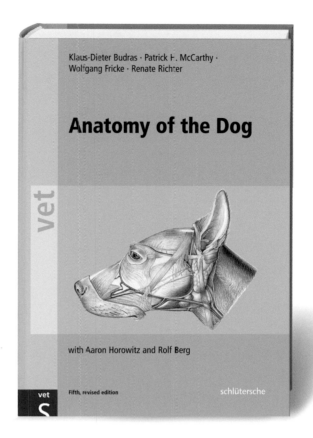

Already acknowledged by students and teachers as an essential resource for learning and
revision, this book will also be a valuable reference for qualified practitioners.

- Fully illustrated with color line diagrams, including unique three-dimensional
  cross-sectional anatomy, together with radiographs and ultrasound scans
- Includes topographic and surface anatomy
- Tabular appendices of relational and functional anatomy
- New section on computed tomography

Authors

Klaus-Dieter Budras, DVM, PhD, Professor em., University of Berlin, Germany
Patrick H. McCarthy, DVM, PhD, Professor em., University of Sydney, Australia
Rolf Berg, DVM, PhD, Professor, Ross University, St. Kitts, West Indies
Aaron Horowitz, DVM, PhD, JD, Professor, Ross University, St. Kitts, West Indies
Wolfgang Fricke, medical illustrator, University of Berlin, Germany
Renate Richter, medical illustrator, University of Berlin, Germany

"If the practicing veterinarians have not bought an anatomy book since veterinary school, this
book is highly recommended; this is a book that one would be proud to use as a teaching tool
with clients."
JAVMA – American Veterinary Medical Association

"A region with which I was very familiar from a surgical standpoint thus became more
comprehensible.
[...] Showing the clinical relevance of anatomy in such a way is a powerful tool for stimulating
students' interest. [...] In addition to putting anatomical structures into clinical perspective, the
text provides a brief but effective guide to dissection."
The Veterinary Record

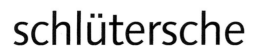
schlütersche

Subject to change.

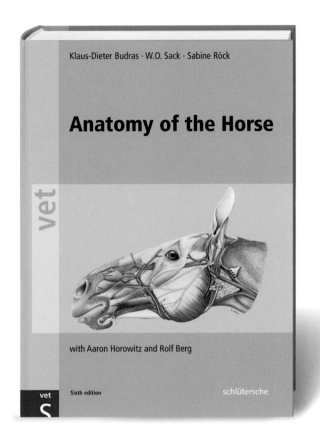

Klaus-Dieter Budras ·
W. O. Sack · Sabine Röck

Anatomy
of the Horse

with Aaron Horowitz and Rolf Berg

Sixth edition

2011. 208 pp., 56 large-sized color plates
and 229 illustrations, radiographs, drawings
and photographs, 9 ¾ x 13 ½", hardcover
ISBN 978-3-89993-666-7

Anatomy of the Horse has been accepted as a highly successful text-atlas of equine anatomy.
The chapters on functional anatomy of this present 6th edition have been totally revised and
include new chapters on the eye, abdomen, female reproduction and ultrasonography and
especially orthopaedics.

- Fully illustrated with color line diagrams, including unique three-dimensional
  cross-sectional anatomy, together with radiographs and ultrasound scans
- Includes topographic and surface anatomy
- Tabular appendices of relational and functional anatomy

Authors

Klaus-Dieter Budras, DVM., Ph.D., Professor em. of Anatomy, University of Berlin, Germany
Sabine Röck, Medical Illustrator, Berlin
W.O. Sack, DVM, Ph.D., Professor em., Cornell University
Aaron Horowitz, DVM, PhD, JD, Professor, Ross University, St. Kitts, West Indies
Rolf Berg, DVM, PhD, Professor, Ross University, St. Kitts, West Indies

"The aim of the authors has been admirably achieved. The textbook is already acknowledged
as an essential resource for students and teachers and will be an essential reference book for
veterinary practitioners and horse lovers in the English-speaking world."
JAVMA – American Veterinary Medical Association

"In conclusion, I am able to recommend this book to all students and doctors of veterinary
medicine, as well as to all those who have an interest in horse anatomy and equine practice."
Veterinaski Arhiv – Journal of the Faculty of Veterinary Medicine, University of Zagreb

Subject to change.

schlütersche